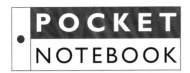

POCKET
NOTEBOOK

Pocket
PEDIATRICS

Third Edition

T0199863

Edited by

PARITOSH PRASAD, MD, DTM&H
Attending Physician, University of Rochester Medical Center

Associate Authors

UZAIR ADMANI, MD
Resident, University of Rochester Medical Center

PETER BOULOS, MD
Resident, University of Rochester Medical Center

FRANCIS COYNE, MD
Chief Resident, University of Rochester Medical Center

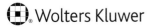 Wolters Kluwer

Philadelphia • Baltimore • New York • London
Buenos Aires • Hong Kong • Sydney • Tokyo

Acquisitions Editor: Robin Najar
Product Developmental Editor: Ashley Fischer
Editorial Coordinator: Blair Jackson
Marketing Manager: Rachel Mante Leung
Production Project Manager: Marian Bellus
Design Coordinator: Joan Wendt
Manufacturing Coordinator: Beth Welsh
Prepress Vendor: Aptara, Inc.

© **2020 Wolters Kluwer.**

Printed in China

Library of Congress Cataloging-in-Publication Data

Names: Prasad, Paritosh. editor. | Admani, Uzair, editor. | Boulos, Peter,
   editor. | Coyne, Francis, editor.
Title: Pocket pediatrics / [edited by] Paritosh Prasad, Uzair Admani, Peter
   Boulos, Francis Coyne.
Other titles: Pocket pediatrics (Prasad)
Description: Third edition. | Philadelphia : Wolters Kluwer, [2020] |
   Includes bibliographical references and index.
Identifiers: LCCN 2019007268 | ISBN 9781975107628
Subjects: | MESH: Pediatrics–methods | Handbook
Classification: LCC RJ61 | NLM WS 39 | DDC 618.92–dc23
LC record available at https://lccn.loc.gov/2019007268

CCS0623

Asim Abbasi, MD
Faculty, University of Rochester Medical Center

Rebecca Abell, DO
Faculty, University of Rochester Medical Center

Sakina Attaar, MD
Resident, University of Rochester Medical Center

Rose Barham, MD
Resident, University of Rochester Medical Center

Shara Bialo, MD
Faculty, University of Rochester Medical Center

Adam Bracken, MD
Resident, University of Rochester Medical Center

Nicole Cifra, MD
Resident, University of Rochester Medical Center

Margaret Connolly, MD
Resident, University of Rochester Medical Center

Maria Cordisco, MD
Faculty, University of Rochester Medical Center

Rita Dadiz, DO
Faculty, University of Rochester Medical Center

Jake Deines, MD
Faculty, University of Rochester Medical Center

Francis Gigliotti, MD
Faculty, University of Rochester Medical Center

Michael Joynt, MD
Faculty, University of Rochester Medical Center

Maha Kaissi, MD
Resident, University of Rochester Medical Center

Emily Krainer, MD
Resident, University of Rochester Medical Center

Julia Lister, MD
Resident, University of Rochester Medical Center

Jeanne Lomas, DO
Faculty, University of Rochester Medical Center

Gregory Mak, MD
Resident, University of Rochester Medical Center

Bethany Marston, MD
Faculty, University of Rochester Medical Center

Caitlin Metzger, MD
Resident, University of Rochester Medical Center

Jonathan Mink, MD
Faculty, University of Rochester Medical Center

Craig Mullen, MD
Faculty, University of Rochester Medical Center

Sylwia Nowak, MD
Resident, University of Rochester Medical Center

Erin Rademacher, MD
Faculty, University of Rochester Medical Center

Justin Rosati, MD
Resident, University of Rochester Medical Center

Maria A. Slack, MD
Faculty, University of Rochester Medical Center

Ajay Tambralli, MD
Resident, University of Rochester Medical Center

Karen Voter, MD
Faculty, University of Rochester Medical Center

Hilary Whelan, MD
Resident, University of Rochester Medical Center

PREFACE

In the eight years since its initial publication, *Pocket Pediatrics* has been put to the test by several new generations of interns and residents. Their input and insight has resulted in this, the third edition of *Pocket Pediatrics*. As ever, we remain committed to creating a highly portable rapid reference for the pediatric health care practitioner in training with a specific emphasis on high-yield information and evidence-based practice.

To that end, this new edition has been completely rewritten from scratch with all updated references and materials.

As before, this handbook is not meant to be a comprehensive treatment of the whole of pediatrics, or even an exhaustive treatment of the specific topics treated within its pages. The topics were chosen because they are believed to represent the core knowledge one would wish to have at one's disposal. The information collected on each topic was selected and organized to present a high-yield overview of each subject by currently training residents revised by actively practicing pediatric attendings. Each section has been rereviewed with an eye to presenting the most up-to-date evidence-based practices and society and association guidelines, with the addition of well in excess of 100 new citations to point interested readers in the direction of more complete treatments of each topic. Where evidence is lacking, we have included accepted best practices as well as expert opinions.

As in the prior editions, great care has been taken to formulate every reference in such a way that each can be searched easily on www.pubmed.gov and should directly take the searcher to the article in question.

We acknowledge as well that this handbook will forever be a work in progress, as our understanding of pediatrics continues to grow and as, day by day, new knowledge about disease processes, new laboratory tests and procedures, and new evidence-based practice guidelines are added to our collective armamentarium. We have endeavored to make the following text as current as possible, but it should never take the place of clinical experience and clinical judgment.

PARITOSH PRASAD, MD, DTM&H

2/2 – secondary to
ABG – arterial blood gas
ABPA – allergic bronchopulmonary aspergillosis
Abx – antibiotics
AD – autosomal dominant
ADR – adverse drug reaction
aka – also known as
AOM – acute otitis media
AR – autosomal recessive
AS – ankylosing spondylitis
ASD – atrial septal defect
Assn – association
AV – atrioventricular
AVM – arterial-venous malformation
AVNRT – AV nodal reenterant tachycardia
AVRT – AV reentrant tachycardia
AVSD – atrioventricular septal defect

BMV – bag-mask ventilation
BPD – bronchopulmonary dysplasia
btwn – between
BZD – benzodiazepine

CAH – congenital adrenal hyperplasia
CF – cystic fibrosis
CHD – congenital heart disease
CMP – complete metabolic panel
CO – cardiac output
CPB – cardiopulmonary bypass
CXR – chest x-ray

d – day
Def – definition
depol – depolarization
Dx or Dz – disease
dz – disease

ECG – electrocardiogram
ED – emergency department
ENT – ear, nose, and throat
EoE – eosinophilic esophagitis
Eos – eosinophils
Epi – epidemiology
ETT – ET tube

FH – family history
FPIES – food-induced enterocolitis syndrome
FTT – failure to thrive

GA – gestational age
GBS – group B streptococcus
GBS – Guillain-Barré syndrome
G-CSF – granulocyte colony–stimulating factor
gen – generation
GERD – gastroesophageal reflux disease
GIR – glucose infusion rate
GTTs – guttae (Latin) for drips

Hb/Hct – hemoglobin/hematocrit
HFNC – high-flow nasal cannula

HPF – high-power field
HR – heart rate
hr – hour
HSCT – hematopoietic stem cell transplant
HSM – hepatosplenomegaly
Hx – history
hyperK – hyperkalemia

I:E ratio – inspiratory:expiratory ratio
ICH – intracranial hemorrhage
ICP – intracranial pressure
INF $_\gamma$ – interferon gamma
irreg – irregular
IUGR – intrauterine growth restriction
IV – intravenous
IVH – intraventricular hemorrhage
IVIG – intravenous immunoglobulin

JVP – jugular venous pressure

LAD – left-axis deflection
LAD – lymphadenopathy
LBBB – left bundle branch block
LBW – low birth weight
LFTs – liver function tests
LLSB – left lower sternal border
LOC – level of consciousness
LR – lactate ringers
LTM – long-term monitoring
LUSB – left upper sternal border
LVH – left ventricular hypertrophy

MAOI – monoamine oxidase inhibitor
Mgmt – management
mo – month
MOA – mechanism of action
Mod – moderate

NAC – N-acetylcysteine
NADPH – nicotinamide adenine dinucleotide phosphate
NEC – necrotizing enterocolitis
Neuts – neutrophils
nml – normal
norm – normal
NS – normal saline

OSA – obstructive sleep apnea

PCOS – polycystic ovarian syndrome
PDA – patent ductus arteriosus
pHTN – pulmonary hypertension
Plts – platelets
PMH – past medical history
PO – per oral (by mouth)
PPROM – premature prolonged rupture of membranes
Pts – patients
PTX – pneumothorax
PVL – periventricular leukomalacia

r/o – rule out
RAD – right-axis deviation

RAE – right atrial enlargement
RBBB – right bundle branch block
RD – registered dietician
resp – respiratory
RF – risk factors
ROM – rupture of membranes
RR – respiratory rate
RVH – right ventricular hypertrophy

SC – subcutaneous
SES – socioeconomic status
Sev – severe
SG – specific gravity
SH – social history
SIADH – syndrome of inappropriate
    antidiuretic hormone
SIDS – sudden infant death syndrome
SMA – spinal muscular atrophy
Staph – staphylococcus
Strep – streptococcus
SVT – supraventricular tachycardia
Sxs – symptoms

TCAs – tricyclic antidepressant
TG – triglycerides
TR – tricuspid regurgitation
TV – tricuspid valve
Tx – treatment

UOP – urine output
URI – upper respiratory infection
US – ultrasound

Vfib – ventricular fibrillation
VLBW – very low birth weight
VT – ventricular tachycardia

w/ – with
WBC – white blood cell count
Wk – week
WPW – Wolff–Parkinson–White

yr – year

CONTENTS

ALLERGY AND IMMUNOLOGY
Sylwia Nowak, Jeanne Lomas, and Maria A. Slack

CARDIOLOGY
Peter Boulos and Michael Joynt

ENDOCRINOLOGY

Rose Barham and Shara Bialo

FLUIDS AND ELECTROLYTES

Hilary Whelan and Erin Rademacher

GASTROENTEROLOGY

Margaret Connolly and Rebecca Abell

HEMATOLOGY
Francis Coyne and Craig Mullen

ONCOLOGY
Francis Coyne and Craig Mullen

GENETIC AND METABOLISM

INFECTIOUS DISEASE

NEUROLOGY
Emily Krainer, Justin Rosati, and Jonathan Mink

PULMONARY
Caitlin Metzger, Peter Boulos, and Karen Voter

RENAL
Julia Lister, Adam Bracken, and Erin Rademacher

RHEUMATOLOGY
Ajay Tambralli and Bethany Marston

NICU
Maha Kaissi and Rita Dadiz

PICU
Uzair Admani and Jake Deines

CLINICAL IMAGES IN PEDIATRIC DERMATOLOGY

Sakina Attaar and Maria Cordisco

(The Harriet Lane Handbook. 21st ed. 2017)

Age	Gross Motor	Visual Motor/ Problem Solving	Language	Social/ Adaptive
1 mo	Raises head from prone position	Visually fixes, follows to midline, has tight grasp	Alerts to sound	Regards face
2 mo	Holds head in midline, lifts chest off table	No longer clenches fists tightly, follows object past midline	Smiles socially (after being stroked or talked to)	Recognizes parent
3 mo	Supports on forearms in prone position, holds head up steadily	Holds hands open at rest, follows in circular fashion, responds to visual threat	Coos	Reaches for familiar people or objects, anticipates feedings
4 mo	Rolls over, supports on wrists, shifts weight	Reaches w/ arms in unison, brings hands to midline	Laughs, orients to voice	Enjoys looking around
6 mo	Sits unsupported, puts feet in mouth in supine position	Unilateral reach, uses raking grasp, transfers objects	Babbles, ah-goo, razz, lateral orientation to bell	Recognizes that someone is a stranger
9 mo	Pivots when sitting, crawls well, pulls to stand, cruises	Uses immature pincer grasp, probes w/ forefinger, holds bottle, throws objects	Says "mama" and "dada" **indiscriminately**, gestures, waves bye-bye, understands "no"	Starts exploring environment, plays gesture games (e.g., pat-a-cake)
12 mo	Walks alone	Uses mature pincer grasp, can make a crayon mark, releases voluntarily	Uses 2 words other than "mama, dada" or proper nouns, jargoning (runs several unintelligible words together w/ tone or inflection) follows one-step command w/ gesture	Imitates actions, comes when called, cooperates w/ dressing
15 mo	Creeps up stairs, walks backward independently	Scribbles in imitation, builds tower of 2 blocks in imitation	Uses 4–6 words, follows one-step command without gesture	Uses spoon and cup
18 mo	Runs, throws objects from standing without falling	Scribbles spontaneously, builds tower of 3 blocks, turns 2 or 3 pages at a time	Mature jargoning (includes intelligible words), 7–10 word vocabulary, knows 5 body parts	Copies parent in tasks, plays in company of other children
2 yr	Walks up and down steps without help	Imitates stroke w/ pencil, builds tower of 7 blocks, turns pages one at a time, removes shoes, pants, etc.	Uses pronouns (I, you, me) inappropriately, follows two-step commands, 50-word vocabulary, uses 2-word sentences	**Parallel play**
3 yr	Can alternate feet going up steps, pedals tricycle	Copies a circle, undresses completely, dresses partially, dries hands if reminded, unbuttons	Uses minimum of 250 words, 3-word sentences, uses plurals, knows all pronouns, repeats 2 digits	Group play, shares toys, takes turns, plays well w/ others, knows full name, ages, gender

| 4 yr | Hops, skips, alternates feet going down steps | Copies a square, buttons clothing, dresses self completely, catches a ball | Knows colors, says song or poem from memory, asks questions | Tells "tall tales," plays cooperatively w/ a group of children |
| 5 yr | Skips alternating feet, jumps over low obstacles | Copies a triangle, ties shoes, spreads w/ knife | Prints first name, asks what a word means | Plays competitive games, abides by rules, likes to help in household tasks |

HEALTHCARE MAINTENANCE

(Bright Futures Guidelines for Health Supervision of Infants, Children, and Adolescents. 4th ed. 2017)

Age	Anticipatory Guidance	Screening
New-born	• Weight gain, feeding • Crib safety (own crib in parents' room, narrow slats w/ sides up, back to bed, no loose bedding) • Rear-facing car seat in back seat • Home safety (smoke detectors, water temp <120°, no smoking) • Emergency phone numbers, CPR	• Newborn genetic screen • Hearing (if not done in hospital) • Postpartum depression • Vision, BP (if risk factors/concerns)
1 mo	• Start supervised "tummy time" • Develop routines, recognizing cues • Calm baby by rocking, talking, swaddling, never shake • Toy safety (caution w/ loops, strings, cords)	• Maternal postpartum depression • TB (if risk factors)
2 mo	• Strategies for ↑ fussiness • Plan for return to school/work • Keep small objects, plastic bags out of reach • Always supervise when on high place or in tub	• Verify hearing screening and rescreen if needed
4 mo	• Put to bed when awake but drowsy, can sleep in crib in own room (lower mattress before begins sitting) • Introduce cereal if child ready • Avoid bottle in bed	• Anemia (if preterm/LBW, not on iron-fortified formula)
6 mo	• Support ↑s in language and cognitive development, read aloud • Introduce cereal, single-ingredient soft foods if ready, limit juice • Clean teeth w/ washcloth/soft brush & water • Home safety (block stairs, cleaning products, heaters, outlet covers, window guards, weapons locked, avoid infant walkers)	• Oral health risk assessment • Lead (if risk factors) • TB (if risk factors)
9 mo	• Discipline (+ reinforcement, distraction, limit use of "no") • Anticipate changing sleep pattern • Be aware of new social skills & separation anxiety • Limit or avoid TV, videos, computers • Provide 3 meals, 2–3 snacks/d; ↑ texture & variety of table foods, introduce cup • Water safety (always be w/i arm's length)	• Structured developmental screen • Oral health risk assessment
12 mo	• Discipline (time out, praise, distraction) • Est. bedtime routine w/ reading, 1 nap/d • Supervise tooth brushing BID w/ fluoride • Encourage self-feeding (avoid small, hard food; choking) • Lock medications, know poison control number	• Anemia, lead
15 mo	• Maintain consistent routine. Present child w/ options, speak in simple clear language • Avoid bottle in bed • Fire safety (lock matches, lighters)	

18 mo	• Support independence but set limits • Daily playtime, read, sing • Anticipate anxiety in new situations • Toilet training (when dry for 2 hr at a time, knows wet/dry/bowel movement, pulls pants up/down)	• Structured developmental screen • Autism-specific screen
2 yr	• Switch to forward-facing car seat w/ harness[a] • Help child express feelings • Encourage play w/ others • Teach personal hygiene, toilet training (above) • Encourage active but safe play: bike helmet, supervise outdoor play, cross street w/ adult • Switch to fat-free milk[b]	• Autism screen • Lead screen • *Dyslipidemia (if risk factors)*
2.5 yr	• Repeat speech w/ correct grammar • Establish family routine including exercise	• Structured developmental screen
3 yr	• Encourage storytelling, imaginative play • Limit media exposure to <2 hr/d, no TV in bedroom • Move furniture away from windows	• Visual acuity measurement
4 yr	• Consider structured learning programs (preschool, museum trips), encourage reading • Teach safety around adults (abuse prevention) • Answer questions about body parts using appropriate terms	• Visual acuity measurement • Audiometry
5–6 yr	• Discuss school experiences • Eat breakfast; fruits and vegetables • 2 cups low-fat milk/dairy/d • 60 min mod to vigorous physical activity/d • Begin flossing daily • Water safety, swimming lessons • Use safety equipment w/ sports	• Visual acuity measurement • Audiometry (6 yr)
7–8 yr	• Once 4'9" can stop using booster seat in car, must use lap and shoulder belt • Ask teacher for evaluation if any concerns • Encourage independence • Discuss rules and consequences • Note and discuss early pubertal changes • Supervise computer use	• Vision screen (8 yr) • Audiometry (8 yr)
9–10 yr	• Encourage self-responsibility, assign chores • Know child's friends and ensure adequate supervision, discuss bullying • Puberty, body image • Counsel about sexual activity • Counsel about avoiding tobacco, alcohol, drugs • Limit nonacademic screen time to 2 hr/d	• Snellen test (10 yr) • Audiometry (10 yr) • Universal lipid screening
11–14 yr	• Begin speaking w/ child alone at clinic visits • 3+ serving low-fat milk/dairy/d • Coping w/ stress, mood changes, nonviolent conflict resolution • Secure alcohol and prescription medications • 13 yo may sit in front seat of car • Caution w/ drivers using any alcohol/drugs	• Snellen (once during time period) • *STI screening (if sexually active)* • *Substance use* • *Lipid screening (if abn b/w 9–11 yo or new risk factors)*
15–17 yr	• Driving safety: limiting night driving, teen driving, wear seat belt • Encourage responsibility, community involvement • Violence prevention, sexual activity, substance use	• Snellen (once during time period) • Fasting lipid profile
18–21 yr	• Planning for the future • Continue discussions regarding violence prevention, sexual activity, substance use	• Snellen (once during time period) • Fasting lipids

[a]*Car Safety Seats: A Guide for Families.* 2012, AAP.
[b]*Pediatrics* 2011;128:S213.

GROWTH & NUTRITION

Principles of Growth & Nutrition (*Bright Futures Guidelines for Health Supervision of Infants, Children, and Adolescents.* 4th ed. 2017)

- Term infants lose up to 10% BW in 1st wk, but should regain by 2 wk
- Exclusively breastfed infants gain weight faster than formula-fed infants for the first few months, this slows ~3 mo
- Feeding is recommended 8–12 times a d initially without going less than 3 hr between feeds
- No free water until 6 mo due to immature kidneys and inability to concentrate
- No cow's milk until 1 yr of age due to risk of iron deficiency. After 1 yr of age, can feed up to a maximum of 24 oz whole cow's milk a day
- Vitamin D: Not in breast milk. Supplement (400 IU daily if breastfed, 200 IU daily if formula fed) until taking >1 L of formula or milk
- Introduce complementary iron-rich (e.g., beans, broccoli, spinach, meats) foods between 4–6 mo, otherwise supplement 1 mg/kg/d iron at **4 mo** in exclusively breastfed infants

Average Growth & Caloric Requirements (Table adapted from *Nelson Textbook of Pediatrics.* 20th ed. 2015)

Age	Average Weight Gain (g/d)	Daily Caloric Allowance* (kcal/kg/d)
Birth–3 mo	25–30	115
3–6 mo	20	110
6–9 mo	15	100
9–12 mo	12	100
1–3 yr	8	100
4–6 yr	6	90–100

*Breast milk and standard formula have ~**20 kcal/oz**

Breastfeeding (*Pediatrics* 2012;129(3):e827–e841)

- AAP recommends exclusive breastfeeding until 6 mo followed by breastfeeding in combination with the introduction of complementary foods until at least 12 months of age. However many choose to breastfeed for longer
- Initial colostrum is high in antibodies and provides immunity boost
- Infant benefits: ↓ rates of AOM, GI infections, NEC, SIDS, asthma, eczema, and ↑IQ
- Maternal benefits: ↓ risk of breast/ovarian cancer, weight loss, cost savings
- Contraindications: Galactosemia or other metabolic disorders, drug abuse (methadone is ok if on maintenance), VZV lesions on breast, HIV, HTLV 1 or 2, untreated tuberculosis. Hepatitis B and C are NOT contraindications
- Mastitis and candidal infections are NOT contraindications; however maternal treatment is necessary

Commonly Used Formulas

Class	Brand Names	Carbohydrate Source	Protein Source	Indications
Term formula	Carnation Good Start; Enfamil w/ Iron; Similac w/ Iron	Lactose	Cow's milk	Appropriate for most infants
Preterm formula	Enfamil 24 Premature; Preemie SMA 24; Similac 24 Special Care	Lactose	Cow's milk	Less than 34 wk gestation; weight less than 1,800 g (3 lb, 15 oz)
Enriched formula	Enfacare; Similac NeoSure	Lactose	Cow's milk	34–36 wk gestation; weight 1,800 g (3 lb, 15 oz) or greater
Soy formula	Enfamil ProSobee; Good Start Soy; Similac Isomil	Corn-based	Soy	Congenital lactase deficiency, galactosemia
Lactose-free formula	Enfamil Lactofree; Similac Sensitive	Corn-based	Cow's milk	Congenital lactase deficiency, primary lactase deficiency, galactosemia, gastroenteritis in at-risk infants

Hypoallergenic formula	Similac Alimentum; Enfamil Nutramigen; Enfamil Pregestimil	Corn or sucrose	Extensively hydrolyzed	Milk-protein allergy
Nonallergenic formula	Elecare; Neocate; Nutramigen AA	Corn or sucrose	Amino acids	Milk-protein allergy
Antireflux formula	Enfamil AR; Similac Sensitive RS	Lactose, thickened w/ rice starch	Cow's milk	Gastroesophageal reflux

AA, arachidonic acid references Nutramigen AA.
(Adapted from Am Fam Physician 2009;79(7):565–570)

FAILURE TO THRIVE (FTT)

(Pediatr Rev, Failure to Thrive: Current Clinical Concepts, 2011)

Overview
- A physical sign of undernutrition, commonly thought of as crossing 2 major percentile lines or having a weight <5th percentile for age
- Most commonly due to caloric insufficiency, only ~10–20% have an identified underlying organic cause
- In malnourishment, weight affected first, then height, and then head circ.
- Ddx:
  - Inadequate caloric intake: Malnourishment can be secondary to food insecurity, incorrect formula prep, motor disfunction, poor breast-milk supply
  - Inadequate absorption: Milk-protein allergy, biliary atresia/liver disease, cystic fibrosis, necrotizing enterocolitis (NEC)/short gut, celiac disease
  - ↑ metabolic demand: Hyperthyroid, growth-hormone deficiency, congenital heart disease, chronic lung disease, chronic infection, genetic abnormality, metabolic disease

Workup
- Detailed birth, family, and social hx. Food diaries to estimate caloric intake
- Physical exam for dysmorphic features, evidence of neglect
- Observe the child feeding
- Pre- and postfeed weights to quantify intake
- Confirm results of newborn screen for hypothyroid, cystic fibrosis
- Lab tests are not generally recommended unless a specific etiology is suspected (e.g., cultures if infectious etiology/sepsis suspected, lead and CBC w/ MCV if lead poisoning suspected, sweat chloride test if cystic fibrosis suspected, celiac screen if celiac is suspected; baseline CBC and electrolytes are often obtained)
- Speech and OT (can assist w/ different bottle nipples, positions, and evaluation of infant's suck and swallow coordination
- Nutrition, lactation, or GI referrals may be helpful

Management
- Outpatient: Close observation, feed 120 kcal/kg/d × (median weight for age/current weight), encourage structured mealtime, concentrate formula to deliver calories if needed
- Inpatient: Indicated when physiologic signs of malnutrition (hypothermia, bradycardia), concern for safety, electrolyte abnormalities, or weight <60% of ideal
  - Initial steps: Observe feeding and latch, calorie counts, pre- and postfeed weights in breastfeeding infants (infant in same clothes, no diaper changes, before and after feed to quantify amt of breast milk delivered)
  - OT and speech consultation if suck/swallow reflex is uncoordinated or there is a concern for aspiration
  - GI consultation may be necessary if infant has been feeding an adequate amt documented during hospitalization but is not gaining weight
- In some cases NG- or G-tube placement may be required to weight restore infant if the above interventions have not been successful. Insulin resistance and metabolic syndrome is a risk that should be considered when nutritionally repleting

VACCINATIONS

- Up-to-date schedules available at: http://www.cdc.gov/vaccines/recs/schedules
- Guide for parents: http://www.cdc.gov/vaccines/spec-grps/parents.htm
- VISs are available at: http://www.cdc.gov/vaccines/pubs/vis/default.htm

Vaccine Safety
- Vaccine Adverse Event Reporting System (VAERS): http://www.vaers.hhs.gov
- Clinically significant event after vaccine admin should be documented in medical record and VAERS form should be completed

Contraindications (https://www.cdc.gov/vaccines/hcp/acip-recs/general-recs/contraindications.html)
- To any vaccine: Anaphylaxis after a previous vaccine dose or component
- Live attenuated vaccines should be administered together or at least 28 d apart
- **MMR:** Pregnancy, known severe immunodeficiency; contains trace amt neomycin
- **IPV:** Contains trace amt of streptomycin, neomycin, and polymyxin-B
- **Varicella:** Pregnancy, known severe immunodeficiency; contains trace amt neomycin, precaution if received antibody-containing product w/i 11 mo
- **Rotavirus:** SCID
- **DTap, Tdap:** Encephalopathy w/i 7 d of admin of previous dose
  - Defer vaccine in pts w/ progressive neurologic disorder (infantile spasms, uncontrolled epilepsy, encephalopathy) until neurologic status clarified
  - Freq boosters may result in Arthus-like rxn; painful swelling shoulder to elbow
- **Hepatitis B vaccine:** Caution in pts w/ severe yeast allergy, allergic rxn rarely occur
- **Influenza (live-attenuated):** Pregnancy, known severe immunodeficiency, certain medical conditions, anaphylactic allergy to eggs
- **Influenza (inactivated):** Anaphylactic allergy to eggs
- **Zoster:** Suppression of cellular immunity, pregnancy

SUDDEN INFANT DEATH SYNDROME (SIDS)

Definition (*AAP Policy Statement: SIDS and Other Sleep-Related Infant Deaths, Pediatrics 2016, e20162938*)
- Unexplained death of an infant <1 yo after thorough evaluation (scene investigation, autopsy, clinical review)

Pathophysiology/Proposed Mechanisms
- Largely unknown
- Some infants w/ SIDS have 5HT transporter gene polymorphism at the ventral medulla → ↓s arousal to hypercarbia/hypoxemia
- Nicotine exposure alters nicotinic acetylcholine receptor expression at brainstem → impairs arousal
- Exogenous stressors, such as positioning

Risk Factors
- Prematurity, LBW, and smoke exposure
- Breastfeeding is a protective factor

Prevention & Risks
- "Back to Sleep" campaign by AAP recommends putting infant to sleep on back every time until 1 yo
- No pillow, stuffed animals, or soft bedding, only firm crib mattress w/ fitted sheet
- If an infant rolls themselves over onto their stomach, it is not necessary to put them back on their back
- Avoid overheating and ventilate room as needed, as this has been shown to be a risk factor in SIDS

SKULL DEFORMITIES

(Pediatrics 2011;128:136; Clin Pediatr (Phila) 2007;46:292)

Principles of Skull Formation & Deformities
- Normally anterior fontanelle will close at 9–18 mo; posterior fontanelle closes at 2 mo
- Skull deformities usually will worsen in 0–4-mo period and stabilize between 4–6 mo, improve after 6 mo

- Etiology is a combination of limited or selective head rotation, supine position (↑ w/ "Back to Sleep" campaigns), rapid growth of skull and gravity

Basic Types
- Plagiocephaly: Asymmetric flattening of occiput w/ anterior displacement of ipsilateral ear, forehead, and cheek resulting in parallelogram shape
- Scaphocephaly/dolichocephaly: ↑ anterior–posterior diameter relative to biparietal diameter, often in premature infants
- Brachycephaly: ↑ biparietal diameter relative to anterior–posterior diameter, symmetric flattening of occiput

Prevention & Treatment
- Tummy time while infant is awake and being observed, and by alternating position of head while sleeping
- Changing infant's head position by moving visual stimuli in relation to the infant so head is turned different ways
- Treatment: Physical therapy for neck stretching if a component of torticollis present or not improved after 2–3 mo
- Helmet therapy if deformity is severe or no improvement by 4–6 mo

Craniosynostosis
- Definition: Premature closure of sutures casing skull deformity
- History of abnormal head shape since birth, varies by which sutures prematurely fuse
- Most common single-suture synostosis is sagittal craniosynostosis, which leads to scaphocephaly
- Can result in ↑ICP, which leads to neurologic defects
- Warrants immediate referral to neurosurgery
- Treatment is w/ helmet and/or surgery

Features Distinguishing (**left**) Deformational Plagiocephaly From (**right**) Unilambdoid Synostosis

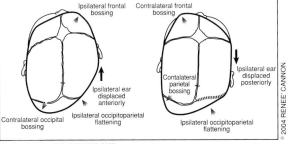

(Am Fam Physician 2004;69(12):2863–2287)

LEAD SCREENING AND TOXICITY

(Pediatrics 2016;138(1):e20161493; CDC, Lead, updated 2017)

Screening
- Recommended at **1 yr** and **2 yr** well-child visits in children who are at high risk (≥25% of houses built before 1960 or a prevalence ≥5% of blood lead ≥5 μg/dL)
- ~5% of children between 12–24 mo will have elevated lead levels
- Additional lead levels at different ages may be indicated if risk factors exist (e.g., sibling w/ elevated lead level, pica behaviors)

Risks
- Homes built before 1978
- Home recently renovated (w/i past 6 mo)
- Sibling w/ elevated lead level
- Some methods of alternative medicine can ↑ risk of lead toxicity (if ceramics, for example, are involved)
- Developmental delay, pica

Pathogenesis
- Neurotoxin that interferes w/ cell migration during brain development
- Children more at risk due to immature blood–brain barrier
- Basophilic stippling apparent on histology (due to inhibition of pyrimidine 5-nucleosidase causing RNA aggregates)
- ↓ protoporphyrin → microcytic anemia

Symptoms
- Primarily asymptomatic
- Vomiting, anorexia, abdominal pain/colic
- Intermittent lethargy, irritability
- In severe cases: Encephalopathy, headache, coma, convulsions

Prevention
- Wash children's hands and toys
- Prevent children from playing in soil
- Take shoes off at door to prevent soil being brought in, clean floors regularly
- Limit exposure to lead-based paint jewelry, and imported food likely to be contaminated by lead

Treatment/Approach (CDC, Recommended Actions Based on Blood Lead Levels, 2018)
- Confirmatory venous sample usually recommended if elevated level on capillary sample
- For any elevated level (≥5): Obtain environmental history, provide education regarding risk reduction and nutrition
- ↑ calcium and iron in diet (prevent lead absorption)
- Assess developmental milestones
- Lead levels >10 must be reported to local health department

Recommendations for Confirmed Venous Lead Levels		
Level (µg/dL)	Recommendations	Follow-up level
<5	• Routine assessment of nutritional and developmental milestones • Anticipatory guidance about common sources of lead exposure	
5–9	• Routine assessment of nutritional and developmental milestones • Environmental assessment of detailed history to identify potential sources of lead exposure • Nutritional counseling related to calcium and iron intake	1–3 mo
10–19	• Routine assessment of nutritional and developmental milestones • Environmental assessment of detailed history and environmental investigation including home visit to identify potential sources of lead exposure • Nutritional counseling related to calcium and iron intake; consider lab work to assess iron status	1 wk–1 mo
20–44	• Complete history and physical exam • Neurodevelopmental assessment • Environmental investigation of the home and lead hazard reduction • Lab work: Iron status and hemoglobin or hematocrit • Abdominal x-ray (w/ bowel decontamination if indicated)	1 wk–1 mo
45–69	• Complete history and physical exam • Complete neurological exam including neurodevelopmental assessment • Environmental investigation of the home and lead hazard reduction • Lab work: Iron status and hemoglobin or hematocrit • Abdominal x-ray (w/ bowel decontamination if indicated) • Oral chelation therapy; consider hospitalization, if lead-safe environment cannot be assured	45–59 →48 hr 60–69 →24 hr
≥70	• Hospitalize and commence chelation therapy in conjunction w/ consultation w/ a medical toxicologist or a pediatric environmental health specialty unit • Proceed w/ additional actions according to interventions for BLLs between 45–69 µg/dL	Urgently as emergency test

Adapted from CDC, Recommended Actions Based on Blood Lead Level, 2017. Retrieved from https://www.cdc.gov/nceh/lead/acclpp/actions_blls.html

DEVELOPMENTAL DELAY

Differential Diagnosis
- Hearing loss
- Lead poisoning
- Genetic disorders (fragile X or Rett)
- Seizure disorder (consider EEG)
- PKU
- Fetal alcohol syndrome

Surveillance & Screening *(American Academy of Pediatrics; Council on Children w/ Disabilities: Surveillance and Screening Policy Statement, 2006)*
- Screening for developmental milestones at each visit starting at birth
- Standardized developmental screening is recommended at 9-, 18-, and 30-mo visits
- Commonly used screening tools: Ages & Stages Questionnaire, M-CHAT (autism specific)

Treatment
- Early intervention referral and evaluation if concern for developmental delay (federally funded for children ages 0–3). If patient is eligible for services, they can receive occupational therapy, speech therapy, physical therapy, or other interventions by appropriate professionals to assist the child developmentally
- Treatment of any medical or psychiatric comorbidities
- Child will transition to school-based services on child's 3rd birthday

DSM-5 Criteria: Autism Spectrum Disorder (ASD) *(Adapted from DSM-5, Carpenter, MUSC Center for Disease Control and Prevention, Autism Spectrum Disorder Diagnostic Criteria)*
- Persistent deficits in social communication and social interaction across contexts, as manifested by the following, currently or by history:
  - Abnormal social-emotional reciprocity (e.g., failure of normal back and forth conversation, reduced sharing of interests, emotions, or affect, failure to initiate or respond to social interactions)
  - Deficits in nonverbal communicative behaviors used for social interaction (e.g., poorly integrated verbal and nonverbal communication, abnormalities in eye contact/body language/gestures, lack of facial expressions and nonverbal communication)
  - Deficits in developing, maintaining, and understanding relationships (e.g., difficulty adjusting behavior to suit various social contexts, difficulty sharing imaginative play or making friends, absence of interest in peers)
- Restricted, repetitive patterns of behavior, interests, or activities as manifested by at least two of the following:
  - Stereotyped or repetitive speech, motor movements, or use of objects
  - Insistence on Sameness (IOS), inflexible adherence to routines, ritualized patterns of verbal or nonverbal behavior, or excessive resistance to change
  - Highly restricted, fixated interests that are abnormal in intensity or focus
  - Hyper or hyporeactivity to sensory input or unusual interest in sensory aspects of environment
- Symptoms must be present in early childhood
- Symptoms together limit and impair everyday functioning (e.g., socially, occupationally, nutritionally)
- Symptoms not better explained by intellectual disability or global developmental delay

OVERWEIGHT AND OBESITY

Definitions
Adult:
- Overweight = Body mass index (BMI) between 25–30
- Obese = BMI >30
- Morbid obesity = BMI >40
Pediatric:
- Overweight = BMI ≥85th percentile
- Obese = BMI ≥95th percentile

Complications (Pediatrics 2005;116:473)
- Respiratory: Obstructive sleep apnea
- Cardiovascular: Hypertension, hypercholesterolemia, coronary artery disease as an adult
- GI: Reflux, gallbladder disease, nonalcoholic fatty liver disease
- Endocrine: Type 2 diabetes, PCOS, metabolic syndrome (↑ waist circ + 2 of following: ↑ triglycerides, ↓ HDL, HTN, insulin resistance)
- Orthopedic: Slipped capital femoral epiphysis (SCFE), osteoarthritis as an adult
- Neuro: Pseudotumor cerebri/idiopathic intracranial hypertension

Screening
- AAP and CDC recommend screening annually for children >2 yr of age w/ BMI

Treatment (*Recommendations for Treatment of Child and Adolescent Overweight and Obesity, Pediatrics, 2007*)
- Evidence-based treatment is generally limited for treatment of obesity
- ↓ in energy intake, but not <1,200 kcal has been shown to be effective in short term; however many children regain weight
  - ↓ sugary beverages or soft drinks
  - Limit television to <1–2 hr/d, no TV for children <2 yo
  - Reinforce importance of breakfast: Skipping breakfast is more common in children w/ obesity
  - Programs using self or parental monitoring of intake and parental modeling
  - Contingency management (e.g., must play outside before watching TV)
- Two drugs have FDA approval for obese children:
  - Sibutramine, a serotonin reuptake inhibitor, is approved for ≥16 yr
  - Orlistat, an enteric lipase inhibitor, is approved for ≥12 yr
- Gastric bypass surgery is rarely used and requires an extensive psychological and medical evaluation in addition to at least 6 mo in a behavior treatment program

EATING DISORDERS

(DSM-5, American Psychiatric Association, Feeding and Eating Disorders, 2013; Academy for Eating Disorders, Medical Care Standards Guide. 3rd ed. 2016)

Anorexia Nervosa
- Restriction of energy intake relative to requirements, leading to a significantly LBW in the context of age, sex, developmental trajectory, and physical health
- Intense fear of gaining weight or becoming fat, and the use of behaviors to prevent weight gain
- Presence of body image disturbance

Bulimia Nervosa
- Recurrent episodes of binge eating (defined as eating in a discrete period of time, a larger amt than most would eat, and a sense of lack of control over eating during the episode)
- Recurrent inappropriate compensatory behaviors in order to prevent weight gain (vomiting, laxatives, diuretics, other medications, fasting, or excessive exercise)
- Presence of body image disturbance

Binge Eating Disorder
- Recurrent episodes of binge eating (as previously described)
- Marked distress regarding binge eating
- Binge eating is not associated w/ the recurrent use of inappropriate compensatory behavior as in bulimia nervosa

Avoidant Restrictive Food Intake Disorder (ARFID)
- A lack of interest in eating or food; avoidance based on the sensory characteristics of food or concern about aversive consequences of eating as manifested by persistent failure to meet appropriate nutritional and/or energy needs
- The eating disturbance does not occur w/ another eating disorder, and there is no evidence of body image disturbance
- The eating disturbance is not attributable to a concurrent medical condition/disorder or the severity of the eating disturbance exceeds that routinely associated w/ the condition or disorder and warrants additional clinical attention

Major DSM-5 Changes
- ARFID and binge eating disorder as new diagnoses
- Elimination of a minimum weight for diagnosis of anorexia nervosa

Medical Complications & Management
- Refeeding syndrome: Occurs during weight restoration as a result of ↑ use of ATP leading to hypophosphatemia. Treated w/ oral supplementation to prevent severe metabolic derangements
  - Hypokalemia, hypoglycemia, and hypomagnesemia can also be seen
  - Clinical features of refeeding syndrome are edema, heart or respiratory failure, muscle weakness
  - Risk factors: Severe malnutrition or rapid weight loss, postbariatric surgery, previous refeeding syndrome
  - Prevention/treatment: Monitoring of electrolytes w/ oral supplementation being the preferred method of correction. Phosphate will nadir at 3–7 d. Consider inpatient refeeding or slower rate of caloric ↑ if at high risk
- Amenorrhea occurs as a result of ↓LH/FSH. DEXA scan indicated for amenorrhea >6 mo. OCPs are not recommended to induce menstruation, and can have a harmful effect on bone density
- Hyponatremia and hypochloremia as a result of purging can lead to metabolic acidosis
- Bradycardia and hypotension can be indicative of malnutrition. Prolonged QT and CHF can lead to sudden cardiac death in severe cases. Avoid large boluses of fluids
- Mallory–Weiss tears: Tears in mucosal lining due to persistent vomiting. Can lead to esophageal rupture
- Russell sign: Calluses on knuckles as a result of purging

CONTRACEPTION/GYNECOLOGY

(American Academy of Pediatrics, Policy Statement on Contraception for Adolescents, 2014; CDC, US Medical Eligibility Criteria for Contraceptive Use, 2010)

Basic Concepts of Pediatric Gynecology
- Setting expectations for confidentiality is important. If a pediatric patient (<18 yo) reports sexual abuse, healthcare providers are required to report to CPS
- While providers aren't required to share sexual health information w/ a patient's parents, certain tests and treatments may be visible to parents via insurance paperwork
- Encourage patients to discuss sexual health w/ a parent or trusted adult as appropriate
- Counsel on most effective contraceptive options first; long acting reversible contraceptives (LARC)
- For reference, unprotected sexual contact will yield an 85% pregnancy rate in 1 yr

Intrauterine Device (IUD)
- Copper IUDs can lead to heavier bleeding. Approved up to 10 yr
- Hormonal (levonorgestrel) leads to lighter bleeding or amenorrhea in most patients. Approved up to 5 or 3 yr depending on product
- Risk of ectopic pregnancy is lower than without contraception; however since IUDs are so effective at preventing pregnancy, confirmed pregnancies are more likely to be ectopic in women w/ IUDs
- Can be used in nulliparous women
- Contraindicated only if active pelvic infection
- Considered one of the most effective methods of birth control (<1% pregnancy rate)

Progestin Implant
- Placed in upper arm
- Patients often experience irregular bleeding initially, which usually resolves in 6 mo. ~25% of implant users discontinue w/i a year w/ irregular bleeding being the most common cause. Can give oral contraceptives in addition to implant to control spotting/bleeding. (Contraception 2006;74(4):287–289)
- Considered one of the most effective methods of birth control (<1% pregnancy rate)
- Barrier protection needed for 1st wk or after placement

Injectable
- Medroxyprogesterone injections every 3 mo
- Side effects include weight gain, ↓ bone density and delayed return of fertility w/ discontinuation (up to a year)
- Due to ↓ in bone density, vitamin D and calcium are recommended
- Requires adherence to injection schedule, w/ 6% pregnancy w/i a year of typical use

Oral Contraception
- Up to 8% failure rate w/ typical use <1% failure rate w/ perfect use
- Estrogen-containing contraception:
  - ↑ risk of thrombosis and is contraindicated in patients w/ clotting disorders, migraines w/ aura or focal neurologic signs (↑ risk of stroke), uncontrolled hypertension, and patients who smoke if 35 yr and older
  - Protective against endometrial and ovarian cancer
  - Metabolized hepatically, therefore certain medications can ↓ effectiveness such as rifampin and anticonvulsants
  - Can be helpful in patients w/ PCOS, because the mechanism of action is inhibition of ovulation
- Progestin-only OCPs:
  - Mechanism of action is thickening of cervical mucous
  - Different side-effect profile, can be used in individuals w/ risk factors of thrombus
  - Safe in breastfeeding mothers

Emergency Contraception
- Levonorgestrel 1.5 mg ("Plan B") or ulipristal 30 mg ("Ella") can be administered without a prescription at any pharmacy
- Prevents ovulation and follicular development. No known effects on implantation
- Indicated w/i 72 hr of unprotected sex is preferred (75%+ ↓ in pregnancy). Can be effective for up to 120 hr
- Copper IUD can also be used as emergency contraception device

Sexually Transmitted Infections: Prevention & Screening (CDC Treatment Guidelines, Sexually Transmitted Infections, 2015)
- Minors can consent to their own care for sexually transmitted infections without parental notification
- **Barrier protection** (e.g., condoms) should be recommended to all individuals at risk for STIs including those using LARC
- **Annual testing** is recommended for chlamydia and gonorrhea in all sexually active women <25 and in individuals w/ HIV
- **Collection:** Chlamydia and gonorrhea can be diagnosed by self-collected urine specimen. "Vaginitis probe" test for bacterial vaginosis (Gardnerella), Candida, and Trichomoniasis. This can be collected vaginally by the patient
- **HIV testing** should also be offered to all adolescents confidentially w/ frequency of repeat testing based on risk

Human Papillomavirus (HPV) & Cervical Cancer
- **HPV vaccine** indicated for **all patients regardless of sexual activity** to protect against cervical cancer, anogenital cancer, and oropharyngeal cancer. Vaccine series is 2 doses or if started before 15th birthday w/ a minimum of 5 mo between doses. Individuals who are immunocompromised or started series on 15th birthday or later need 3 doses: 4 wk between doses 1–2, 12 wk between doses 2–3, 5 mo between doses 1–3 (CDC 2017 Immunization Schedule)
- **Pap smears:** Indicated in all patients 21–65 yo by USPSTF every 3 yr. In women 30–65 yo, can space to ever 5 yr if used in conjunction w/ HPV testing

Sexually Transmitted & Pelvic Infections: Treatment (CDC Treatment Guidelines, Sexually Transmitted Infections, 2015)
- **Chlamydia:** Azithromycin 1-g PO as a single dose. USPSTF recommends test of cure for women 3 mo after treatment
- **Gonorrhea (including pharyngeal):** Ceftriaxone 250-mg IM as single dose. USPSTF recommends test of cure for women 3 mo after treatment
- **Syphilis:** Benzathine penicillin G, dose and duration dependent on stage
- **Bacterial vaginosis:** 500-mg metronidazole BID × 7 d (cannot use alcohol while taking)
- **Trichomoniasis:** 2 g of metronidazole or tinidazole as single dose. If persistent, 2-g metronidazole × 7 d
- **Candida:** 150-mg PO fluconazole as single dose
- **Pelvic inflammatory disease:** 2-g IV cefotetan q12 hr & 100-mg doxycycline PO/IV q12 hr OR 2-g IV cefoxitin & 100-mg doxycycline q12 h

Viral Upper Respiratory Infections

- Typical course lasts 7–10 d, hospitalization is rarely needed
- Symptoms include congestion, cough, fevers are usually low grade
- Treatment is symptomatic: Hydration, rest, antipyretic for fevers and comfort. Cough suppressants are not recommended in children as they have poor evidence for efficacy
- Period of improvement followed by period of worsened illness can be an indication for secondary bacterial pneumonia
- Viral bronchiolitis and can be more problematic due to relatively small airway anatomy. Hospitalization is sometimes needed for hydration or oxygen administration, and symptoms peak at 4–5 d

Urinary Tract Infection (AAP, Urinary Tract Infection: Clinical Practice Guidelines, 2016)

- Symptoms include burning during urination, ↑ in urinary frequency, abdominal pain, nausea, vomiting, and fever (fever is most likely the presenting complaint in infants)
- Risk factors: Female sex, constipation, vesicoureteral reflux
- Management:
  - Antibiotic choice may vary by local susceptibilities. Amoxicillin, cephalexin, nitrofurantoin, and trimethoprim-sulfa are common options. Treatment duration is **7–14 d**
  - Febrile infants w/ UTIs should have renal and bladder ultrasonography to evaluate for anatomic abnormalities. If this reveals hydronephrosis, a voiding cystourethrogram (VCUG) is indicated
  - Treatment thresholds: >50,000 colonies of a single organism on cathed urine specimen, >100,000 colonies on "clean catch", or >10,000 if accompanied by WBC >10/high-powered field. **Cathed specimen is recommended for febrile infants or other ill-appearing children.** Urinalysis w/ +leukocyte esterase and +nitrites is indicative of a UTI
- Prevention: Treatment of constipation, prophylactic antibiotics if 3 febrile UTIs in 6 mo or 4 total UTIs in 1 yr (trimethoprim-sulfa or nitrofurantoin)

Toilet Training & Nocturnal Enuresis (AAP, Toilet Training: Guidelines for Parents, 1999; International Children's Continence Society, UpToDate, Nocturnal Enuresis in Children, 2018)

- The AAP recommends a **child-centered** approach to toilet training, w/ training beginning when child shows signs of readiness such as sphincter control (remains dry for several hours), ability to follow instructions, imitation of behaviors, and desire for independence. This usually occurs ~24–30 mo
  - Parents are encouraged to use positive reinforcement and reassurance when teaching child to use the toilet, and take care not to overcorrect accidents
  - Continence while sleeping (naps and night) occur later than daytime continence (thus diapers should still be used)
- Enuresis is defined as episodes of urinary incontinence at age ≥5 in the absence of other symptoms
- Primary enuresis = when children have never had a period of nighttime dryness (80%); secondary enuresis = enuresis after a period of nighttime dryness (20%), often occurs after stressful event or change
- Epidemiology: 16% of children aged 5 have enuresis, 10% at age 7, 5% at age 10
- Management and treatment: Enuresis usually resolves by itself, and reassurance and education may be sufficient. Sticker charts and motivational tools can also be used, as can enuresis alarms and desmopressin is sometimes used, especially when children are older and are highly concerned about their enuresis (e.g., sleepovers)

Musculoskeletal Injuries (Pediatr Rev. 2013;34:366; Curr Rev Musculoskelet Med. 2008;3-4:190; Pediatr Emerg Care. 2016;32:452)

- Nursemaid's elbow: Caused by pulling of the child's arm by the hand or wrist. The elbow becomes dislocated and nearby tissue moves into the joint space, causing pain. Child will hold arm **slightly bend w/ palm facing inward**, and will **resist movement**. This can be reduced by hyperpronation, or supination followed by flexion

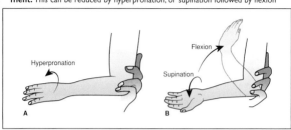

From Tintinalli JE, Stapczynski JS, Ma OJ, Yealy DM, Meckler GD, Cline DM. *Tintinalli's Emergency Medicine: A Comprehensive Study Guide.* 8th ed. 2015: McGraw-Hill Education.

- Supracondylar fracture of the humerus: Most common at ages 6 and 7 because the supracondylar area is undergoing remodeling causing a more slender cortex. 95% of these fractures are **posteriorly displaced**. Caused by hyperextension and fall on outstretched hand, and has high risk of neovascular compromise
- "Toddler's fracture": Oblique, nondisplaced fracture of the distal 1/3 of the tibia, common in children 1–3 yr. Cause is usually rotational but low impact. Patients refuse to bear weight on affected leg
- **Concussions** (Pediatrics 2018;142:3074)
  - Due to biokinetics of acceleration–deceleration and rotational forces
  - For children, highest risk of concussion in high school is football
  - Symptoms can include fogginess, difficulty concentrating, confusion, irritability, drowsiness or sleep difficulty. LOC is uncommon
  - Workup includes detailed history and physical. Imaging is not recommended unless another injury is suspected, as concussions do not indicate a structural disturbance. If during a sports game, standardized score such as SCAT2 or BESS can be helpful in determining return to play
  - Treatment is physical and cognitive rest w/ gradual return to normal activities. Symptoms usually last 7–10 d

Attention Deficit Hyperactivity Disorder (CDC, Attention-Deficit/Hyperactivity Disorder (ADHD), 2017)

- Diagnosis of ADHD necessitates impairment in **2 settings**
- **Vanderbilt** questionnaires for parents and teachers can be helpful in tracking symptoms over time and monitoring for treatment effectiveness
- Behavioral therapy and medications vary by age
  - Ages 4–5: Behavioral training for parents, methylphenidate
  - Ages 6–11: Stimulates are most effective, then atomoxetine, then guanfacine ER, then clonidine ER
  - Ages 12–18: Behavioral and medications offered together
- Side effects of stimulants can include appetite suppression, sleep disturbances, irritability, ↑ heart rate (screen for early sudden cardiac death in family first)

INITIAL ASSESSMENT/TRAUMA EXAM

(Rosen's EM Concepts and Clinical Practice. 9th ed. 2018;2042–2057)

PRIMARY SURVEY

A—Airway
- Ensure patency (ask patient name, assess speech, and WOB), stabilize c spine
- Assess for signs of obstruction (i.e., gurgling, stridor)
  - Can use jaw thrust or chin lift if needed; avoid head tilt for c-spine protection
  - Clear airway of debris (loose teeth, blood, vomitus, etc.)
  - Utilize airway adjuncts as needed
- If unable to maintain airway, intubate or initiate bag-mask ventilation (BMV)
  - Indications for definite airway-impending obstruction (i.e., burns, penetrating injury); respiratory insufficiency; multisystem trauma w/ shock; GCS <9 or penetrating cranial injury

B—Breathing & Ventilation
- Assessment: Equal and adequate chest rise; respiratory rate; auscultation; assess trachea
- Mgmt: High-flow O_2 if needed; consider BMV as bridge to intubation if needed

C—Circulation & Hemorrhage Control
- Assessment: Perfusion (cap refill, extremities, pulses); vital signs
  - Assess for and control sources of hemorrhage
- Mgmt
  - Access: 2 large-bore IVs else I/O if needed; obtain labs including type and screen and VBG
  - NS bolus 20 mL/kg, repeat up to ×3; transfuse blood for hemorrhagic losses

D—Disability Assessment
- Assessment: LOC, GCS score; pupil size + reactivity; extremity movement; posturing[a]

Glasgow Coma Scale (GCS)		
Eye Opening	**Verbal**	**Motor**
4 = spontaneous	5 = oriented	6 = obeys commands
3 = to verbal stimuli	4 = confused	5 = localizes pain
2 = to pain	3 = inappropriate words	4 = withdraws from pain
1 = none	2 = incoherent	3 = flexion/decorticate
	1 = none	2 = extension/decerebrate
		1 = none

[a]Posturing – flexor = decorticate; extensor = decerebrate (worse, indicates brainstem injury)

- Mgmt: Manage seizures (BZDs), treat hypoglycemia (D50), treat ICP
  - For increased ICP: Elevate head of bed, analgesia + sedation; 3% saline (10 mL/kg) or mannitol (0.25–0.5 g/kg); neurosurgery consult

E—Events, Exposure
- Expose patient completely and log roll for complete exam; maintain normothermia

F—FAST & Family
- If trained and concern for significant blunt abdominal trauma, consider performing FAST Exam (high sensitivity for traumatic free fluid in peritoneum and pericardium). If perforating abdominal trauma, obtain STAT CT abdomen/pelvis
- Don't forget to update family

SECONDARY SURVEY

AMPLE History
- A: Allergies
- M: Medications
- P: PMH
- L: Last meal
- E: Events and environment

HEAD/NECK TRAUMA

- Initial assessment as above; look for any obvious injuries; GCS; detailed neuro exam
- Red flags for intracranial injury (ICI): Prolonged LOC, seizures, vomiting, amnesia, lethargy, signs of skull fracture or cephalohematoma, abnormal findings on neuro exam (Emerg Med 2013;23:190–199)
  - If any concerning features, obtain STAT CT head w/o contrast
  - If any findings of ↑ ICP, manage as discussed on prior page

Cervical Spine Injury (CSI)

- Children are at higher risk of c-spine and ligamentous injuries than adults; often associated with head injuries
- Clinical decision rules (Who do I obtain imaging in?)
  - **NEXUS Criteria:** >83% Se in systematic reviews (in **adults,** ↓ in peds) (Ann Emerg Med 1998;32(4):461)
    - RFs for CSI: Focal neuro deficit, midline spinal tenderness, altered LOC, intoxication, present, distracting injury present
    - If any of the following, consider radiographs. Else, c spine can be cleared
  - **PECARN:** Having 1 of below is 98% Se and 26% Sp for CSI in children (Ann Emerg Med 2010;58(2):145–155)
    - RFs for CSI: AMS, focal neuro deficit, neck pain (>2 yo), torticollis, substantial torso injury, high-risk mechanism (diving, >55 mph MVC, ejected from car, death in same crash), PMH RF for CSI (Hx of trisomy 21, connective tissue Dx, juvenile RA, etc.)
    - If any of the above, consider imaging (radiographs to start, CT if needed or high-risk mechanism of injury)
- Mgmt of CSI: Apply c collar on arrival, image per PECARN or NEXUS criteria, further mgmt depends on imaging results

Blunt Head Injury (BHI)

- Trauma is the most common cause of pediatric death; largely due to head injury
- Goal of clinical assessment to assess for risk of ICI and obtain imaging if needed
- Mgmt: Initially ABCs; then general exam
- History: Ask about mechanism (height, speed, restraining or safety devices) and sxs (LOC, amnesia, confusion, vomiting, headache, general behavior)
- Clinical decision tool: **PECARN Algorithm** (Lancet 2009;374:1160)
  - Indications for imaging (4% risk of ICI*): GCS <14 or AMS; focal neuroabnormalities; skull fracture on exam (<2 yo) or signs of basilar skull fracture (BSF) (>2 yo) → 4% risk of ICI
  - Other RFs (0.9% risk of ICI*): Observe for 4–6 hr, consider imaging
    - >2 yo: LOC, severe mechanism, vomiting, severe headache
    - <2 yo: LOC, severe mechanism, nonfrontal scalp hematoma, Δ behavior
  - If none of the above → do not image, <0.05% risk of ICI
- Other clinical-decision rules include CATCH and CHALICE: which were not as Se in meta-analysis
- Assuming imaging not indicated or negative, manage for concussion (PCP follow-up, graduated return to play, brain rest, etc.)

* Refers to clinically significant ICI (requiring neurosurgical intervention or prolonged hospitalization)

RESPIRATORY EMERGENCIES

ASTHMA EXACERBATION

- Initial assessment: Physical px (wheezing, RR, retractions, ability to talk); oxygen saturation
  - Consider CXR if any localized findings on exam or history concerning for pneumonia
- Triggers: Infections (URTIs, pneumonia), allergens, stress, cold air/change, exercise, smoke
- Mgmt:
  - O_2 prn, goal sats >92%
  - Bronchodilators: Albuterol/ipratropium nebs (duonebs) q20 min × 3 initially
    - NOTE: MDIs with spacer may decrease LOS as compared to nebulization (Cochrane 2014;CD000052)
  - If inadequate response, start continuous albuterol 0.5 mg/kg/hr (max 20 mg/hr)

- Steroids: Multiple options
  - IV: Solu-Medrol 2 mg/kg (max 80 mg) loading dose
  - PO: Prednisolone 1 mg/kg/d BID (max 40 mg) × 3–5 d or dexamethasone 0.6 mg/kg (max 12 mg) × 1 (equivalent in studies – ↓ nausea, and only 1 dose) (Ann Emerg Med 2016;67:593)
- If ongoing, IV magnesium sulfate 50 mg/kg (max 2 g) IV × 1 (watch out for hypotension)
- If ongoing symptoms, will require PICU consultation and admission
  - Consider terbutaline 0.01 mL/kg (of 1 mg/mL solution) max 0.4 mg subcu
    - Can also consider epinephrine 0.01 mL/kg (of 1 mg/mL solution) max 0.4 mg IM
  - Can consider continuous terbutaline – 10 mcg/kg over 10 min (max 500 mcg) bolus then 0.4 mcg/kg/min continuous (increase by 0.5 mcg/kg/min q30 min to max 4 mcg/kg/min)
  - If heading toward intubation, can try ketamine 2 mg/kg bolus + 2–3 mg/kg/hr; can prevent intubation in severe asthma (J Emerg Med 2006;30:163)
  - Consider HeliOx: ↓ density of gas → laminar flow → can ↓ work of breathing and prevent extubation (Pediatric Crit Care 2005;6(2):204)
  - Consider BiPAP: Start at 10/5 and escalate prn for improved work of breathing
    - Can ↓ WOB, ↑ ventilation, and prevent intubation (Pediatric Pulm 2011;46:949)
    - Consider simultaneous ketamine or precedex to help with tolerance
- **If all else fails**, intubate via RSI using ketamine (can help with bronchospasm) and your choice of paralytic
  - NOTE: Important to adjust I:E ratio and monitor RR on ventilator to match physiologic prolonged E time to minimize risk of auto-PEEP and PTX

ANAPHYLAXIS

(Tintinalli's Emergency Medicine. 7th ed. 2011;177:180)

- Clinical criteria
  - Acute onset (min to hr) with involvement of skin and/or mucosal tissue (hives, itching, swollen lips/uvula/tongue) + 1 of following:
    - Respiratory compromise (wheeze/bronchospasm, stridor, hoarseness, dyspnea, etc.)
    - Reduced blood pressure or signs of end-organ dysfunction (i.e., syncope, incontinence)
  - OR 2 of the following after exposure to likely allergen for patient: Skin/mucosal involvement; respiratory sxs; shock; persistent GI symptoms
- Mgmt:
  - Remove allergen; ABCDs; place on monitor; O₂ prn; establish IV access
  - IM epinephrine 0.01 mg/kg of 1:1,000 (0.01 mL/kg); max 0.3 mg; repeat q5–15 min if needed
    - NOTE: A repeat dose will often be needed
  - H1 blocker: Diphenhydramine 1.25 mg/kg (max 50 mg) IV
  - H2 blocker: Ranitidine 0.5–1 mg/kg (max 50 mg) IV
  - Albuterol prn for bronchospasm; NS bolus prn for hypotension
  - Monitor for at least 2–3 hr after dose of Epi prior to discharge
  - Can give IV Solu-Medrol for theoretical latent phase of response; no evidence to support this
  - Discharge with EpiPen (0.3 mg for >30 kg, 0.15 mg/Jr dose for 15–30 kg)

UPPER AIRWAY OBSTRUCTION/STRIDOR

(Nelson Textbook of Pediatrics. 20th ed. 2016;2031–2036;
Atlas of Pediatric Physical Diagnosis. 7th ed. 2018;868–915)

Croup

- Epi: Usually 3 mo–5 yo, most common at 2 yo; M > F; disease of late fall + winter
- Causes – Parainfluenza (75%), influenza, RSV, adenovirus, mycoplasma (rare), previously Hib
- Sxs: "Barking" cough, hoarseness, inspiratory stridor; low-grade fever; agitation, crying
- Px: Hoarse cough, inflamed nasopharynx, ↑ WOB, hypoxia (bad sign)
- Img (if obtained): XR can show "steeple sign"/subglottic narrowing (not very Se, can be seen at baseline). Diagnosis is primarily clinical and does not require imaging
- Mgmt: Dexamethasone 0.6 mg/kg (max 10 mg) (↓ LOS, ↑ sleep)
  - Racemic epi nebs 0.05 mg/kg prn for stridor at rest (minimum 4 hr obs post rac epi required)

Epiglottitis
- Epi: Rare now, usually 6–12 yo
- Causes – Hib; *H. influenzae* (nontypeable), GAS, *S. aureus*
- Sxs: **Toxic appearing,** high fever, sore throat, **rapidly progressive respiratory distress**
- Px: Tripoding, drooling (80%); ↑ WOB; stridor is a late and bad sign; cherry-red swollen epiglottis
- Img: CXR shows "thumb sign"
- Mgmt: AIRWAY EMERGENCY (may require intubation, should have specialists [anesthesia, ENT] at bedside), humidified O_2 prn. Obtain IV access if no impending airway issues, start IV ABX (vanc + CTX). Don't lie patient down, let parents hold child for maximum comfort (airway can worsen when fussy or agitated)

Retropharyngeal Abscess
- Epi: 3–4 yo
- Causes: GAS, *S. aureus*; respiratory anaerobes
- Sxs: Sudden high fever, toxicity, drooling, "hot potato voice," ↑ WOB in pt with URI Sxs prior
- Px: Pain with movement of neck; stertor; ↑ WOB; pharynx asymmetrically swollen
- Img: XR (lateral neck) shows widened prevertebral soft tissue (poor Se)
- Mgmt: Manage airway as needed, ENT consult (may require drainage), consider CT scan, start IV ABX (unasyn or clinda)

Foreign Body Aspiration
- Always on differential for acute onset respiratory distress; esp w/o other URI Sxs
- Sxs: Sudden coughing/choking w/o signs of illness; tachypnea
- Px: Focal wheezing or ↓ air movement, stridor
- Mgmt: If severe sxs + history → back blows, Heimlich; call pulm for possible rigid bronch
  - If unsure/stable → obtain lateral neck XR + CXR + R and L lateral decubitus films (evaluate for air trapping – side with obstruction will not collapse as much when child lies on that side)

CARDIOVASCULAR EMERGENCIES

SHOCK

- Shock = inability of body to deliver adequate oxygen to meet metabolic demands of vital organs and tissues (whether this is due to perfusion, lack of oxygen, or increased demand) (*Nelson Textbook of Pediatrics.* 20th ed. 2016;516–517)
- See page *** in reference section for normal VS by age

Types of Shock
- Should consider all etiologies of shock as they do occur with relative frequency in pediatrics (Peds EM 2010;30:622)

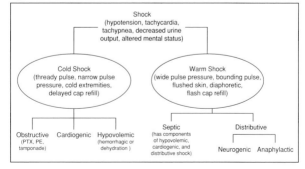

- Obstructive ← PTX, PE, tamponade
  - Clinical sxs: Distended neck veins, pulsus paradoxus, etc.
- Cardiogenic ← Cardiomyopathy, ischemic insult, etc.
  - Clinical sxs: Peripheral edema, pulmonary edema, elevated JVP
- Hypovolemic ← Hemorrhage, increased insensible losses/decreased intake
  - Clinical sxs: Dry mucous membranes, dry skin, etc.
- Septic ← Infection (bacterial, viral, fungal, etc.)
  - Clinical sxs: Usually have signs of infection (fever, ↑ WBC, localizing sxs for infection)
- Neurogenic ← Spinal trauma/shock
- Anaphylactic
  - Clinical sxs: Usually with assoc. stridor/respiratory symptoms, peripheral flushing, wheezing

Management of Shock

- Initial eval: Px (assess ABCs), VS, CBC, CMP, lactate, can consider VBG, blood cultures, consider UA + urine culture; imaging as indicated by exam; establish access (2 large-bore IVs)
- Increase/restore intravascular volume
  - NS boluses 20 mL/kg pushed rapidly, repeated up to 3 times
  - Monitor for signs of fluid overload (esp if any cardiac history)
- Assess for etiologies of shock and then treat appropriately
  - If septic, start broad-spectrum antibiotics right away (initial choice varies by institution)
  - If obstructive, resolve obstruction (decompress, drain effusion, anticoagulate/lyse, etc.)
  - If cardiogenic, be gentle with IVF and call PICU as patient may need inotropic agents or advanced therapies
  - If hemorrhagic, give blood
  - If anaphylactic, see **Anaphylactic Shock** on page***
- If remain in shock despite fluid resuscitations, can start pressors peripherally in consultation with PICU
  - Cold shock → start with epinephrine 0.05–1 mcg/kg/min
  - Warm shock → start with norepinephrine 0.1–1 mcg/kg/min
  - May require arterial line or central access if remain critically ill, or intubation if there are concerns regarding mental status or airway
- Continually reassess mgmt and patient
  - Further/advanced treatment of shock is discussed in PICU

SVT

- Most common nonsinus pediatric arrhythmia
- Cause: Accessory pathway (50%) vs. nodal reentry (20%) vs. ectopic atrial foci (15%) (*Cardiac Electrophysiology.* 7th ed. 2018;1030–1044)
- ECG: Narrow complex (<0.08 s), regular R-R, unvarying tachycardia with HR > 180 (children) or >220 (infants); P-waves absent (*Rosen's Emergency Medicine.* 9th ed. 2018;2099:2145)

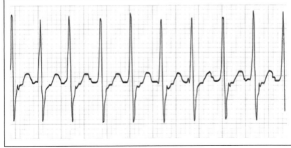

From Allen HD, Shaddy RE, Penny DJ, et al. *Moss and Adams' Heart Disease in Infants, Children, and Adolescents.* 9th ed. Philadelphia, PA: Wolters Kluwer; 2016.

- Sxs: Very non-Sp in children – fatigue, dizziness, palpitations; infants → fussiness/crying
- Mgmt
  - Initial: Assess hemodynamic stability, obtain ECG, obtain IV access

- **Stable** → put on monitor + apply AED pads; try **vagal maneuvers** (ice to face, Valsalva, knees to chest); else **adenosine** 0.1 mg/kg (max 6 mg); repeat in 3 min with double the dose (max 12 mg) (via 3-way stop cock, followed by rapid NS flush); if refractory → **sync cardioversion**
  - If remains refractory → call Peds Cards; consider **amiodarone** 5 mg/kg (max 300 mg) over 20–60 min
  - Or procainamide 15 mg/kg IV over 30–60 min (do not use with amiodarone)
- **Unstable/signs of shock** → **synchronized cardioversion** 0.5–1 J/kg; repeat with 2 J/kg if needed; sedate if possible

BRUE/BRIEF RESOLVED UNEXPLAINED EVENTS (FORMERLY ALTE)

(Pediatrics 2016;137:e1–e32)

- Def: An event occurring in infant <1 yo when observer reports sudden, **brief (<1 min)**, and now **completely resolved** episode of >1 of following: Cyanosis or pallor; absent, decreased, or irregular breathing; marked change in tone; altered level of responsiveness
  - For diagnosis of BRUE to be made, workup must be completely negative
- Workup (obtain H&P, additional workup per exam) → determine if high or low risk
  - High-risk groups: <2 mo, <32 wk GA, recurrent events
  - Low-risk groups: Opposite of above + <1 min event, no concerning findings on H&P
- Etiologies: No cause found in 50% of cases; most common causes = GERD, seizure, lower respiratory tract infection
  - Others: Child abuse, arrhythmia, infection (i.e., pertussis, URI, PNA), seizures, congenital/genetic, breath-holding spells, OSA, congenital or acquired heart disease, hypoglycemia, sepsis
- Mgmt if deemed to be low risk – Educate parents re: BRUE, offer CPR training, monitor for ~4 hr; arrange for close follow-up
  - NOTE: Labs, imaging, and admission are not required for most BRUEs
- Mgmt if deemed to be high risk – Workup as appropriate, will likely require admission for workup
- Prognosis: Studies show no correlation between BRUE/ALTE and SIDS

NEUROLOGIC EMERGENCIES

SEIZURES/STATUS EPILEPTICUS

- Status epilepticus = continuous seizures or intermittent seizures w/o complete recovery for >30 min
- Etiologies: Idiopathic (24%), febrile (24%), CNS infection, trauma, intoxication, metabolic, neoplasm, neurocutaneous syndrome, shunt malfxn (if Hx)
- Mgmt
  1. Assess + manage ABCs (with focus on airway); obtain access + labs (BG, CBC, CMP, Ca, Mag, tox studies prn; anticonvulsant levels prn, blood cultures); place patient on side (prevent aspiration); O_2 prn
  2. Start with BZDs: **IV/IM lorazepam** 0.05–0.1 mg/kg (max 2 mg) OR **PR diazepam** 0.5 mg/kg (max 20 mg) OR **buccal midazolam** 0.5 mg/kg (may work better than PR diazepam) (Lancet 2005;366:205–210); repeat 5 min prn (IM as good as IV). Trial at least 2 doses prior to escalating
  3. If any concern for infectious component/possible meningitis, start CTX 50 mg/kg (max 2 g); lack of LP should not delay antibiotics
  4. If refractory: 1. Load **fosphenytoin** 20 mg/kg (PE equivalent) @ 3 mg/kg/min (max 150 mg/min); 2. Load **levetiracetam** 20 mg/kg @ 5 mg/kg/min; 3. Consider **phenobarbital** 15–20 mg/kg @ 1 mg/kg/min and ICU admission
     - NOTE: If remains refractory after fosphenytoin load, will likely require intubation

FEBRILE SEIZURES

(Rosen's EM Concepts and Clinical Practice. 9th ed. 2018;2058–2068)

- Def: Seizure accompanied by fever w/o evidence of CNS infection in patient with no prior Hx of seizures
- Epi: 6 mo–5 yo; RF is rate of change of fever not degree of fever;

- Types
  - Simple: Single, <15 min, nonfocal or tonic-clonic
  - Complex: Recurrent (>1 in 24 hr), >15 min, focal, occur outside typical age range
- Mgmt: If ongoing >10 min, treat as above with BZDs; if resolved...
  - Simple → control fever, monitor; no workup needed
  - Complex → consider neuro consult; may require imaging + EEG (possibly as OP)
  - Indications for LP (Pediatrics 2011;127(2):389) – Meningeal signs of ill-appearing, <1 yo, and unvaccinated or s/p recent antibiotic treatment, consider in <6 mo since true febrile seizures are rare at that age
- Prognosis: 33% will have febrile seizure in the future; 1–2% risk of epilepsy (0.5–1% in gen pop)
  - RFs for recurrence: FH, <18 mo, lower fever or short duration of fever prior to seizure

HEADACHES/MIGRAINES

- Evaluation: Pattern/onset, activity @ onset, location, relieving factors, prior history of headaches, recent trauma, neuro exam
- Red flags: Sudden onset, severe onset, activity associated, trauma associated, focal neuro abnormalities
- If concerned: Initial test = CT head to r/o acute intracranial pathology
- Migraine sxs: Headache assoc. w/ n/v, photophobia, phonophobia, sometimes abd pain
- Mgmt of migraines: Consider 20 mL/kg NS bolus; promethazine 0.15 mg/kg (max 10 mg, works better than ketorolac); ketorolac (0.5 mg/kg max 30 mg) (Ann Emerg Med 2004;43:256–262)
  - If ongoing, can consider dose metoclopramide 0.2 mg/kg (max 10 mg) and diphenhydramine 1 mg/kg (max 50 mg)

SURGICAL EMERGENCIES

APPENDICITIS

- Cause: Obstruction of appendix from inflammation, fecolith, or enlarged lymph node
- Epi: Most common indication for emergent abdominal surgery in children; up to 8% of acute abdominal pain in children
- Pathophysiology of pain
  - Initial obstruction → stretching of hollow organ → stimulation of visceral nerves → initial referred pain of T10 dermatome (**periumbilical**)
  - As inflammation progresses → local peritoneal irritation → somatic nerve stimulation → **RLQ pain** and can eventually progress to **peritonitis**
- Clinical sxs → periumbilical pain migrating to RLQ, anorexia, vomiting (after onset of pain), pain with movement (peritonitis)
- Px findings
  - Peritoneal signs (pain with shaking, walking, jumping, bumps during car ride)
  - Not validated in peds – Rovsing sign (pain in RLQ with palpation of LLQ), psoas sign (↑ RLQ pain with extension of R thigh), obturator sign (↑ RLQ pain with flexion and internal rotation of R hip)
- Clinical decision rule: Pediatric appendicitis score (Pediatrics 2008; 153:278–282)
  - Assign 1 point for: Anorexia, fever, nausea/vomiting, WBC >10,000, ANC >7,500, migration of pain to RLQ
  - Assign 2 points for: RLQ pain to coughing/percussion/hopping, tenderness over R iliac fossa

Score	Risk of Appe	Mgmt
<2	2%	Unlikely Appe, 99% NPV
3–6	8–38%	Further workup, serial exams
> = 7	78–96%	Urgent imaging, surg consult

- Workup
  - Labs: CBC, BMP
  - Imaging
    - Abd US: Up to 98% Se **IF** appendix is visualized – first choice unless urgent imaging indicated – look for noncompressible, fluid-filled appendix >6 mm
    - CT abd w/ contrast (94–100% Se, 93–100% Sp) – if US fails to r/o appendicitis or high clinical concern
- Mgmt: NPO, mIVF, surgical consult for appendectomy, broad-spectrum ABX if evidence of perforation or sepsis
  - New evidence – ABX alone may be sufficient therapy – primarily studied in adults – small study, but RCT to ABX 1st vs. surgery → ABX patients had decreased LOS and only 13% eventually required appendectomy (Ann Emerg Med 2017;70:1–11.e9)
- Complications
  - Perforation – Consider when signs of peritonitis or evidence on imaging – up to 25% of pts
    - Risk: Not as time dependent as previously thought, OK to wait up to 24 hr prior to procedure if needed (Journal of Pediatric Surgery 2018;396–405)
    - Tx: Start IV zosyn immediately, urgent surgical consult for immediate resection

---

INTUSSUSCEPTION

(Academic Radiology 2017;24:521–529)

- Pathophys: Telescoping of part of intestine into itself; most commonly ileocolic
- Cause: Mostly idiopathic, although up to 25% will have pathologic lead points
  - Lead points – Meckel (most common), viral infections, enteric infections, reactive lymphoid hyperplasia. Rarely polyps, lymphoma, AVMs, HSP, CF, HUS
- Epi: 6–36 mo; most common cause of SBO in this age
  - NOTE: Outside this age range, should have high concern for pathologic lead point
- Clinical → sudden onset, intermittent, severe, crampy pain with drawing up of legs toward abdomen; inconsolable; 15–20 min intervals; vomiting; bloody stool (50%)
- Diagnosis – Ultrasound – 97.9% Se, 97.8% Sp, nearly 100% NPV – looking for "target sign"
  - Consider KUB (to look for perforation or evidence of obstruction) – 48% Se, 21% Sp
    - NOTE: If symptoms resolve, may have spontaneously resolved → imaging will be negative
- Tx
  - If any concerning sxs or imaging for perforation → surgical consult for possible ex lap
  - Else, can try pneumatic reduction by radiology (83% success rate); liquid reduction not as successful and has more complications
    - NOTE: >3.5 cm intussusception → more likely to require surgical mgmt

---

INGESTIONS/TOXIDROMES

(Peds In Review 2017;38:207–220)

- Initial assessment: Take thorough history from available information sources (substances patient had access to, medicines kept at home, prior history of substance use, medications, timing, potential dose)
  - Tox-specific Px: ABCs, VS, neuro exam (LOC, pupil exam, tone/reflexes), mucous membranes, lungs, abdomen, skin (diaphoresis, flushing, impaired perfusion, track marks, etc.)
  - Labs: CMP, APAP level, ASA level, urine drug screen; ECG; consider VBG
- Sxs and the drugs that cause them
  - Miosis ← cholinergics, clonidine, carbamates, opioids, organophosphates, phenothiazines, pilocarpine, hypnotics
  - Mydriasis ← sympathomimetics, anticholinergics, withdrawal syndromes
  - Coma ← lead, lithium, EtOH, TCAs, thallium, heroin, arsenic, antidepressants, anticonvulsants, antipsychotics, antihistamines, risperidone, insulin, CO, clonidine
  - Seizures ← organophosphates, TCAs, insulin, sympathomimetics, cocaine, amphetamines, anticholinergics, methanol, PCP, BZD withdrawal, bupropion, EtOH withdrawal, lithium, lead
  - Hypoglycemia ← oral hypoglycemics, β-blockers, insulin, ethanol, salicylates

ACETAMINOPHEN INGESTION

- Epi: 1/3 of all ingestion-related visits; intentional or due to unintentional use of combination products
- Sxs → vague abdominal pain, nausea, vomiting
- Workup – LFTs, BMP, PT/INR, APAP level @4 hr after ingestion
- Tx: If <2 hr since ingestion, can consider charcoal 1 g/kg (max 50 g) po; NAC if above treatment line on Rumack–Matthew nomogram (to the R) (total 300 mg/kg given over 21 hr, see manufacturer dosing recommendation for protocol)
  - NOTE: 20% risk of anaphylactoid reaction with NAC – monitor closely, may require anti histamines and even epi

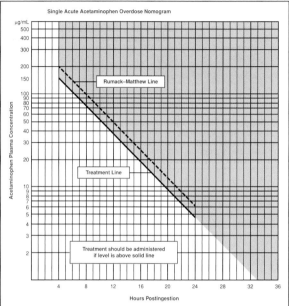

Single Acute Acetaminophen Overdose Nomogram

ASPIRIN INGESTION

- Sxs → vomiting, tinnitus, tachypnea, hyperpnea, tachycardia; if severe → mental status changes, delirium, agitation, and even seizures
- Workup: ASA level as above (peaks at 2 hr post ingestion), BMP with AGMA
- Tx: If level >30 mg/dL → urinary alkalization; >90 mg/dL → **hemodialysis**

ECG CHANGES IN TOXIC INGESTIONS

- Widened QRS (>100 msec) = abnormal; requires therapy due to risk of ventricular dysrhythmia
  - Causes: Local anesthetics, bupropion, carbamazepine, class Ia/Ic antiarrhythmics, cocaine, diphenhydramine, lamotrigine, quinidine, TCAs
  - Tx: IV sodium bicarbonate (disrupts sodium channel blockade) 1–2 mEq/kg bolus followed by 150 mEq in sodium bicarbonate in 1 L D5 @ 1.5–2 × maintenance; serial ECG and VBGs
- QTc prolongation (>500 msec)
  - Causes: Antipsychotics, class Ia/Ic/III antiarrhythmics, fluoroquinolones, macrolides, methadone, ondansetron, SSRIs, SNRIs

- Tx: Stop offending agent; check lytes and replete prn for goal Mag >2, goal iCa >2, and goal K 4
  - If torsades → Mag if HDS, else defibrillation

TOXIDROMES

(Harriet Lane, 21st ed. 2018;20–29)

- Anticholinergics → delirium, psychosis, paranoia, dilated pupils, thirst, hyperthermia, ↑ HR, urinary retention
  - Causes: Antihistamines, phenothiazines, scopolamine, TCAs, antipsychotics, anti-PD meds
  - Diagnosis: Physostigmine challenge 0.02 mg/kg repeat q5–10 min until effect (max total dose 2 mg) and monitor for sx improvement
  - Tx (if positive challenge): Supportive mgmt with hydration, BZDs prn for agitation, consider repeat physostigmine if sxs unresponsive to supportive care
- β-blockers → coma, seizures, AMS, hallucinations, bradycardia, AV block, CHF, hTN, respiratory depression, hypoglycemia
  - Tx: Glucagon
- CCBs → seizures, coma, dysarthria, lethargy, confusion, bradycardia, AV conduction block, widened QRS, hTN, pulmonary edema, hyperglycemia
  - Tx: CaCl 10%
- Cholinergic (muscarinic) → salivation, lacrimation, urination, defecation, ↑ HR, emesis, bronchospasm
  - Causes: Organophosphates
- Cholinergic (nicotinic) → Muscle fasciculations, paralysis, ↑ HR, ↑ BP
  - Causes: Tobacco, black-widow venom, insecticides
- Opiates → sedation, constricted pupils, hypoventilation, ↓ BP
  - Causes: opioids, dextromethorphan
  - Tx: Naloxone 0.1 mg/kg/dose (max dose 2 mg) repeat q2–3 min prn if effect seen
- Sympathomimetics → agitation, dilated pupils, ↑ HR, ↓ BP, moist skin
  - Causes: amphetamines, cocaine, albuterol, caffeine, PCP, ephedrine, LSD, MDMA
  - Tx: Supportive care
- Sedative/Hypnotic → ↓ mental status, normal pupils, ↓ BP
  - Causes: BZDs, barbiturates, EtOH, ethylene glycol, methanol
  - Tx
    - BZDs: Can consider flumazenil if acute ingestion, high risk of seizures in patients on chronic BZD therapy
    - EtOH: Supportive care
    - Ethylene glycol/methanol → fomepizole
- Serotonergic → confusion, flushing, ↑ HR, shivering, hyperreflexia, muscle rigidity, clonus
  - Causes: SSRIs, MAOIs, tramadol, TCAs, St John's Wort, trazodone
  - Tx: Supportive care; BZDs prn for agitation; cyproheptadine (antidote) if needed

ED PROCEDURES

PROCEDURAL SEDATION

- Goal: Administer sedative/dissociative agent + analgesic → alleviate pain, anxiety, and suffering during minor medical procedures while maintaining spontaneous cardiore-spiratory function
- Equipment needed: Monitors (ECG, oximetry, BP, CO_2 capnography); O_2 cannula + BVM + advanced airway equipment; drugs (see below)
- Choices of agents

Choice of Agents

Ketamine[a] IV 1–2 mg/kg bolus; then 0.5 mg/kg q15 min prn (ADRs – sympathomimetic, n/v, emergence rxn, laryngospasm, strange dreams)

Ketamine[a] IV 1–2 mg/kg; repeat 0.5 mg/kg q5–15 min prn

Etomidate 0.2 mg/kg IV (minimal resp depression)

Midazolam 0.05 mg/kg IV (0.02 mg/kg if w/ fentanyl) (ADRs – vomiting, resp depression, hypotension)

Propofol 0.5–1.5 mg/kg IV (repeat 0.5 mg/kg q5 min prn) (ADRs – CV + resp depression)[b]

Intranasal Sedatives
(Use IV preparation and split volume between nares, administer via atomizer)
Midazolam 0.4 mg/kg (max 10 mg)
Dexmedetomidine 1 µg/kg[c]
Fentanyl 1.5 mcg/kg (max 100 mcg)

[a]Has both sedative + analgesic properties
[b]No analgesic properties, good for sedation but not for painful procedures
[c]Some evidence to show improved success rate with procedure such as MRI over intranasal versed
(Anesth Clin Pharmacol 2017;33(2):236)

LACERATION REPAIR

(Peds EM 2010;9:1)

1. Irrigate wound thoroughly with NS using jet lavage (the more fluid the better!)
2. Check patient's tetanus status and obtain history regarding mechanism of injury
3. Assess wound – Site of wound? Active bleeding? Signs of infection? Time of injury? Can edges be approximated easily? Any concern for foreign body? Is it the result of a bite? Any neurovascular injury? Any tendon or deep structure injury?
   • If wound overlying joint space, need to r/o injury to joint capsule
   • If active bleeding, obtain hemostasis via pressure; if refractory → call specialist
   • If signs of infection → consider delayed primary closure; start ABX
   • If wound old (>6–10 hr) → consider delayed primary closure
   • If any concern for foreign body → low threshold to obtain imaging; irrigate extensively
   • If result of bite injury, see below
   • If any concern for tendon damage or neurovascular injury (i.e., on hand), consult specialist
4. Laceration repair
   • In young child/large or complex laceration, consider procedural sedation (above)
   • Anesthetize – Apply topical immediately (×30 min), followed by subcu prior to repair (below)

Topical (Agent – Onset – Administration – Notes)	Subcutaneous (Agent – Onset – Duration – Max Dose)
EMLA or LMX – 30–60 min – apply to intact skin – avoid use in <3 mo)	• Bupivacaine – 10 min – 200 min – 3 mg/kg
LET – 20 min – can apply to open dermis – avoid if concerned about perfusion	• Lidocaine – 5 min – 100 min – 4 mg/kg[*] • Lidocaine + Epi – 5 min – 120 min – 7 mg/kg

[*]NOTE: Lidocaine 1% = 10 mg/mL → 4 mg/kg = 4 mL/kg of 1% solution

   • Consider repair via adhesives for small wounds or facial wounds
   • Suture types (see next page for size and duration based on location of wound)

Nonabsorbable	Absorbable (Suture – Time to 50% – Complete Absorption Time)
Ethilon Silk Ethibond	• Vicryl rapide – 5 d – 42 d • Monocryl – 1 wk – 91–119 d • Fast gut – 7 d – 21–42 d • Chromic gut – 3–4 wk – 90 d

   • NOTE: No evidence to show different cosmetic result or infection rate with absorbable sutures

5. Postrepair care
   • Dress wound; advise to keep clean; avoid sun exposure
   • No evidence to support topical antibiotics or vit E; can use emollient after stitches are removed for scar prevention
   • Suture size + duration based on location of wound

Location	Size	Removal Time
Scalp	4-0–5-0	5–7 d
Face	6-0	3–5 d
Eyebrow	5-0–6-0	4–5 d
Lip	6-0	3–5 d
Trunk/Extremity	4-0–5-0	6–8 d
Hands/Feet	4-0–5-0	7–10 d

Bite Wounds

- Etiology: Dogs (90%), cats (5–10%), humans (2–3%), rodents (2–3%)
- Infection risk: Dogs (5–10%), humans (18%), cats (50%)
- Mgmt:
  - Aggressive irrigation + debridement
  - Assess need for rabies prophylaxis (consider IG for stray dogs that cannot be observed)
  - Contraindications for primary closure: Cat or human bite, puncture/deep wounds, hand or foot bites, bites involving genitalia or face, signs of infection
  - Tx: Primary closure if able, ABX prophylaxis (augmentin 22.5 mg/kg/d BID max 875 mg BID or bactrim + clinda)

ALLERGIC RHINITIS

(Ann Allergy Asthma Immunol 2013;111:446–451; Ann Allergy Asthma Immunol 2010;104:13–29; Ann Allergy Asthma Immunol 2009;103:373–380; J Allergy Clin Immunol Pract 2013;1:214–226; Pediatric Allergy. 3rd ed. 2016:210–218)

- Mucosal inflammation induced by IgE-mediated immune response to specific allergens
- Most common triggers: Animal dander, pollens, house dust mites, cockroach, mold
- Risk factors: Family history of allergy, higher SES, maternal smoke exposure, air pollution

Evaluation

- **History:** Rhinorrhea, congestion, cough, nasal, eye or throat itching
- **Exam:** Shiners, Dennie–Morgan lines, injected sclera with irritation, transverse nasal crease, pale and boggy nasal mucosa
- **Diagnosis:** Often clinical diagnosis is sufficient
  - Nasal smear looking for eosinophils
  - Skin prick testing, specific IgE measurement in blood (significant only w/ clinical sxs)
  - Gold standard: Nasal provocation challenge (not practical)
  - Consider sleep study to assess for OSA (Ann Allergy Asthma Immunol 2015;115:96–102)
  - Differential: Acute or chronic sinusitis, adenoid hypertrophy, nonallergic (vasomotor, episodic, infectious, gustatory), rhinitis medicamentosa (long-term use of decongestants)

Treatment

- Allergen avoidance: Requires trigger identification (skin testing, serum-specific IgE)
  - HEPA filter (pollen), impermeable bedding covers (house dust mites), ↓ moisture-prone areas (keep rooms at ideal humidity levels if possible)
- Antihistamines: 2nd gen (loratadine, fexofenadine, cetirizine, desloratadine, levocetirizine)
  - 1st gen (diphenhydramine, hydroxyzine)
  - Side effects higher with 1st gen; sedation, anticholinergic effects
- Intranasal corticosteroids (fluticasone, mometasone, budesonide)
  - Most effective maintenance for nasal congestion; side effects: nasal irritation, epistaxis
- Mast cell stabilizers (intranasal cromolyn)
  - Most effective prophylaxis, not widely used 2/2 frequent dosing
- Intranasal antihistamines (olopatadine, azelastine)
  - Effective for acute symptoms; side effects: bitter taste
- Immunotherapy (J Allergy Clin Immunol Pract 2014;2:332–340)
  - Consider when above ineffective, side effects limiting, or triggers difficult to avoid
  - Subcutaneous (injections): All aero-allergens
  - Sublingual (tablets): Grass for ages >5 yr, ragweed and house dust mite for ages >18
  - Limitations: Requires allergist referral, not well studied in children <5, poor adherence

SINUSITIS

(J Allergy Clin Immunol Pract 2013;1:205–211; Pediatric Allergy. 3rd ed. 2016:228–237)

- Inflammation of one or more paranasal sinuses
- Classified as acute, subacute, chronic, or recurrent (>4 episodes in 1 yr)
- Risk factors: Current allergic rhinitis, grass pollen hypersensitivity; association with asthma

Evaluation

- **History:** Rhinorrhea, headache, congestion, facial pain/fullness
- **Exam:** Sinus tenderness, purulent drainage in nasal cavity or posterior nasopharynx
- **Imaging:** X-ray if uncertain or recurrent, CT noncon if severe, immunocompromised, or suspect complications
- **Lab:** Nasal cultures if chronic or refractory, consider skin/serum IgE testing if environmental allergies result in greater severity and frequency
- **Diagnosis:** Often clinical diagnosis is sufficient

- Bacterial, viral, prolonged URI, rhinitis, turbinate or adenoid hypertrophy, CF, GERD w/ nasopharyngeal reflux, dental caries/abscess, primary ciliary dyskinesia (Kartagener)

Treatment
- Acute
  - Symptom duration <10 d and not worsening, likely viral etiology
- Analgesics &/or decongestants; use caution as little/no evidence for use in children & possible serious harm. Available studies suggest no use <2, no use <6, or not at all (Can Fam Physician 2009;55(11):1081–1083; JAMA 2007;297(8):800–801; Cochrane Database Syst Rev 2012;2:CD004976)
  - Symptom duration >10 d or worsening, likely bacterial etiology
    - Watchful waiting for reliable patients
    - First line: Amoxicillin or amoxicillin clavulanate
    - Analgesics &/or decongestants as above
- Subacute, chronic, recurrent
  - Nasal cultures can guide antibiotic choice
  - Nasal saline irrigations useful
  - Failed medical therapy, consider surgical management (ENT referral)
  - Consider workup for cystic fibrosis, primary ciliary dyskinesia, ABPA, Churg–Strauss

LOWER AIRWAY

Refer to Pulmonary section 13-2 and ED section 2-3 for anaphylaxis

FOOD ALLERGIES

OVERVIEW AND EVALUATION FOR FOOD ALLERGIES

(Ann Allergy Asthma Immunol 2016;117:452–454; Ann Allergy Asthma Immunol 2016;117:468–471; Ann Allergy Asthma Immunol 2014;112:121–125; J Allergy Clin Immunol Pract 2016;4:215–220; J Allergy Clin Immunol Pract 2015;3:1–11; J Allergy Clin Immunol Pract 2015;3:833–840; *Pediatric Allergy.* 3rd ed. 2016:371–376; *Harriet Lane.* 20th ed. 2012:338)

- Most often allergy to food protein, allergy to chemical/food additive uncommon
- Common (IgE-mediated) triggers: Milk, soy, egg, peanuts, tree nuts, wheat, fish, shellfish
- Common (non–IgE-mediated) triggers: Milk, soy, oat, rice
- Risk factors: Eczema (mod–sev), fam hx of food allergies, environmental allergies, asthma
- **Types:** IgE-mediated w/ acute onset of symptoms (within 30 min) vs. non–IgE-mediated with delayed or chronic symptoms

Evaluation
- **History:** Clinical symptoms occur reproducibly on exposure of a given food. Focus history points on timing in relation to ingestion, possible causal foods, food handling/preparation, additional factors around same time (illness, aspirin, exercise)
  - Symptoms include urticarial rash, rhinitis, wheezing, SOB, nausea, dysphagia, abdominal pain/cramps, vomiting, diarrhea, blood in stool
- **Exam:**
  - Skin: Acute urticaria, angioedema, atopic dermatitis
  - Respiratory: Rhinitis, wheezing, dyspnea, resp distress
  - Cardio/general: Lethargy, pallor, hypotension; FTT if chronic
- **Lab/Other:**
  - Skin-prick tests and/or allergen-specific serum IgE blood work to identify triggering foods
    - Serum IgE useful when unable to do skin testing due to skin conditions (severe atopic dermatitis, dermatographism) or unable to stop antihistamines for testing
- **Diagnosis:**
  - Gold standard: Double-blind, placebo-controlled, medically supervised oral food challenge
    - If no clinical history, skin prick or serum testing does not confirm allergy
    - To verify clinical reactivity to specific food allergen
    - Test periodically for resolution of allergy

- Differential: Anaphylaxis or other allergic reaction from another exposure (insect sting, drug); food intolerance (nonimmunologic); toxic/bacterial reaction to spoiled food; pharmacologic reaction to food

Treatment
- Allergen avoidance is basis of prevention
- Careful ingredient label reading, avoiding cross-contamination, nutritionist involvement
- Antihistamines, corticosteroids for less severe symptoms, EpiPen for anaphylaxis
  - Food elimination diets useful in suspected non–IgE-mediated chronic reactions (i.e., food protein–induced enterocolitis syndrome [FPIES])
    - To verify clinical reactivity to specific food allergen
    - Test for resolution of allergy

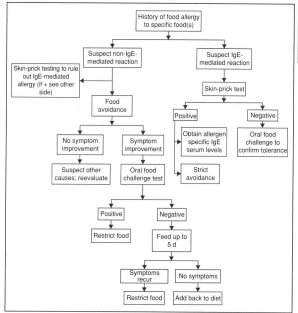

ORAL ALLERGY SYNDROME

(Ann Allergy Asthma Immunol 2010;104:101–108; Pediatric Allergy. 3rd ed. 2016:409–413)

- IgE-mediated food allergy due to cross-reaction of food proteins and pollen
- Examples: Birch tree and apple/pear/peach/almond; ragweed and banana/melon

Evaluation
- **History:** Symptoms (mucosal itching) localized to oropharynx after ingestion of fresh fruits & vegetables in patients with rhinitis
- **Lab/Other:** Skin-prick tests & serum-specific IgE levels to identify triggering pollens
  - Better clinical correlation if fresh fruit & vegetable extract used but not standardized
- **Diagnosis:** Often clinical diagnosis is sufficient
  - Differential: Contact urticaria/dermatitis, food allergy, EoE, burning mouth syndrome

Treatment
- Avoid trigger fresh fruits & vegetables, heated forms generally tolerated
- Oral antihistamines to relieve mild symptoms

FOOD PROTEIN–INDUCED PROCTOCOLITIS

(Allergy Asthma Proc 2015;36:172–184; *Pediatric Allergy*. 3rd ed. 2016:392–398)

- More commonly known as cow's milk protein allergy of infancy, typically seen in infancy
- Non–IgE-mediated food hypersensitivity localized to rectum and distal sigmoid colon

Evaluation
- **History:** Blood-streaked stools NOT associated with growth problems or FTT
  - Most common triggering foods: Milk, soy
- **Diagnosis:** Often clinical diagnosis is sufficient
  - Skin testing most often NEGATIVE (non–IgE-mediated)
  - Differential: Anal fissure, infection, FPIES or food protein–induced enteropathy (more severe), necrotizing enterocolitis

Treatment
- Triggering food avoidance w/ reintroduction of offending food after 12 mo of age
  - Breastfed: Maternal avoidance of milk (→ soy)
  - Formula-fed: Casein hydrolysate formula

FOOD PROTEIN–INDUCED ENTEROCOLITIS SYNDROME (FPIES)

(Allergy Asthma Proc 2015;36:172–184; Ann Allergy Asthma Immunol 2017;118:411–418; J Allergy Clin Immunol Pract 2013;1:317–322; J Allergy Clin Immunol Pract 2013;1:343–349)

- **Non–IgE-mediated food hypersensitivity,** typically seen in infancy

Evaluation
- **History:** Most common triggering foods: **milk and soy** for liquids, **oat and rice** for solids
  - Acute: Profuse vomiting, dehydration; delayed 1–4 hr after ingestion of trigger food
    - Commonly present to ED for acute vomiting → require IV fluid resuscitation
- Chronic: Food is ingested regularly in diet (cow's milk–based formula, etc.), chronic diarrhea, mucus or blood in stools, FTT
- Lab: CBC/diff (may show ↑ WBC w/ ↑ neuts, ↑ eos, ↑ plts, ↓ Hb/Hct)
- **Diagnosis:** Often clinical diagnosis is sufficient
  - Skin testing typically NEGATIVE (non–IgE-mediated)
  - Differential: Food protein–induced proctocolitis, eosinophilic GI disorders, sepsis in acute episodes, infectious gastroenteritis, necrotizing enterocolitis

Treatment
- Triggering food avoidance and reevaluation in 12–18 mo
- Delayed introduction of common trigger foods, work closely with RD

EOSINOPHILIC ESOPHAGITIS (EoE)

(Ann Allergy Asthma Immunol 2014;112:397–403; Ann Allergy Asthma Immunol 2007;98:207–215; J Allergy Clin Immunol Pract 2017;5:369–375; J Allergy Clin Immunol Pract 2013;1:332–340)

- Eosinophil-predominant inflammation of esophagus

Evaluation
- **History:** Food aversion, gagging in younger children, abdominal pain, GERD/indigestion, vomiting, dysphagia, or food impaction in older children
  - Can be triggered by multiple foods, possibly aeroallergens
  - Some is entirely PPI-responsive (not driven by foods)
- **Diagnosis:** EGD (w/ biopsy) showing >15 eosinophils/HPF at more than one location
  - Differential: GERD, infectious esophagitis (candida, etc.), esophageal dysmotility

Treatment
- Goal of therapy: Relieve symptoms and prevent disease progression
- Allergy testing for trigger foods, elimination diets (empiric or skin testing–based)
- Fluticasone (sprayed and swallowed) or oral viscous budesonide

CUTANEOUS/SKIN DISORDERS

ATOPIC DERMATITIS

(Ann Allergy Asthma Immunol 2015;114:6–11; J Allergy Clin Immunol Pract 2017;5: 1519–1531; J Allergy Clin Immunol Pract 2014;2:361–369; J Allergy Clin Immunol Pract 2014;2:388–395; J Allergy Clin Immunol Pract 2013;1:22–28; J Allergy Clin Immunol Pract 2013;1:142–151; Pediatric Allergy. 3rd ed. 2016:438–457)

- Characterized by defective epidermal barrier and cutaneous inflammation

Evaluation
- **History: Pruritus**, papulovesicular & erythematous lesions + excoriation & serous exudate
  - Common triggers: Climate, irritants (chemicals, fabrics, fragrances), microbes/ infection (staph, HSV), aeroallergens (dander, dust mites), ~1/3 of pts w/ food-related triggers
- **Exam:**
  - Infants: Erythematous, scaly lesions on face/cheeks, scalp, extensor surfaces
  - Children: Plaques in flexural areas
  - Adolescents: Localized and lichenified skin changes, mainly on hands and feet
- **Lab/Other:**
  - Skin prick &/or allergen-specific IgE blood work recommended in moderate to severe cases or those w/ history of exacerbation by specific environmental exposures or foods
  - SCORAD system severity classification
- **Diagnosis:** Often clinical diagnosis is sufficient
  - Differential: Allergic contact/irritant dermatitis, psoriasis, tinea (like nummular eczema)

Treatment
- Restore skin hydration
  - Frequent use of bland emollients (petroleum jelly, vaseline, aquaphor)
    - Multiple times per day & immediately after bath
- Reduce inflammation
  - Topical corticosteroids
    - Low (hydrocortisone) to medium potency (triamcinolone) for 7 d for flares
    - Higher potency (fluocinonide, betamethasone) if severe flare → taper w/ ↓ potency
    - Avoid use in groin, axilla, face
  - Topical calcineurin inhibitors (tacrolimus, pimecrolimus), 2nd line w/ derm consult
- Bleach baths, wet wraps
- Identification and elimination of potential triggers
- Infection (superinfection, coinfection):
  - Mild or limited: Topical bacitracin, mupirocin (avoid Neosporin due to contact dermatitis)
  - Moderate: Oral cephalexin or clindamycin empirically for 2 wk or longer
  - Severe: IV antistaphylococcal antibiotic, IV, or PO antiviral (for eczema herpeticum)

URTICARIA

(Am Fam Physician 2017;95:717–724; Ann Allergy Asthma Immunol 2017;118:500–504; Ann Allergy Asthma Immunol 2008;100:181–188; Ann Allergy Asthma Immunol 2008;100:403–412; J Allergy Clin Immunol Pract 2014;2:434–438; Pediatric Allergy. 3rd ed. 2016:458–466)

- Spontaneously erupting, pruritic wheals (hive) with central pallor due to variety of triggers; however, can be idiopathic
- **Can be associated with angioedema**
- **Types:**
  - Acute vs. chronic (persistent or recurring for at least 6 wk)
  - Physical: Caused/reproduced by specific physical stimuli
  - Cholinergic: Caused by heat, exertion, or emotional upset
  - Contact: Caused by skin contact with allergen or chemical

Evaluation
- **History:** Identify onset of symptoms, frequency and duration of lesions (come & go), chronicity of symptoms, potential physical triggers, exacerbating factors, signs associated with lesions (angioedema), personal and family history of urticaria or atopy
  - Systemic symptoms rare unless hives attributable to an allergic trigger (food, etc.)

- **Exam:** Skin lesions as described above
- **Diagnosis:** Often clinical diagnosis is sufficient
  - Physical provocation test for physical urticaria (scratch on arm/upper back produces hive)
  - Differential: Viral exanthem, atopic/contact dermatitis, drug eruptions, serum sickness

Treatment
- Consider omalizumab for chronic urticaria refractory to H1-antihistamine (J Allergy Clin Immunol Pract 2017;5:1489–1499)

HEREDITARY ANGIODEMA

(Ann Allergy Asthma Immunol 2010;104:193–204; Ann Allergy Asthma Immunol 2009; 102:366–372; Immunol Allergy Clin N Am 2017;37:541–556; Immunol Allergy Clin N Am 2017;37:557–570; Immunol Allergy Clin N Am 2017;37:585–595; J Allergy Clin Immunol Pract 2013;1:427–432)

- Most angioedema in children is histamine-mediated (see above) and accompanied by hives
- Hereditary angioedema is **bradykinin-mediated** (due to unregulated C1-inhibitor protein function causing excess bradykinin production, vascular leak, and swelling)

Evaluation
- **History:** Recurrent episodes (w/o urticaria) of face, larynx, abdomen, extremities, genitals

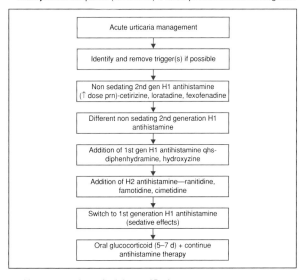

- May or may not have a family history: AD inheritance or spontaneous mutation
- One or more of the following: Recurrent swelling, unexplained recurrent abdominal pain, history of laryngeal edema, serpentine rash prior to attack
- **Lab:** Serum C4 level for screening; if ↓ send C1-inhibitor protein and function
- Differential: Histamine-mediated angioedema, ACE-I–induced angioedema (common in adults), idiopathic angioedema

Treatment
- Not responsive to antihistamines and corticosteroids
- Acute attack
  - Plasma-derived (pd) C1-INH (can be self-administered, IV)
  - Bradykinin receptor antagonist (icatibant, SC)
  - Kallikrein inhibitor (ecallantide, SC)

- Prophylactic therapy
  - **C1-INH every 3–4 d–preferred due to side effect profile and efficacy**
  - Anabolic androgens (danazol, stanozolol)
  - Antifibrinolytics (aminocaproic acid, tranexamic acid)
- Short-term prophylaxis
  - C1-INH (1–6 hr prior to procedures)
  - Icatibant (selective bradykinin receptor antagonist)
  - Fresh–frozen plasma (1–2 hr prior to procedures)
  - High-dose androgens (start 5 d prior and continue 5 d after procedures)

CONTACT DERMATITIS

(Ann Allergy Asthma Immunol 2014;113:9–12; J Allergy Clin Immunol Pract 2015;3:652–658; J Allergy Clin Immunol Pract 2015;3:661–667; J Allergy Clin Immunol Pract 2015;3:S1–S39)

- Inflammatory reaction of skin caused by direct contact with an irritant or allergic substance

Evaluation
- **History:**
  - Irritants: Sharply demarcated erythema and superficial edema at site of contact, burning or stinging, appear within minutes to hours after exposure–**poison ivy**
  - Allergens: Ill-defined lesions that extend beyond area of contact, intensely pruritic, appear 24–72 hr after exposure
    - Most common allergen triggers include plants (poison ivy), metals (nickel jewelry), topical antibiotics (neomycin sulfate), and fragrances
- **Diagnosis:** Often clinical diagnosis is sufficient
  - Patch test (small concentration of diluted known allergen applied to upper back and evaluated 48 & 96 hr later)–done in allergy or dermatology office
  - Differential: Atopic dermatitis, latex allergy, psoriasis, drug eruption
    - Irritant dermatitis (nonimmune-mediated): Cleaning/industrial solvents, acids, bases

Treatment
- Identify and remove offending agent
- Moderate (triamcinolone) to highly potent (clobetasol, betamethasone) topical steroids
- Wet dressings with Burlow solution
- Oral corticosteroids for refractory or prolonged episodes
- Antibiotic ointment (mupirocin), only if concurrent infection present

OTHER

DRUG ALLERGIES

(Ann Allergy Asthma Immunol 2014;112:404–412; J Allergy Clin Immunol Pract 2017;5:577–586; J Allergy Clin Immunol Pract 2017;5:711–717; J Allergy Clin Immunol Pract 2014;2:3–12)

- Hypersensitivity reaction to a medication
- **Types:** IgE (drug-specific antibody) vs. non–IgE-mediated (serum sickness, SJS, TEN, DRESS)

Evaluation
- **History:** Most often cutaneous findings, also bronchospasm, GI symptoms, or anaphylaxis
- Diagnosis: Skin prick or intradermal testing (validated for penicillin only)

Treatment
- For skin test–negative patients: Graded drug challenge for remote (>10 yr) or vague reaction histories as having low risk of reaction
- Drug desensitization (temporary) in immediate, IgE-mediated allergy, for whom skin testing is positive, unavailable, or no acceptable alternative medications available

LATEX ALLERGY

(Ann Allergy Asthma Immunol 2012;109;160–165; Eur J Dermatol 2016;26;523–530; J Allergy Clin Immunol Pract 2017;5;1212–1216; J Occup Health 2016;58;138–144)

- Non–IgE-mediated contact dermatitis vs. IgE-mediated (urticaria, rhinitis, anaphylaxis)
- Cross-reactivity between latex and certain fruits (avocado, banana, kiwi, chestnut)
- Common sources: Toys, balloons, cleaning gloves, condoms, swim caps, pacifiers, erasers

Evaluation
- **History**: Often clinical diagnosis is sufficient
- **Diagnosis**: No commercial skin prick test reagent available
- **Differential**: Irritant contact dermatitis

Treatment
- Avoidance of latex

INSECT STING ALLERGY

(Ann Allergy Asthma Immunol 2017;118:28–54; J Allergy Clin Immunol Pract 2015;3:315–322; J Allergy Clin Immunol Pract 2015;3:324–328; J Allergy Clin Immunol Pract 2015;3:331–334)

- IgE-mediated response against insect venom proteins
- Common stinging insects: Order Hymenoptera, includes families Apidae (bees), Vespidae (yellow jacket, yellow hornet, wasp), Formicidae (fire ants)
- Allergy to salivary proteins of biting insects (order Diptera and Hemiptera like mosquitoes or kissing bugs, respectively) uncommon
- **Types**:
  - Large local reactions (<10 cm of swelling continuous with sting site)
  - Systemic cutaneous reaction localized to skin only (urticaria, angioedema)
  - Systemic reaction w/ multiple organ involvement (anaphylaxis) very rare in children
  - Skeeter syndrome: Large local reactions often misdiagnosed as cellulitis; unlikely, if time frame of symptoms is <24 hr (J Allergy Clin Immunol Pract 2015;3:316)
- **Diagnosis:**
  - Testing generally not indicated for large local reactions unless repeat or patient concern
  - Skin prick testing available although cross-reactivity & cross-sensitization high especially between hornet and yellow jacket
    - Testing may be negative after a serious sting reaction; retest in 3–6 wk
  - Differential—Other causes of anaphylaxis, toxic reaction to sting, mastocytosis, cellulitis

Treatment
- Allergen avoidance
- Mild local reactions: Analgesics, cold compresses
- Large local reactions: As above, and antihistamines for pruritus
- Cutaneous systemic reactions: Antihistamines
- Severe systemic reactions: Epinephrine
- Immunotherapy indicated for children >16 yr with cutaneous systemic reactions and all children with history of anaphylaxis/systemic reaction

IMMUNOLOGY

APPROACH TO THE CHILD WITH RECURRENT INFECTIONS

(Ann Allergy Asthma Immunol 2017;119:299–303; Ann Allergy Asthma Immunol 2017;118:655–663; Pediatric Allergy. 3rd ed. 2016:63–69)

- Maternal antibodies protect infant until 6–9 mo. Children w/ normally functioning immune systems can develop 6–8 URIs/yr in 1st 5 yr of life

Identifying Children with Increased Infection Susceptibility

Frequency	Severity	Opportunistic Infections	Other Factors to Consider
• >6 new infections/yr • >2 pneumonias/yr • Recurrent tissue/ organ abscesses • Increasing frequency of acute otitis media in children >2 yo • >2 serious sinus infections/yr despite medical and/or surgical management • Chronic/ recurrent infections without other explanation	• Failed antibiotic treatment for >2 mo • Sepsis in absence of known risk • Mastoiditis • Pneumonia with empyema • Bacterial arthritis, meningitis, osteomyelitis • Resistant superficial or oral candidiasis	• PCP pneumonia • Mucocutaneous candidiasis • Invasive fungal infection • Invasive Neisseria spp infection • Pseudomonas sepsis	• Infections at multiple anatomic locations • Anatomic or physiologic features that suggest complex syndrome (DiGeorge, Wiskott-Aldrich, dysmotile cilia syndromes, cystic fibrosis) • Failure to thrive • Family history of immunodeficiency, early unexplained death • Lack of other epidemiologic reasoning (daycare, school-age siblings, smoke exposure, atopy)

Screening Diagnostic Studies

Suspected Abnormality	Diagnostic Studies
General	• CBC and differential • CMP • Skin prick and serum IgE levels if applicable • HIV testing if appropriate • Microbial cultures if applicable
Antibody/B-cell/Humoral Immunity	• Quantitative immunoglobulins with reference to age (IgG, IgA, IgM, IgE) • Antibody (titers) to previously administered immunization
T-cell/Cellular Immunity	• Lymphocyte count • T-lymphocyte enumeration (CD3, CD4, CD8) • HIV serology and viral load (ELISA/Western blot/PCR)
Complement	• Total hemolytic complement (CH_{50}) • Individual complement components measured if CH_{50} low or absent
Phagocytic	• Neutrophil count • Neutrophil oxidative burst assay (DHR)

ANTIBODY/B-CELL IMMUNODEFICIENCY

(Ann Allergy Asthma Immunol 2007;98:1–9; J Allergy Clin Immunol Pract 2016;4: 1076–1081; Pediatric Allergy. 3rd ed. 2016;71–79)

Select Disorders	Overview	Typical Clinical Findings	Management
Selective IgA deficiency	• Most common primary immu-nodeficiency • Significantly decreased (<7 mg/dL) or absent serum IgA in absence of other immuno-deficiency in children >4 yr	• Most are asymptomatic • Typically: Young child with recurrent sinusitis, otitis media, &/or pneumonia	• If asymptomatic, no treatment • Must screen blood products for IgA antibodies to prevent infusion reactions • Consider IgG therapy if prophylactic antibiotics trial fails to prevent recurrent infections

| X-linked agamma-globulinemia | • X-linked recessive
• Defect in signal transducing Bruton tyrosine kinase | • Absent tonsils and lymph nodes
• Recurrent bacterial and viral infections including enteroviral meningo-encephalitis and vaccine-associated paralytic poliomyelitis | • Prophylactic antibiotics
• IgG replacement |
| Common variable immunodeficiency | • Late onset, 10–30 yo | • Recurrent sinopulmonary bacterial infections
• Increased risk of autoimmune diseases, cytopenias, lymphoma | • Prophylactic antibiotics
• IgG replacement |

T-CELL/CELLULAR IMMUNODEFICIENCY

(Am J Med Genet 2017;173A:2366–2372; J Clin Immunol 2017;37:626–637; Pediatric Allergy. 3rd ed. 2016:80–89)

Select Disorders	Overview	Typical Clinical Findings	Management
Severe combined immunodeficiency (SCID)	• Profound deficiency of T- and B-cells • Most common form: X-linked • Often defective IL-2RG	• Recurrent infections with common and opportunistic organisms, recurrent fevers, chronic diarrhea, failure to thrive • Common early finding: Persistent mucocutaneous candidiasis • Lymphopenia	• Emergency • Most common curative therapy for all forms: HSC transplant • In adenosine deaminase deficiency, treat with PEG-ADA (enzyme replacement therapy) • Irradiated, CMV-negative, leukore-duced blood products if needed
DiGeorge syndrome	• Heterozygous chromosomal deletion of chromosome 22q11.2	• Hypoplastic thymus, cardiac anomalies, hypocalcemia (parathyroid hypoplasia), facial dysmorphisms • Recurrent viral and fungal infections depending on the degree of T-cell deficiency	• Depends on phenotype and age at diagnosis • Thymic or HSC transplant in certain phenotypes
Wiskott–Aldrich syndrome	• X-linked disease • Mutations in WAS protein involved in cytoskeleton reorganization	• Young male with immune deficiency, thrombocytopenia with small platelets, eczematous dermatitis	• Prophylactic trimethoprim-sulfamethoxazole and acyclovir • IVIG therapy • Definitive therapy: HSCT

PHAGOCYTIC DEFICIENCY

(Adv Ther 2017;34:2543–2557; Ann Allergy Asthma Immunol 2016;117:285–289; *Pediatric Allergy*. 3rd ed. 2016:101–111)

Select Disorders	Overview	Typical Clinical Findings	Management
Chédiak–Higashi syndrome	• Mutations in lysosomal trafficking regulator gene • Giant azurophilic granules in polymorphonuclear cells	• Oculocutaneous albinism, pyogenic infections (staph and strep), neurodegeneration • Late-onset hemophagocytic syndrome-like accelerated phase	• HSC transplant to halt recurring accelerated phase
Chronic Granulomatous Disease	• X-linked recessive mostly • Mutations in phagocytic NADPH oxidase and absent respiratory burst in neutrophils	• Granuloma formation in tissue, recurrent life-threatening catalase-positive bacterial and fungal infections (Staph skin abscesses, Serratia lymphadenitis, infections with *Nocardia*, *Burkholderia*, *Aspergillus*)	• Standard of care: trimethoprim-sulfamethoxazole and itraconazole; INFy • Recombinant G-CSF to raise neutrophil counts • -HSC transplant is curative
Leukocyte adhesion deficiency	• Mutations in adhesion molecules on neutrophils (neutrophils unable to leave circulation)	• Recurrent bacterial sinopulmonary and skin infections, poor wound healing, delayed umbilical cord separation • Neutrophilia in the absence of infection	• Recombinant G-CSF • HSC transplant
Hyper-IgE syndrome	• Impaired neutrophil recruitment to infection sites • Impaired Th17 cell response	• Recurrent staph infections (cold abscesses), severe eczema in early infancy, pneumonia, coarse facies over time, retained primary teeth, scoliosis, hyperextensibility • Chronic mucocutaneous candidiasis	• Antibiotic therapy to treat infection • Prophylactic trimethoprim-sulfamethoxazole and itraconazole
Mucocutaneous candidiasis	• Persistent or recurrent mucocutaneous candidal infections affecting nails, skin, and mucosa	• Chronic noninvasive candidiasis of nail, skin, oral mucosa resistant to topical therapies	• 1st line treatment: Fluconazole • Severe cases: Amphotericin

(*Pediatric Allergy*. 3rd ed. 2016:90–99)

Select Disorders	Overview	Typical Clinical Findings	Management
Complement	• Classified based on affected path: classical, alternative, lectin pathway, or inhibitors of these pathways	• Varied depending on pathway • Classic complement: Recurrent infections with (encapsulated) pneumococcus and *H. flu*; association with autoimmune diseases • Alternative path: Systemic neisserial infections	• Antibiotic therapy for treatment &/or prophylaxis • No commercially available replacement complement components available

ECG BASICS

(Park's Pediatric Cardiology. 6th ed. 2014, Ch 3)

- Standard (12-lead) ECG: 6 precordial leads (V1–V6), 3 bipolar limb leads (I, II, III), and 3 unipolar limb leads (aVR, aVL, aVF)
  - Paper speed 25 mm/s → small box = 0.04 s; large box = 5 small boxes = 0.20 s
  - Voltage 10 mm/mV → 1 mm = 0.1 mV

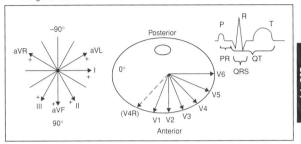

- P-wave: Atrial depol; QRS complex: Ventricular depol; T-wave: Ventricular depol

APPROACH TO ECG INTERPRETATION

(Park's Pediatric Cardiology. 6th ed. 2014, Ch 3)

- Critical to have a systematic approach, check paper speed and voltage:
  - Rate: 300 ÷ # of large boxes btwn R-waves. If rhythm irreg count R-waves across strip x 6
  - Rhythm: Regular (consistent R–R intervals) vs. irregular? Sinus? (nml P-axis: + in II, III, & aVF, no Δ in P-morphology, QRS after every P; constant PR)
    - Respiratory variation (aka sinus arrhythmia) is a normal finding
    - >2.5-mm wide P in II and/or biphasic in V1 = L atrial enlargement
    - >2.5-mm high P in II = R atrial enlargement
  - Axis: Nml axis is **based on age**; look for + R-waves in limb leads. Lead I = 0° & aVF = 90°

R-Waves in I	R-Wave in aVF	Degrees	Axis	Causes
(+)	(+)	0 to 90	Normal	
(+)	(−)	0 to −90	LAD	LVH, LBBB, myocardial dz
(−)	(+)	90 to 180	RAD	RVH, RBBB
(−)	(−)	−90 to −180	Extreme RAD	RAD is normal in neonates

- Intervals: Assess for prolongation/shortening and elevation/depression
  - PR: Prolonged = 1° AV block. Short w/ WPW, ectopic pacemaker, glycogen storage dz
  - QRS: Long if >0.08 ms if <8 yr or >0.10 ms if >8 yr; due to any non–His-Purkinje conduction: LBBB, RBBB, ventricular rhythm, fascicular block, WPW, hyperK, meds
  - QT: Start of Q to end of T; correct for HR w/ Bazett formula (QTc = QT/√RR)
- R-waves: R:S ratio initially >1 in V1/V2, and <1 in V5/V6. ~3 yr R:S ratio becomes <1 in V1/V2 and >1 in V5/V6. Some have juvenile pattern until 8–12 yo (Heart 2005;91:1626)
  - RVH criteria: RAD, R-wave in V1 > age norm, S in V6 > age norm, upright T-wave in V1 in pt <12 yr, rSR' pattern in V1, where R' > R & ≥5 mm
- T-waves: Δ w/ age. 1st 3 d up in V1–V3, then inverts. Δ back during childhood starting w/ V3 → V1. T-wave in V5/V6 should be + at all ages (Heart 2005;91:1626)

ECG Parameters by Age					
Age	HR	PR Interval	QRS Axis (°)	QRS Interval	QTc Limit
0–1 wk	90–160	0.08–0.15	60–180	0.03–0.08	<0.49
1 wk–2 mo	100–180	0.08–0.15	45–160	0.03–0.08	<0.49
2–6 mo	105–185	0.08–0.15	0–135	0.03–0.08	<0.49
6 mo–1 yr	110–170	0.07–0.16	0–135	0.03–0.08	<0.45
1–8 yr	90–165 (1–2 yr) 65–140 (>2 yr)	0.09–0.17	0–110	0.04–0.08	<0.45
8–16 yr	60–130	0.09–0.17	−15–110	0.04–0.09	<0.45
>16 yr	50–120	0.12–0.20	−15–110	0.05–0.10	<0.45

CONDUCTION ABNORMALITIES

ARRHYTHMIAS

(Moss & Adams. 8th ed. 2013, Ch 18)

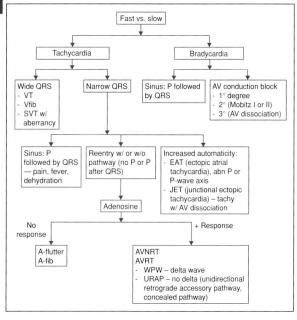

BRADYARRHYTHMIAS

(Park's Pediatric Cardiology. 6th ed. 2014, Ch 24–25)

Sinus Bradycardia
• HR <80 in infants or <60 in children
• Causes: Usually benign but can be assoc w/ ↑ ICP (Cushing triad), resp distress, electrolyte imbalance, hypothermia, hypothyroidism, meds, long QT syndrome
• Treatment = None necessary in absence of symptoms or hemodynamic compromise

AV Block
- **1° AV block:** Prolonged PR interval with QRS following each P
  - Causes: Normal variant, ↑ vagal tone, fever, hyperK, digoxin, endocardial abscess, myocarditis (Lyme, diphtheria, rheumatic, viral), structural anomalies (AVSD, ASD, Ebstein)
- **2° AV block:** 2 types, Mobitz I & II. Cannot distinguish when 2:1 block
  - Mobitz I (Wenckebach): Progressive PR prolongation with eventual dropped QRS
    - ↑ refractory period of AV node. Typically benign
  - Mobitz II: Consistent PR with intermittently dropped QRS
    - Dysfunction at bundle of His. Can progress to 3° block, may require pacemaker
- **3° AV block:** Complete heart block (CHB)/complete AV dissociation
  - Congenital CHB: Assoc. with TGA, maternal SLE (1 in 60 risk), maternal anti-Ro Ab (1 in 20 risk), Lyme dz, rheumatic fever, diphtheria, KD, cardiac surgery, others
  - Clinical presentation may be Stokes–Adams attacks (syncopal attacks)
  - Tx: Temp pacing (transvenous/transcutaneous), atropine, isoproterenol, pacemaker

TACHYARRHYTHMIAS

(Heart Diseases in Children: A Pediatrician's Guide. 2011, Ch 32; Moss & Adams. 8th ed. 2013, Ch 18)

Sinus Tachycardia (HR >160 in infants or >140 in children)
- Typically benign: Can be caused by pain, fever (each 1°C ↑ in body temp → ~9.6 bpm ↑ in HR), dehydration, hypoxia, anemia, hyperthyroidism, shock, drugs, thrombosis, others
- Tx: Reverse underlying cause

Supraventricular Tachycardia (SVT)
- 2 main types: AVRT and AVNRT. A flutter, a fib, junctional tachycardias, & others also classify as SVT but less common in pediatrics
- Narrow QRS, regular rhythm, usually cannot see P-waves
- Can classify by RP interval (short vs. long, i.e., short RP in orthodromic AVNRT)
- Sxs: Abrupt onset palpitations, ± chest pain, near-syncope, syncope, dyspnea
  - **AVRT** (AV reentrant tachycardia): Due to accessory pathway – most common SVT in infants & children. 25% of AVRT accessory pathways capable of bidirectional conduction – seen on resting ECG as Delta wave or short PR, aka **Wolff–Parkinson–White syndrome** (WPW)
    - 10–30% of WPW associated with structural CHD → echo indicated
    - Danger from concurrent rapidly conducting SVT (i.e., a fib/flutter) with accessory pathway capable of conducting rapidly → direct ventricular depol at 300+ bpm
  - **AVNRT** (AV nodal reentrant tachycardia): Reentrant circuit within AV node. Most common SVT in adolescents. Difficult to distinguish from AVRT on ECG
- Treatment of SVT
  - Stable: Vagal maneuvers, adenosine (rapid IV push with saline chase w/ stopcock)
  - Unstable: Synchronized cardioversion (0.5–1 J/kg), cardiology consult
  - Prevention of SVT: Depends on etiology, β-blockers tend to be 1st line (other AV nodal blockers, digoxin, CCB may be used) over other antiarrhythmic agents, ablation

Increased Automaticity
- Foci other than SA node driving rhythm, not reentry
  - Ectopic or multifocal atrial tachycardia: Nonsinus P-waves, possible varying morphology
  - Junctional ectopic tachycardia (JET) – Foci in/near AV junction – often seen postop (especially post ToF repair, <72 hr)
  - Atrial flutter: "saw-tooth" flutter waves ~300 bpm. Associated w/ atrial enlargement, myocarditis, postop CHD repair, muscular dystrophy. Also seen in healthy newborns

Atrial Fibrillation
- Irregularly irregular, can occur after alcohol binge, mitral regurgitation, other causes of LAE
- Tx: AV-node blocking agents if needed (unnecessary if normal HR)

VENTRICULAR ARRHYTHMIAS

(Park's Pediatric Cardiology. 6th ed. 2014, Ch 18 & 24)

Ventricular Tachyarrhythmias
- **Ventricular tachycardia:** Rapid (>120), wide complex, discordant (opposite facing) T-waves
  - Monomorphic (same QRS) vs. polymorphic vs. bidirectional vs. Torsades de pointes (TdP)
    - Must differentiate from SVT with aberrant (BBB) conduction as tx varies
  - Can be life threatening if degenerates to ventricular fibrillation
  - Causes: LQTS (Romano-Ward, Jervell & Lange-Nielsen), hypoMg, ARVD, Brugada, CPVT, noncompaction, postop, myocarditis, Chagas, infarct, hypo/hyperK, drugs (Rx/illicit)
  - Treatment: If symptomatic must treat urgently with synchronized DCCV (0.5–1 J/kg), if conscious/asymptomatic, IV push amiodarone and/or lidocaine can be used. IV Mg for TdP

Ventricular Fibrillation
- Chaotic, irregular ventricular contractions w/o effective circulation
  - Treatment: Immediate CPR, **defibrillation** as soon as possible (2 J/kg)

SYNCOPE

(Pediatr Rev 2000;21:384; Pediatr Rev 2000;21:201)

- Sudden, often brief, LOC and postural tone due to ↓ cerebral blood flow

Differential Diagnosis
- Breath-holding spells: Incidence of 4.6%, primarily 1–5 yr of age, strong FH
  - Provoked by pain, anger, or frustration; normal physical and neuro exam
  - Cyanotic type (80%): Peaks at 2 yr and resolves by 5
    - Prodrome of crying → forced expiration → apnea, may have clonic jerks and brady
  - Pallid type (20%): Preceded by frustration, pain, sudden startle, or minor trauma
    - Initial quieting and breath holding → pallor → LOC and loss of muscle tone
    - Ocular compression test: ≥3 s of asystole → pallid syncope (+ need normal EEG)
- Neurocardiogenic (vasovagal): ~75% of syncopal spells. 2/2 to dysautonomia, often with FH
  - Usually in adolescents; prolonged standing, warm environments, showers may trigger
  - Prodrome: Nausea, diaphoresis, light headedness, or yawning
- Other: Neuropsych, migraine, seizure, panic, ↓BG, paroxysmal vertigo, cough, POTS

Cardiac Syncope
- Arrhythmogenic: Prolonged QT, WPW, heart block, sick sinus syndrome, SVT
- Structural: HOCM, severe aortic/pulmonic stenosis, pHTN, anomalous coronary, myxomas

Evaluation
- Physical exam with focus on cardiac and neuro exam with orthostatic VS
- ↑ concern for cardiac etiology w/ syncope at rest, during exercise (HOCM), associated chest pain, without warning/prodrome, FH of: sudden death, deafness, CHD, early MI, arrhythmia
- Further workup w/ ECG, Holter, exercise testing, echo; tilt-table test now rarely performed
- **Treatment** for cardiac causes of syncope involve antiarrhythmics, RF ablation, ± pacemaker

APPROACH TO HEART MURMURS

(Pediatr Rev 2007;28:e19)

- Sound heard by passage of blood causing vibration of normal structures vs. structural defect
- ~1% of population with structural heart lesion

Murmurs

- Identify timing in cardiac cycle, intensity, location, pitch, quality, duration
  - Intensity grading: Systolic murmurs graded on scale 1–6; diastolic 1–4 (no thrill w/ diastolic)
    - 1 – soft, difficult to hear; 2 – easily heard, not loud; 3 – loud, no thrill; 4 – loud + thrill; 5 – thrill + audible w/ stethoscope just touching; 6 – audible without contact
  - RUSB – aortic region, LUSB – pulmonic region, LLSB – tricuspid region, apex – mitral region

Complimentary Exam Findings

- Observation for syndromic appearance, central cyanosis, breathing, JVP
- Palpation for thrills and PMI
- Pulse exam: Bounding (↑ pulse pressure; PDA, AR, hyperthyroid, AVF), pulsus parvus (weak)/tardus (late) in AS, unequal pulses (coarctation)
- Auscultation for split S2 (single S2 raises concern for CHD), gallops, rubs (pericarditis)
- Abdominal exam: Hepatosplenomegaly (CHF), pulsatile liver (TR)

Innocent Murmurs *(Heart Diseases in Children: A Pediatrician's Guide. 2011, Ch 1)*

- Suggestive qualities: Asymptomatic pt, split S2 w/ resp variation, grade 1–2/6, systolic
- **Still murmur:** Most common innocent murmur, caused by turbulent flow in LVOT
  - Vibratory, "musical," systolic, "hockey-stick" ↓ L sternal border → L chest. ↑ w/ supine
- **Flow murmur:** Turbulent flow across aortic (RUSB) or pulmonic (LUSB) valves
  - Soft, medium frequency, blowing, systolic, cresc–decresc, no ejection click
  - Can be a secondary finding of pathologic lesion: ASD, TAPVR, AI, PDA, systemic AVM
- **Peripheral pulmonic stenosis (PPS):** Cause: relatively small branch PAs w/ sharp branching
  - Systolic, LUSB with radiation to bi/l axilla, low/mod pitch
  - Should resolve at ~8 wk. If not consider syndromic (Williams, Alagille, Noonan, Rubella)

Pathologic Murmurs *(Heart Diseases in Children: A Pediatrician's Guide. 2011, Ch 1; Moss & Adams. 8th ed. 2013, Ch 5)*

- **Systolic:** Louder than innocent murmurs (3+), often holosystolic, ejection vs. regurgitant
  - Holosystolic: Obscure S1, high-pressure → low-pressure flow
    - VSD (LSB, ↑ freq = ↓ size), MR (apex, blowing), TR (LLSB, blowing), PDA (machine-like)
  - Late systolic: MR from valve prolapse (MVP), preceded by midsystolic click, apex, blowing
  - Ejection murmurs (AS, PS): Presence of ejection click, may have diastolic component, abnl split S2, evidence of CHF (hepatomegaly, JVD), cresc–decresc
- **Diastolic:** Always pathologic (except venous hum – continuous, supraclavicular)
  - Early: Begin immediately after S2, typically decresc, 2/2 incompetent semilunar valve
    - AR/AI: High pitched, best heard w/ pt leaning forward, L midsternal border → apex
    - PR: Lower pitched, LUSB/L midsternal border → LLSB
  - Mid: Rumble, cresc–decresc, best heard w/ bell, ↑ flow across AV valves (MS/TS)
    - Austin–Flint murmur: Similar sound heard at apex 2/2 severe AR
  - Late (Presystolic): Cresc, also 2/2 stenosed AV valve during atrial contraction
- **Continuous:** Harsh machinelike murmur classic for PDA

Further Evaluation

- Echo is gold standard to assess cardiac structure; ancillary testing w/ ECG or CXR may be helpful; some suggest referral to pediatric cardiology before imaging

CONGENITAL HEART DISEASE

INFECTIVE ENDOCARDITIS PROPHYLAXIS

(Circulation 2007;116:1736–1754)

- Updated AHA guidelines endorsed by IDSA and Pediatric Infectious Disease Society
- "Prophylaxis for dental procedures should be recommended only for patients with underlying cardiac conditions associated with the highest risk of adverse outcome from infective endocarditis."

- Cardiac conditions for which dental ppx indicated per AHA guidelines:
  - Prosthetic valve, previous IE, history of cardiac transplant with valvulopathy
  - **Congenital heart disease:**
    - Unrepaired cyanotic lesions including palliative shunts/conduits
    - Completely repaired with prosthetic material or device for 6 mo postop
    - Repaired with residual defects at or adjacent to site with prosthetic material or device

---

OBSTRUCTIVE LESIONS

(Park's Pediatric Cardiology. 6th ed. 2014, Ch 13; Pediatric Cardiology: The Essential Pocket Guide. 3rd ed. 2014, Ch 5)

Coarctation of the Aorta (CoA) *(Moss & Adams. 8th ed. 2013, Ch 47)*
- Narrowing of aorta, usually distal to L subclavian art opposite ductus arteriosus
  - Narrowing can be discrete or diffuse
- M > F, assoc. w/ Turner, bicuspid aortic valve (≥50%), and circle of Willis aneurysms
- **Evaluation:**
  - History: If severe defect with hypoplastic arch may present in acute heart failure, can also present in infancy in outpatient setting with vague complaints (classically headache)
  - Exam: Murmurs over L back along spine, strong radial pulse in infant, SBP in UE > LE by 20+ mmHg, weak or delayed femoral/LE pulses
  - ECG: Normal or possibly LVH in older children or ↑ R-sided forces in neonates
  - CXR: Poststenotic dilation may be seen as "figure of 8," rib notching also possible
  - Echo: Necessary to assess for presence and degree of poststenotic dilation
- **Treatment:**
  - Surgically vs. transcatheter balloon dilation. ↑ risk aneurysms, restenosis w/ cath repair

Pulmonary Stenosis *(Moss & Adams. 8th ed. 2013, Ch 40)*
- Valvular PS accounts for ~8% of all CHD
- Cyanosis from PS is due to ASD with R → L flow
- **Types:**
  - Valvular: 90%. Leaflet fusion/thickening with small orifice and poststenotic dilation
    - Assoc. with Noonan syndrome
  - Subvalvular (infundibular): Rarely isolated, typically with large VSD as in TOF
  - Supravalvular: Narrowing of pulm trunk, its bifurcation, and/or peripheral branches
    - Syndromes w/ periph PS: Williams, Noonan, Alagille, EDS, congenital rubella
      - See description in innocent murmurs section
- **Evaluation:**
  - History: Critical PS ductal-dependent, otherwise usually asymptomatic. Mod–severe lesions may present w/ fatigue & exercise intolerance
  - Exam: Cresc–decresc SEM @ LUSB & L upper back ± click. Louder/longer/later peaking w/ ↑ stenosis unless ↓ CO. P2 intensity ↓ w/ ↑ stenosis. ± RV thrill
  - ECG: Normal to RAD, RVH to RVH with strain
  - CXR: Might see bulge at L upper cardiac border 2/2 to poststenotic dilation
  - Echo: Assessment of anatomy, transstenotic pressure gradient, velocity across stenosis
- **Treatment:**
  - Tx of choice is balloon dilation. Surgery only necessary in severe cases, unfavorable anatomy for cath, or syndromic patients with dysplastic valves

Aortic Stenosis *(Moss & Adams. 8th ed. 2013, Ch 46)*
- **Types:** All result in LVOT obstruction
  - Valvular: Most common (~71%), 2/2 bicuspid, unicuspid, or stenotic tricuspid valve
    - Critical AS (rare) typically valvular, ductal dependent, likely associated HLHS
  - Subvalvular: Discrete stenosis vs. LVOT "tunnel" stenosis (i.e., HCM)
  - Supravalvular: Assn w/ Williams syndrome
- **Evaluation:**
  - History: CHF/shock possible but rare in infancy. Usually incidentally found or w/ murmur
  - Exam: Harsh-ejection cresc–descresc murmur at RUSB, ejection click, S2 split is narrow or paradoxical with ↑ stenosis, radiation to neck
    - Prominent murmur at birth as opposed to most other lesions (identified later)
  - ECG: Normal to LVH ± strain
  - CXR: Normal to cardiomegaly w/ LV dilatation

- Echo: Necessary to assess for presence of VSD, AV valve structure and chordae attachment
- **Treatment:**
  - Tx of choice is balloon dilation. Surgery only necessary in severe cases

---

ACYANOTIC LESIONS

(Park's Pediatric Cardiology. 6th ed. 2014, Ch 11; Pediatric Cardiology: The Essential Pocket Guide. 3rd ed. 2014, Ch 4)

Atrial Septal Defects *(Heart Diseases in Children: A Pediatrician's Guide*, 2011, Ch 6)
- Distinguished from PFO: Small opening or potential opening in area of fossa ovalis
- Magnitude and direction of shunt determined by size of defect and compliance of ventricles
- **Types:**
  - Ostium secundum defect (can be very difficult to distinguish from PFO)
  - Ostium primum defect: Form of AV septal or AV canal defect
  - Sinus venosus ASD: Associated with partial anomalous pulm venous return
  - Common atrium: Entire septum missing, associated with MV prolapse
- **Evaluation:**
  - History: Large defects – CHF, FTT, recurrent pulm infxn; small/mod defects usually w/o sxs
  - Exam: Prominent RV impulse & S_1, wide fixed split S_2; SEM at LUSB (can also hear TR)
  - ECG: Normal to RAD; incomplete RBBB, RAE, RVH
  - CXR: ↑ pulm vascular markings, possible cardiomegaly and prominent PA
  - Echo: Shunt seen on color doppler, dilated RA/RV, possible L septal deviation
- **Treatment:**
  - Small and mod secundum defects found in infancy tend to close spont before age 2
    - If defect remains open after consider percutaneous closure with occlusion device
  - Sinus venosus & primum defects do not close spontaneously, surgery around 1 yr

Ventricular Septal Defects *(Heart Diseases in Children: A Pediatrician's Guide*, 2011, Ch 7)
- Most common congenital cardiac defect. High (left) → low (right) pressure shunt
- **Types:** May also occur as a combination of any of the following types
  - Inlet (directly beneath AV valves)
  - Outlet (gives rise to great vessels)
  - Perimembranous (junction btwn inlet and outlet, 70% cases)
  - Muscular (btwn LV and RV, 20% cases)
- **Evaluation:**
  - History: Most w/o sxs & heard on routine exam; larger defects present with pulm edema, tachypnea, ↑WOB, FTT, recurrent pulm infxn, easy fatigability
  - Exam: Usually only holosystolic murmur; larger defects with ↑WOB, hepatomegaly, dynamic laterally displaced LV impulse, ± systolic thrill & apical (MV) diastolic rumble
  - ECG: Small defects – normal; large – LAE/LVH → biV hypertrophy (suggests Eisenmenger)
  - CXR: Small defects – normal; large – cardiomegaly & pulm vascular congestion
  - Echo: Gold standard to assess size & number of VSDs present ± possible associated defects
- **Treatment:** Muscular VSDs usually close spontaneously
  - Initially medical: Diuretics, afterload reduction, inotropic agents (digoxin)
  - Surgical vs. catheter closure before 1 yr for: Large defect, FTT, failed medical tx, Qp:Qs ≥2
  - Encourage dental hygiene but no dental ppx needed

AV Canal Defects *(Heart Diseases in Children: A Pediatrician's Guide*, 2011, Ch 9)
- Also known as AV septal defect (AVSD) and endocardial cushion defect, ~5% of CHD
- Commonly associated with trisomy 21
  - ~40–45% of T21 with CHD and ~40–45% of all CHD in T21 is AV canal defect

- **Types:** All have ASD
  - Complete: ASD + VSD + single AV valve on common annulus (no separate MV/TV)
    - Unbalanced = common AV valve favors one side → hypoplastic opposite ventricle
  - Intermediate: Same as complete but separate valves (w/ bridged leaflets) on same annulus
  - Partial: ASD + MV cleft (→ MR), no VSD, separate AV valves w/ associated annulus
  - Transitional: Same as partial + inlet VSD
- **Evaluation:**
  - History: Clinically present similar to VSD
  - Exam: Murmurs of ASD, VSD; active precordium. ± gallop
  - ECG: Prolonged PR, superior axis ($-60°$ to $-150°$). RVH + superior axis should raise suspicion
  - CXR: Cardiomegaly & pulm vascular congestion, proportional to degree of shunting
  - Echo: Necessary to assess for presence of VSD, AV valve structure and chordae attachment
- **Treatment:**
  - Surgery is indicated for all forms due to risk of Eisenmenger (done at ~6–12 wo)
    - Patch closure (cath avoided due to valve proximity) + valve reconstruction
  - Medical therapy for those with signs/symptoms of CHF
  - Unbalanced defects treated as single ventricles with staged Fontan

Patent Ductus Arteriosus (PDA) *(Heart Diseases in Children: A Pediatrician's Guide, 2011, Ch 8)*

- Persistent (fetal) connection of aorta → PA. Clinically similar in presentation to VSD
- ↑ risk w/: Prematurity, ↑ altitude, perinatal hypoxemia, maternal rubella
- **Evaluation:**
  - History: Preemies present d 3–7 w/ resp distress, apnea/brady, inability to wean vent
  - Exam: Cont machinery murmur at LUSB, hyperactive precordium, wide pulse pressure
  - ECG: Most likely normal but can have evidence of LVH
  - CXR: Same as VSD, pulm congestion w/ large PDA
  - Echo: Necessary to confirm dx and assess for LA & LV dilation
- **Treatment:**
  - In a preterm infant can use either indomethacin or ibuprofen
    - Surgical closure necessary if symptomatic and failed medical therapy
  - Can await spont closure in asymptomatic infant
  - Closure at 6–12 mo if no spont closure by transcatheter occlusion (coil vs. Amplatzer)
  - Large PDA w/ CHF requires urgent closure via transcatheter approach

---

CYANOTIC LESIONS

(Park's Pediatric Cardiology. 6th ed. 2014, Ch 14; Moss & Adams. 8th ed. 2013, Ch 38–44, 48–49)

Evaluation of the Cyanotic Child *(Pediatr Clin North Am 2004;51:999)*

- Cardiac causes include the 5 Ts (transposition of great arteries [TGA], tetralogy of Fallot [ToF], total anomalous pulm venous return [TAPVR], truncus arteriosus, tricuspid atresia), critical pulm stenosis/atresia, Ebstein anomaly, L to R shunt w/ pulm edema, single-ventricle physiology, low cardiac-output states
- **Types:**
  - Central cyanosis: ↓ arterial O_2 content
  - Peripheral cyanosis (Nl PaO_2): Cold exposure, Raynaud, polycythemia, early shock
  - Differential cyanosis (pink upper body, cyanotic lower): R → L shunt, PDA
  - Reverse differential (upper body cyanotic, pink lower): TGA, interrupted arch, critical CoA
  - Harlequin condition (1 quadrant or ½ of body cyanotic): Vasomotor instability

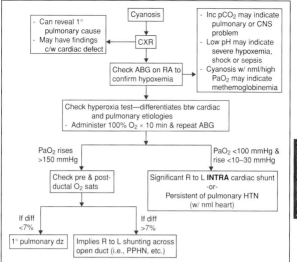

- **Prostaglandins to maintain PDA indicated with failed hyperoxia test**

Tricuspid Atresia (Nelson Textbook of Pediatrics. 20th ed. Ch 430.4)
- Failure of TV to form → hypoplastic RV & PS. 25% also have TGA. **Atrial shunt necessary**
- Degree of cyanosis/hypoxemia depends on patency of duct, size of VSD, presence of TGA (↓ hypoxia with TGA), and overall RVOT obstruction
- **Evaluation:**
  - History: Severely cyanotic as an infant (rarely present later). + TGA = pulm overcirculation
  - Exam: Single S_2, ± VSD and/or PDA murmur, hepatomegaly
  - ECG: LAD or superior axis; RAE, LVH
  - CXR: Can appear normal, mild cardiomegaly; usually ↓ pulm vasculature (↑ w/ TGA)
  - Echo: Diagnostic; also assesses degree of pulm obstruction, TGA, atrial shunt restriction
- **Treatment:** Initial focus to maintain shunting (PGE₁/septostomy). Palliative surgical correction with staged Fontan (single ventricle) (Thorax 1971;26(3):240–248)

Truncus Arteriosus (Heart Diseases in Children: A Pediatrician's Guide, 2011, Ch 20)
- Single great vessel overlying large VSD to PA & aorta. 40% w/ DiGeorge, 25% w/ R arch
- **Evaluation:**
  - History: Cyanosis & signs/symptoms of CHF due to pulm overcirculation from L to R shunt. 15% w/ interrupted arch have ductal dependent LE flow
  - Exam: Precordial bulge. **Loud single S2**; ± SEM, **click**; ± regurg murmur; ↑ pulse pressure
  - ECG: Biventricular hypertrophy
  - CXR: Cardiomegaly, prominent ascending aorta, ↑ **pulm vasculature**, ± **right arch**
  - Echo: Similar to ToF but w/o separate PA, valve w/ 1–6 leaflets (usually 3 or 4)
- **Treatment:**
  - Early surgical repair preferable but will require upsize of valved conduit (RV → PA)
  - Long-term survival dependent on truncal valve function

Tetralogy of Fallot (ToF) (Heart Diseases in Children: A Pediatrician's Guide, 2011, Ch 13)
- Most common cyanotic CHD. (1) VSD, (2) overriding aorta, (3) RVOT obstruction, (4) RVH
- Degree of cyanosis = degree of RVOT obstruction
  - Ductal/MAPCA dependent w/ severe PS/atresia
    - MAPCA = major aortopulm collateral arteries (systemic → pulm)
- If aortic annulus overlies RV by >50% this may be referred to as **DORV (double outlet RV)**

- **Evaluation:**
  - History: Hypercyanotic (Tet) spells w/ tachypnea, dyspnea, intense cyanosis. Life threatening
    - Rare <9–12 mo
    - ↑ RVOT obstruction or ↓ SVR = ↑ R → L shunting (↑ hypoxemia)
  - Exam: Harsh SEM at LUSB, loud single S2; ECG w/ RAD, RVH
  - ECG: RVH with RBBB common postop
  - CXR: "Boot-shaped" heart, nml heart size, ↓ pulm vasculature
  - Echo: Doppler for evaluation of degree of PS
- **Treatment** (Ann Thorac Surg 1995;60(6 Suppl):S592–S596)
  - Close inpatient monitoring after birth until ductus closure
  - Surgically (at ~6 mo) with repair of RV outflow tract obstruction and closure of VSD
    - Pulm regurg common postop → significant ↑ in risk of ventric arrhythmias
  - Tet spells: Volume, O₂, ↑ SVR (squat/knee-chest, α-agonists), morphine, β-blockers, severe cases may require percutaneous stenting of RVOT

Transposition of the Great Arteries (TGA) (Ann Thorac Surg 1984;38(5):438–443)
- Aorta arises from the RV & PA from the LV → communication btwn systemic & pulm circulation (VSD, PFO, ASD, PDA) necessary
- 3:1 male predisposition
- **Types:** D-transposition (*dextro*, aorta ant & to right of PA) vs. I-transposition (*levo*, left of PA)
- **Evaluation:**
  - History: Persistent cyanosis from birth
  - Exam: Tachypnea w/o retractions, single loud S2; no murmur w/o other defect, cyanosis
  - ECG: RAD, RVH (RV supporting systemic flow)
  - CXR: "Egg on string"; ↑ pulm vasculature
  - Echo: Anteriorly rising aorta + posterior PA. Assess for VSD (40%)
- **Treatment:** Maintain shunting (prostaglandins, balloon atrial septostomy) & definitive repair with surgical arterial switch in 1st 2 wk (prev atrial switch or Mustard procedure)

Tetralogy of Fallot

1. VSD 3. RVOT obstruction
2. Overriding aorta 4. RVH

Transposition of the great arteries

1. Aorta from RV, pulmonary artery from LV
2. Intact ventricular septum 3. PDA

Truncus arteriosus

1. Common arterial trunk (Aorta + PA)
2. VSD

Tricuspid atresia

1. Tricuspid atresia 3. Pulmonary stenosis
2. VSD 4. Hypoplastic RV

Courtesy of Elena Grant, 2012.

Total Anomalous Pulmonary Venous Return (TAPVR) (Ann Thorac Surg 2002;74(5):1616–1620)
- Total or partial return of pulm veins to R-side circulation (RA or systemic vein)
- Clinical presentation dependent on presence/**degree of pulm venous obstruction**
- **Types:** Supracardiac (SVC), infracardiac (IVC, portal, or hepatic vein), or intracardiac (RA or coronary sinus), mixed. Infradiaphragmatic drainage frequently has PV obstruction
- **Evaluation:**
  - History: With PV obstruction – acutely ill w/i hr after birth/without – typically no sxs
  - Exam: ↑ RV impulse; fixed, split S2; SEM at LUSB; middiastolic rumble LLSB
  - ECG: RAD, RVH, ± RAE
  - CXR: "Snowman sign" with nonobstructed supracardiac drainage. Edema present
  - Echo: Dilated R chambers, relative L heart hypoplasia, can evaluate for PV obstruction
- **Treatment:** Obstructed TAPVR requires emergent surgery soon after birth. Prostaglandin use controversial, typically not recommended for obstructed TAPVR

Pulmonary Atresia
- Clinically resembles tricuspid atresia with primary differences being: normal QRS axis, ±TR on exam or echo, ±RV-coronary fistula
  - Wide variety of dz; some require Fontan while 2-ventricle physiology possible for others
- Tx: Maintain shunt → Fontan vs. valvotomy w/ valvuloplasty (preferable to maintain 2-ventricle physiology) vs. combination of both

Ebstein Anomaly
- Inferior displacement of TV w/ RV atrialization. Often with TR; atrial shunt present. RF – in utero lithium exposure.
- **Evaluation:**
  - History: Severe cases p/w neonatal cyanosis, older kids usually p/w murmur, SVT, dyspnea
  - Exam: Widely split S_1 and S_2 + S_3 and S_4. TR murmur
  - ECG: Tall/broad P-waves, RBBB; 20% assn w/ WPW ECG Δs
  - CXR: Can have extreme cardiomegaly w/ balloon shape, ↓ pulm vasculature
  - Echo: Assess degree of tricuspid apical displacement (correlates with survival)
- **Treatment:** Severe cases need palliative surgery. Less severe cases can be observed

Hypoplastic Left Heart Syndrome (HLHS) (NEJM 1983;308:23–26)
- Group of anomalies w/ varying degrees of hypoplastic LV, LVOT, mitral and/or aortic valve atresia, arch hypoplasia (~75% with CoA)
- **Evaluation:**
  - History: Infants present with critical illness w/in first few hr, ductal dependent
  - Exam: ↑ RV impulse; single loud S2, PDA closure → cardiogenic shock
- **Treatment:** Norwood → hemi-Fontan → Fontan. ↑↑ surgical risk

MISCELLANEOUS LESIONS

(Nelson Textbook of Pediatrics. 20th ed., Ch 432; Pediatrics 2006;117;e333; Pediatr Rev 2010;31:e1)

Anomalous Coronary Arteries
- Anomalous left coronary artery from the pulmonary artery (**ALCAPA**)
  - PA pressures fall after birth → compromised L coronary artery (LCA) perfusion pressure
  - Collaterals form btwn R coronary (RCA); flow: aorta → RCA → LCA → PA (AVM-like)
  - LV infarction → fibrosis → LV dilation/MV incompetence
  - Signs/symptoms: Recurrent episodes of discomfort, irritability, diaphoresis, dyspnea, + gallop on exam, older pts w/ many coronary collaterals may p/w angina w/ exertion, CHF
    - ECG: ST elevation w/ episodes of deep anterolateral Q-waves in completed infarcts
      - Classic finding is deep Q-wave in aVL
    - Diagnosis: Can be seen on doppler echo, gold standard: coronary angiography, ↑ trop
    - Treatment: Surgical reimplant on aorta, tx for CHF, CABG, may require transplant

- Other congenital coronary lesions: Anomalous RCA off PA, coronary AVM, myocardial bridge
- Coronary anatomy: Aorta → RCA & LCA. LCA → LAD (L anterior descending) & LCx (L circumflex). On ECG, LAD = anteroseptal leads (V1–V5), LCx (V5–V6, I, aVL), RCA (II, III, aVF)
  - **Pediatric chest pain rarely cardiac (<5%),** anomalous coronary is a possible cardiac cause; others: MVP, pericarditis, coronary spasm, dissection, coronary aneurysm, HOCM, ↑ HR

Vascular Ring & Sling (Park's Pediatric Cardiology. 6th ed. 2014, Ch 16)
- Group of rare anomalies of great vessels that cause breathing and/or feeding difficulty
- **Types:** Below are those requiring surgery & cause both breathing and swallowing difficulty
  - Double aortic arch: Most common, 2 arches completely encircle trachea/esophagus
  - R arch w/ L ductus or ligamentum arteriosum arising from aberrant L subclavian
  - Anomalous L PA from R PA causing a "vascular sling"

Dextrocardia (Pediatric Cardiology: The Essential Pocket Guide. 3rd ed. 2014, Ch 7)
- Dextrocardia refers to the heart being located on the R side of the chest
- **Types:**
  - Situs inversus: IVC/R atrium/liver on L; stomach/aorta/L atrium on R; "mirror image"
    - Strong assn w/ Kartagener syndrome (~40%). Situs inversus can occur w/ L heart
  - Dextroversion (assn: VSD, PS, & L-TGA) & dextroposition (extrinsic displacement, i.e., CDH)
    - Situs solitus (normal organ position) present with these types

CARDIAC PROCEDURES & POST-OPERATIVE COURSE

COMMON CHD SURGERIES

(The Washington Manual Cardiology Subspecialty Consult. 2nd ed. 2009, Ch 15; Chest Radiographic Interpretation in Pediatric Cardiac Patients. 2010, Ch 4)

Procedure	Condition(s)	Description	Timing, Special Considerations
Arterial Switch (Jatene)	D-TGA	Restore anatomic arrangement with transection of aorta and PA and reimplantation in correct position	1st 2 wk; requires coronary reimplantation. Previous surgery was atrial switch (Mustard/Senning)
Modified B–T Shunt	Many, CHD w/ ↓ pulm flow	Artificial tube (usually Gore-Tex) shunt from subclavian art → R PA	Classic B–T is subclavian directly attached to ipsilateral PA
Norwood	Pre-Fontan (stage 1)	Aorta transposed on to pulm trunk (neo-aorta), PA flow by Sano or B–T	Neonatal, hypoplastic arch is augmented with allograft patch
Sano	Pre-Fontan (stage 1)	Artificial tube shunt from RV → PA	Neonatal
Damus–Kaye–Stansel	D-TGA (+ coronaries not amenable to translocation) & stage I Norwood in HLHS	PA transected, end attached to LV then attached to aorta. + RV → PA conduit	1–2 yr; similar to Rastelli, ↑↑ mortality vs. arterial switch
Bidirectional Glenn (BDG)	Pre-Fontan (stage 2), Ebstein	SVC → ipsilateral PA	3–6 mo. Older prn for Ebstein to ↓ RV volume load ("1.5 ventricle")
Hemi-Fontan	Pre-Fontan (stage 2) but not in Ebstein	SVC → ipsilateral PA utilizing section of atrial tissue in anticipation of intracardiac Fontan	Same as BDG

Fontan	Any CHD with functionally single ventricle (i.e., HLHS, tricusp atresia, etc.)	3 stages: 1) B-T/ Norwood/Sano; 2) BDG or hemi-Fontan; 3) Fontan, IVC → PA + RA fenestration (pop-off)	Stage: 1) neonatal; 2) 3–6 mo; 3) 1–3 yr. Fontan procedure can be extracardiac or intra-atrial
Rastelli	RVOT obstruction + VSD + D-TGA (or DORV or others w/ overriding aorta)	VSD repaired with tunnel from LV into aorta. RV → PA conduit placed	>1 yr (palliative shunt, i.e., B–T placed in interim); poor outcomes, other options: Nikaidoh/REV
PA Banding	Any w/ ↑ pulm blood flow & inability to perform 1° repair in present state/age	Radio-opaque band placed around mid-PA trunk	1–3 mo; protects pulm vascular bed from ↑ flow & "conditions" LV. 1° repair preferable if possible
Ross Procedure	Valvular AS	Pulm valve moved to aortic position & pulm valve replaced w/ allograft	To be done if balloon valvuloplasty fails or if severe AR after balloon

PREOPERATIVE CHD CONSIDERATIONS

(Moss & Adams. 8th ed. 2013, Ch 20)

- L → R shunts: Typically closure is indicated (ASD, VSD) if Qp:Qs ≥2:1
  - $Qp:Qs = (SaO_2 - SvO_2)/(SpvO_2 - SpaO_2)$
- See previous "Cyanotic Lesions" section for algorithm of initial evaluation of cyanosis
  - Hyperoxia test, CXR, echo, pre- & postductal sats
    - If + or unable to definitively dx, **start prostaglandin infusion**. May require intubation
    - PGE₁ side effects: Hypotension, apnea, hyperpyrexia, bone pain, tissue friability
- **HLHS:** Most can be managed on room air w/ close monitoring preop. Start PGE₁
  - ABG & lactate measured at regular intervals
  - Restrictive atrial septum managed w/ emergent balloon septostomy after birth
  - Furosemide use prn, feeds should be parenteral to ↓ risk of NEC
  - Intubation for respiratory distress or hemodynamic compromise
  - Norwood stage 1 should be performed during 1st wk if possible
    - Alternative is hybrid technique with PA banding + endovascular PDA stenting
- **D-TGA:** Start PGE₁ after birth
  - Atrial septostomy for ↓ O₂ sat (–<75%), significant cyanosis afterwards → 1° repair ASAP
- **Truncus arteriosus:** Typically managed on room air
  - Preop concerns 2/2 diastolic hypotension (↓ coronary, renal, mesenteric perfusion)
    - Worsens as PVR ↓ after birth → ↑ Qp:Qs; significant ↑ in Qp → 1° repair ASAP
- **TAPVR:** With significant obstruction, primary objective is immediate surgery
  - Without significant obstruction, diuretics can be used for pulm edema
- **ToF:** Many centers do 1° repair in infancy including neonatal period for ↑ RVOT obstruction
  - Also common to perform systemic → pulm shunt to allow growth prior to repair
- **CoA:** Severe cases w/ PDA closure may p/w obstructive shock and ↓ organ perfusion
  - Tx: PGE₁, inotropes, intubation, correcting organ hypoperfusion states
- **Bidirectional Glenn:** Preoperative evaluation should ensure PVR not significantly ↑
- **Fontan:** Preop risk factors (high-risk operation) include ↑ PVR/PA pressure, distorted PAs (usually from previous surgeries), LVEF <60% or ↑ LV diastolic pressure, AV valve regurg, presence of MAPCAs (should be occluded preop)

POSTOPERATIVE CONSIDERATIONS

(Moss & Adams. 8th ed. 2013, Ch 20 & 49)

- Initial evaluation of postoperative CHD patient:
  - Length of CPB, aortic clamping, length of hypothermic arrest, active GTTs, residual defects, bleeding, anesthetics administered, pacing lines present, vascular access, drains
    - Prolonged deep hypothermia associated with neurologic injury
    - Prolonged aortic cross-clamping can result in myocardial reperfusion injury
    - 6–12 hr post-CPB associated with inflammatory reduction in CO

- Bleeding: Risk after CPB is significant, typically 2/2 platelet dysfunction or ↓ fibrinogen
  - Upon admission postop obtain: CBC, fibrinogen, PT/INR, PTT
  - Initial tx for postop bleeding: Platelet transfusions and cryoprecipitate, RBCs prn to ↑ Hct
    - Continued blood loss w/ normal coag studies should prompt eval of surgical source
- **HLHS**, post-Norwood: Maintain Qp:Qs as close to 1:1 as possible (usually by modifying FiO_2), inotropic support usually needed
- **D-TGA**, post-ASO: Echo to assess regional wall motion abnormalities (↓ coronary perfusion), + nitroglycerin to ↑ coronary perfusion, inotropic support needed 2/2 deconditioned LV
  - Vent arrythmias & ↓ CO should prompt evaluation of ↓ coronary flow
  - LeCompte maneuver may cause aortic obstruction, branch pulm artery stenosis
- **Truncus arteriosus:** Hemodynamic compromise 2/2 truncal valve insufficiency, PH, ventricular dysfunction. May require significant inotropic support & iNO for PH
- **TAPVR:** Primary postop complication is PH, peaks 6–12 h postop
  - Will need ↑↑ sedation/analgesia through this initial period, also iNO
- Systemic → Pulm shunts: Postop complications include ↓ diastolic BP & ↑ Qp
  - Improves in 24–48 hr (with PDA closure), inotropes to ↑ diastolic BP until then
    - May require shunt downsize
  - Sudden hypoxemia may indicate **shunt failure** (vs. PH vs. ↓ SVR), can result in cardiac arrest
    - Emergent echo + inotropes to ↑ SVR → endovascular or surgical shunt repair
    - Prevention with low-dose heparin
- **ToF:** Neonatal repairs can require significant inotropic support. High risk for JET
  - Frequent desats can be residual ASD intended as "pop off"
- **AVSD:** Major risk is severe PH, ↓ incidence w/ early repair which is now routine
  - Tx w/ iNO effective if severe PH occurs or there is high risk
- **CoA:** Intraop aorta is cross-clamped for ~15–30 min (↓ coronary O_2 supply) w/o CPB
  - May require vasodilators in early postop course, typically well tolerated
  - Assess LE strength early postop, possible spinal cord ischemia (rare)
- **Hypoplastic/interrupted arch:** ↑↑ postop bleeding risk 2/2 aortic suture lines
  - Ensure available blood products to manage bleeding if occurs. ↑ BP can cause dehiscence
    - HTN managed in 1st 24 hr w/ BB (esmolol or labetalol); 24–48 hr w/ ACE-Is
- **Bidirectional Glenn:** Overventilated (↓ $PaCO_2$) → ↓ cerebral blood flow → SVC flow → ↓ pulm flow → hypoxemia. Postop $PaCO_2$ goal is 40–50 (keep pH >7.3). Elevate HOB. Postop SVC catheter in place and can infuse nitroglycerin through to ↓ PVR
  - Post-BDG headaches (aka "Glenn head") can be treated w/ morphine, tylenol, NSAIDs
- **Fontan:** Highly dependent on adequate PA filling pressures (need adequate volume)
  - Nonfenestrated patients at high risk of ↑ Fontan pressures → persistent pleural effusions
    - These effusions can result in protein losing enteropathy (poor prognosis)
  - Fenestrations, if too large, may cause ↓ O_2 sat
  - Acute liver failure can occur in 1st wk postop, thought 2/2 ↓ CO & hypoperfusion

---

INTERVENTIONAL CARDIOLOGY

(Park's Pediatric Cardiology. 6th ed. 2014, Ch 7; Circulation 2011;123:2607–2652)

Diagnostic Cardiac Catheterization

- Indications: When noninvasive tests do not provide necessary data for ideal management
- Common uses: Measurement of pressure gradients (AS, PS, AR, PR), assess complications of prior surgery (i.e., shunts, conduits, baffles), assess coronary anatomy (i.e., KD), preop planning, identify aortopulmonary collaterals (aka MAPCAs: ToF, pulm atresia), many others
- Complications: Arrhythmia, perforation, structure injury, hemorrhage, infection, renal injury
- Peri-cath considerations: Obtain baseline ECG, labs (coags, CBC, type/screen, blood gas to correct acidosis pre/post), hold digoxin to ↓ risk of arrhythmia

Therapeutic Cardiac Catheterization
- Rashkind atrial septostomy: Augments PFO/ASD to allow for preop stabilization in CHD
- Balloon valvuloplasty: Relieve obstruction of stenotic valves
- Balloon angioplasty ± stenting as primary repair of CoA, branch PA stenoses
- Closure devices for nonsurgical closure of ASD, VSD, PDA, MAPCAs
- Transcatheter valve replacement of pulm valve in postop CHD patients
- Fetal interventions (i.e., AS balloon angioplasty in an effort to prevent progression to HLHS)

CONGESTIVE HEART FAILURE

(Heart 2002;88:198; Park's Pediatric Cardiology. 6th ed. 2014, Ch 27; Nelson Textbook of Pediatrics. 20th ed. Ch 442)

- Syndrome in which: heart unable to meet metabolic needs, cardiac output (CO) unable to keep up w/ venous return, or a combination of the 2
  - Accounts for ~10% of pediatric heart transplant, w/ DCM as most common cause

Pathophysiology
- Preload = loading force on heart (venous return) that stretches myocardial fibers, which (to a point) → ↑ contractility and ↑ CO (Frank-Starling law)
- As filling pressures ↑ beyond point of maximal contractile response, contraction becomes increasingly inefficient → ↓ CO
- As tissue perfusion impaired 2/2 ↓CO, RAAS activated → ↑ renal Na/H_2O retention → ↑ extracellular volume and preload
- RAAS activation also → ↑ afterload against which heart must work → further congestion

Etiologies (Can J Cardiol 2017;33:1342–1433)
- **Increased demand for CO** (high-output heart failure)
  - Hypermetabolic states (hyperthyroidism, anemia, sepsis); valvular insufficiency (inherited or acquired); fluid overload (renal dz or iatrogenic); L → R shunt (PDA, VSD, ASD, etc.)
- **Increased afterload:** AS/PS, CoA, systemic or pulm hypertension
- **Impaired myocardial function/contractility:** Myocarditis, DCM, coronary disease, metabolic abnormalities (i.e., Pompe disease), nutritional or toxic insults (thiamine deficiencies, chemotherapeutics), electrolyte disturbances, dysrhythmias
- **Etiologies by age group:**
  - Neonatal: Severe anemia (hydrops), dysrhythmia (SVT, CHB), CHD, myocarditis, PDA, VSD, bronchopulmonary dysplasia, inherited CM, systemic AVM
  - Infant/toddler: L → R shunt, AVM, ALCAPA, inherited CM, KD, dysrhythmia, myocarditis, valvular dz, postop ventricular dysfunction
  - Child & older: Rheumatic fever, renal dz (HTN), myocarditis, thyroid dz, hemochromatosis, radiation, anthracyclines, IE, CF (R heart failure), inherited CM

Evaluation (Can J Cardiol 2017;33:1342–1433; Moss & Adams. 8th ed. 2013, Ch 73)
- History: Poor feeding, poor weight gain, sweating w/ feeds, poor exercise tolerance, cyanosis, chest pain, nocturnal cough, orthopnea, paroxysmal nocturnal dyspnea
- Exam: May reveal tachycardia or tachypnea, edema less obvious in infants (assess eyelids & sacrum), heart may be enlarged w/ displaced PMI, ± murmur, additional heart sounds (S3, S4), crackles on pulm exam with L heart failure, elevated jugular venous pulsations or enlarged liver seen with R heart failure (which can be secondary to L heart failure)
- ECG: Rarely normal but nonspecific
- CXR: May have cardiac enlargement, pulm edema
- Lab: ↑ BNP (varies by age, no accepted standard), others based on clinical situation (i.e., TSH, HIV)
  - Myocarditis: Workup for myocarditis reviewed separately below
  - Autoimmune: Anti-Ro and La, ANA, RF, ESR, dsDNA, and other autoantibodies
  - Mitochondrial: Carnitine, acyl-carnitine, lactate, glucose, CBC (for neutropenia), urine AA for methylglutaconic aciduria, muscle bx, molecular genetics (Barth syndrome)
- Echo: Necessary to assess cardiac function and for anatomic causes (i.e., ALCAPA)

- Data limited in pediatrics – Equivocal on use of ACE-Is and β-blockers as well as spironolactone
- ACE inhibitors: Retrospective study demonstrating reduced mortality in children w/ DCM compared to standard Rx with digoxin and diuretics (Pediatr Cardiol 1993;14:9)
  - 2 trials in single-ventricle pediatric patients showed no benefit of ACE-Is (Circulation 1997;96:1507–1512; Circulation 2010;122:333–340)
- β-blockers: In children, 2 RCTs have shown improvement of LV fxn, ↑ exercise tolerance & ↓ need for transplant in DCM (Heart 1998;79:337; J Heart Lung Transplant 1999;18:269)
  - Pediatric carvedilol trial: No benefit, possible harm; implied benefit only w/ systemic LV (JAMA 2007;298(10):1171–1179)
- Diuretics: Clear clinical benefit, but no mortality benefit
  - Options – Chlorthiazide, ethacrynic acid, and furosemide
  - Spironolactone: Small RCT in children showed safety & efficacy, no mortality impact
- Digoxin: Long-standing corner stone of pediatric CHF management
  - Studies evaluating efficacy in children show modest benefits in small nonrandomized or unblinded trials in infants w/ VSD
  - ↑ contractility does not consistently correlate with clinical improvement
- **Management of acute CHF** - Exacerbation
  - Diuresis, O_2 prn
  - ↑ contractility w/ inotropes (dopamine, dobutamine, milrinone)
  - ↓ afterload (milrinone, nitroprusside, ACE-Is)

CARDIOMYOPATHIES, PERICARDITIS, & ACQUIRED LESIONS

CARDIOMYOPATHY (CM)

(Nelson Textbook of Pediatrics. 20th ed. Ch 439; Park's Pediatric Cardiology. 6th ed. 2014, Ch 18)

Dilated Cardiomyopathy (DCM)
- **Epidemiology:** Most common CM and cause of cardiac transplantation in children
  - More common M > F, African Americans > Caucasian, and infants (<1 yr) > children
- **Types:** Most commonly idiopathic; secondary causes: myocarditis, doxorubicin, neuromuscular dz (Duchenne, Becker), inborn errors of metabolism, malformation syndromes, familial
- **Evaluation** (Circulation 2006;114:2671)
  - Presenting sx: CHF (89.7%), sudden death (4.9%), exercise intolerance/arrhythmias (2.2%)
    - 3.3% found on routine screening
- **Treatment:** Treat underlying cause, treat CHF as above
  - Immune modulators (cyclosporine, steroids, γ-globulin) used in some pts w/ myocarditis
- **Prognosis** (JAMA 2006;296:1867; Circulation 2006;114:2671)
  - Risk factors for death or need for transplantation: >6 yr and/or CHF at dx, idiopathic cause
  - 1 & 5 yr rate of death or transplantation ~31% and 46%

Hypertrophic Cardiomyopathy (HCM) (Moss & Adams. 8th ed. 2013, Ch 54)
- Complex, relatively common genetic disorder. Can present at any age
- AD inheritance 2/2 mutations in any 1 of 11+ genes
- **Epidemiology:** Most common cause of sudden death in children
  - A prevalence of 1:500 in the general population, most common genetic cardiac disease
- **Types:**
  - Most HCM pts without LVOT obstruction, nomenclature w/ obstruction: HOCM
  - May p/w sudden death, CP, syncope, aortic SEM w/o click, + family hx, ECG Δs
- **Evaluation:**
  - ECG findings in ~95% of cases (LVH, dagger Q-wave in L precordial leads)
  - Echo w/ hypertrophied nondilated LV in absence of other cardiac or systemic dz
  - MRI may show asymmetric LVH undetectable on echo
  - **Screening:** Genetic testing available but clinical screening done w/ imaging (echo, MRI) + ECG

- <12 yr: Screen if symptomatic, malignant fam hx, athlete, signs/sxs
- 12–21 yr: Screening every 12–18 mo
- Genetic testing if gene identified on available assays in affected family member
- **Treatment:**
  - Medical: BB or CCB. Anticoagulants & antiarrhythmics for 2/2 complications (i.e., A fib)
    - Remember, these patients are preload dependent
  - Refractory to medical therapy: Interventional (EtOH septal ablation, dual chamber pacing) & surgical (septal myomectomy). ICD if high risk of sudden death
- **Prognosis:** Overall annual mortality rate is 1%
  - Risk factors for sudden death: Prior hx of cardiac arrest, spontaneous VT, fam hx of sudden death, syncope, hypotension during exercise, and extreme LVH

Restrictive Cardiomyopathy (Heart 2005;91:1199)

- Diastolic dysfunction w/ preserved systolic function + absence of hypertrophy or dilation
- **Types:** Idiopathic, familial, infiltrative (Gaucher, Hurler, amyloid), storage dz (Fabry, glycogen storage, hemochromatosis), hemosiderosis, drugs, radiation
- **Evaluation:**
  - Present with sxs of CHF
  - Exam: Elevated JVP, S3, w/ tachycardia and low pulse volume can be found on exam
  - ECG: Nonspecific ST-T wave Δs; BBB, LVH, & conduction abnormalities can be seen as well
  - CXR: Usually normal cardiac size, pulm congestion often seen
  - Echo: ↑ early diastolic filling velocity, ↓ atrial filling velocity, ↑ ratio of early diastolic filling to atrial filling ratio, and ↓ relaxation time
- **Treatment:** Treat underlying cause
  - Symptomatic therapy includes diuretic for venous congestion, antiarrhythmics or pacemaker for conduction abnormalities, and warfarin for thrombus formation
- **Prognosis:** Worse than in adults. Worse outcomes if p/w pulm venous congestion

PERICARDITIS

(Park's Pediatric Cardiology. 6th ed. 2014, Ch 19; Moss & Adams. 8th ed. 2013, Ch 62; Pediatr Infect Dis J 2006;25:165)

- Inflammation of pericardial layers (parietal & visceral). Can be inflammation alone or w/ effusion (purulent, serosanguineous, or hemorrhagic) ± tamponade
- With purulent pericarditis, effusion can accumulate quickly resulting in R heart failure or tamponade; if develops slowly, greater amount of fluid can be tolerated
- Tamponade = Fluid compresses heart → restricted venous return w/ inspiration → ventricular pressures equalize → septal bowing into LV during filling → ↓↓ CO
  - This is the physiology of "pulsus paradoxus"
- **Types:** Relatively more common in bold
  - Bacterial: **Staph, Strep, Haemophilus, Neisseria,** Tularemia, TB, Bartonella, Actinomyces, Nocardia, Salmonella, Coxiella
  - **Viral:** Enteroviruses (coxsackie B), adenovirus, CMV, VZV, EBV, flu, HIV
  - Parasites: E. histolytica and Echinococcus
  - Fungi: Candida and Aspergillus
  - Other infections: Spirochetes, Mycoplasma, Chlamydia, rickettsiae
  - Noninfectious: **Postsurgical, autoimmune** (JIA, SLE, CTD), toxin mediated, KD
  - Genetic/metabolic: Glycogen storage disease, hypothyroidism, FMF, **uremia**
  - Cancer associated: Leukemia, metastatic or solid tumor, 2/2 chemo or XRT
  - Trauma: Blunt or penetrating or iatrogenic/surgical
- **Evaluation:**
  - History: Pain (can be variable in location/quality) that improves w/ sitting, dyspnea
  - Exam: Pulsus paradoxus (≥10 mmHg drop in SBP w/ inspiration), friction rub, JVD
  - ECG: Diffuse ST elevation, PR depression, ↓ voltage. Electrical alternans w/ effusion
  - CXR: Cardiomegaly (small w/ constrictive pericarditis) w/o pulm vascular congestion
  - Lab: Infectious w/u, BUN, troponin, viral assays, ± autoimmune or malignant eval
    - Pericardial fluid: Cell count, diff, cxs (bacterial, AFB, fungal, viral cxs/PCR), cytology
  - Echo: Gold standard for evaluation of pericardial effusion
- **Treatment:**
  - Pain management and treatment of inflammation with NSAIDs; steroids 2nd line; consider colchicine in older children
  - Pericardiocentesis indicated in tamponade physiology, or if purulent, tuberculous or malignant effusion suspected

ACQUIRED CARDIAC DISEASE

(Park's Pediatric Cardiology. 6th ed. 2014, Ch 19; Pediatric Cardiology: The Essential Pocket Guide. 3rd ed. 2014, Ch 9)

Cardiac Tumors *(Pediatric Cardiology: The Essential Pocket Guide. 3rd ed. 2014, Ch 22)*
- Rare, but if found in children it is more common before 12 mo
  - 1° cardiac tumors in <1 yo are benign 90%, whereas in 1–16 yo 40% malignant
- Numerous rhabdomyomas is strongly associated with tuberous sclerosis
- **Types:**
  - Benign: Rhabdomyoma (50% <12 mo), fibroma, angioma, teratoma, myxoma (rare <1 yr)
  - Malignant: Rhabdomyosarcoma, leiomyosarcoma, angiosarcoma, fibrosarcoma, others
- Present nonspecifically: Arrhythmia, obstruction to flow, ± murmur, ECG Δs, CHF
- Diagnosis typically made by echo. Presence of effusion ↑ likelihood of malignant tumor
- Rhabdomyomas and fibromas may regress spontaneously, more likely in pts <4 yr
- Surgical removal only indicated if inlet or outlet obstruction, arrhythmias, CHF 2/2 to tumor
  - Myxomas, rare in peds, are generally removed

Infective Endocarditis (IE) *(Heart Diseases in Children: A Pediatrician's Guide. 2011, Ch 29)*
- Infection of endocardial lining, usually affects abnormal structures (i.e., congenital valve defects, mechanical valves, patch material, etc.)
- Common concern is 2/2 IE from transient bacteremia from dental procedures
  - See section under CHD re: antibiotic ppx
- **Epidemiology:** Becoming more common with ↑ survival of repaired CHD
  - Incidence ↑↑ in those w/ cardiac risk factors (i.e., CHD): 2,160/100,000 vs. 5/100,000
- **Types:** Gram + organisms remain most common but gram − & fungal on the rise
  - Bacterial organisms: *Strep viridans*, *S. aureus*, CoNS, Enterococcus, HACEK organisms
- **Evaluation:**
  - History: Underlying heart defect, prolonged low-grade fever, fatigue, wt loss, weakness
  - Exam: New murmur, fever, Osler nodes, Janeway lesions, splinter hemorrhages, ± hematuria, ± poor dentition, ± CHF
  - ECG: PR prolongation or 3° block with abscess near atrial conduction pathways
  - Lab: Serial blood cultures, infectious w/u, ESR, CRP, UA
  - Echo: Assess for abscess, vegetation, valve function, dehiscence of prostheses. TEE > TTE
  - Modified Duke criteria
- **Treatment:** Prolonged antimicrobial therapy (typically IV); ~25% may require surgical tx

Kawasaki Disease (KD)
- Systemic vasculitis of unknown etiology – Coronary involvement (arteritis, ectasia, aneurysm) common (20–25%) and #1 cause of M&M
- **Epidemiology:** 80% of cases btwn 6 mo & 5 yr of age
  - M > F; more common in Asian/Pacific Islanders but affects all ethnic groups
- **Evaluation:**
  - History: Fever (≥5 d), hand/foot pain, diffuse rash
  - Exam: Conjunctivitis, maculopapular rash (trunk, extremities), strawberry tongue, cracked lips, palm/sole erythema, periungual desquamation, cervical lymphadenopathy, sinus tach
  - ECG: ± PR prolongation, nonspecific ST-T Δs
  - Lab: Infectious w/u, CBC w/ diff, ESR, CRP, UA, LFTs
  - Echo: Perform early & often (q 2–4 wk until ≥8 wk from onset of fevers)
- **Treatment:** IVIG (given <7–10 d ↓↓ risk of coronary aneurysm), aspirin
  - ± steroids, ± monoclonal Abs, ± additional antiplatelets / warfarin if giant aneurysm develops

Myocarditis *(Nelson Textbook of Pediatrics. 20th ed. Ch 439.5)*
- Acute or chronic myocardial inflammation w/ inflammatory infiltrate & myocyte necrosis
- **Types:** Most common 2/2 viral infection
  - Viral: **Coxsackie B, parvovirus B19**, adenovirus, EBV, CMV, influenza, RSV, HIV, HSV
  - Bacterial: Much loss common; diphtheria, Lyme, mycoplasma, Whipple disease
  - Other infectious causes: Also uncommon; Chagas, rickettsia, fungal
  - Noninfectious: SLE, KD, IBD, thyrotoxic, abx, anthracycline, cocaine, EtOH, many others

- **Evaluation:**
  - History: Variable; ± viral sxs, chest pain, poor feeding, resp distress, malaise, syncope
  - Exam: Evidence of CHF, gallop, tachypnea, ± hepatomegaly, tachy (common), JVD, ± MR
  - ECG: Δs common (~90%); sinus tach, ↓ voltage, PVCs, arrhythmia, prolonged PR & QT
  - CXR: Important for assessment of pulm edema which may be severe, ± cardiomegaly
  - Lab: Troponin, viral cultures, ± autoimmune w/u, infectious w/u
  - Echo: Depressed LV systolic function, may see ↑ wall thickness, MR
  - Other testing: Cardiac MRI & endomyocardial biopsy (not routinely)
- **Treatment:** Supportive, depends on severity
  - Mild: Bedrest, ± O₂, ± po afterload reducers; Severe: Intubation, IV diuretics, inotropes, VAD/ECMO, amiodarone, afterload reduction (nitroprusside), ± steroids/IVIG/antivirals
- **Prognosis:** Mortality rate in neonates can be very high (up to 75% w/ acute sxs reported)
  - Majority of pts outside of neonates completely recover. Up to 25% may need transplant

Rheumatic Heart Disease
- Rheumatic fever is a systemic inflammatory disease after GAS infection (usually pharyngitis)
  - Antibody cross-reaction to myocytes and/or heart valves (usually MV and/or AV) → valve insufficiency and eventually valve stenosis
- **Epidemiology:** Much less common since tx of strep throat w/ abx became routine
  - Remains most common cause of acquired heart disease in children worldwide
- **Evaluation:**
  - Modified Jones criteria: Must have evidence of GAS (anti-DNase B, ASO, or culture) and 2 major criteria or 1 major + 2 minor criteria
    - Major: Carditis, arthritis (migratory), chorea, erythema marginatum, subq nodules
    - Minor: Fever, arthralgia, PR prolongation, ↑ acute phase reactants
  - Echo should be performed to assess valve function and for pericardial effusion
- **Treatment:** Abx for current infection, anti-inflammatory (aspirin preferred, steroids for severe cases w/ valvulitis, CHF), CHF therapy if needed, 2/2 ppx (AHA recommendation)
  - 2° ppx: Penicillin (po daily or IM monthly) until age 21 or for at least 5 yr

HEIGHT

- Avg. height in the U.S.: Female 5′4″ (162 cm), male 5′9″ (175 cm)
- Midparental height = (maternal height + paternal height ± 5 in)/2
- (Add 5″ for male, subtract 5″ for female)
- Genetic potential = midparental height +/− 4 in
- Bone age (L hand 1 view x-ray), should match patient's age and correlate w/ expected growth velocity and puberty
- Growth velocity norms: (From AAFP)

Age	Growth Velocity (per yr)
Birth to 12 mo	23–27 cm (9–11 in)
12–24 mo	10–14 cm (4–6 in)
2–3 yr	8 cm (3 in)
3–5 yr	7 cm (2–3 in)
5 yr to puberty	5–6 cm (2 in)
Puberty:	Girls: 8–12 cm (3–5 in)
(see below for details)	Boys: 10–14 cm (4–6 in)

- Deviations from expected height:

Ddx	Bone Age Appears	Growth Velocity	Puberty	Adult Height
Familial tall stature	Approp	Age approp	Age approp	Tall (consistent w/ mid parental height)
Obesity	Older	Matches older age	Reaches at younger age	Often unaffected; sometimes shorter than expected
Precocious puberty	Older	Matches older age	Reaches at younger age	Likely shorter than expected
Genetic syndrome w/ tall stature	Approp	Depends on syndrome	Age approp if not affected by syndrome	Tall
Familial short stature	Approp	Age approp	Age approp	Short (consistent w/ midparental height)
Constitutional growth delay	Younger	Matches younger age	Reaches at older age	Unaffected (midparental height)
Growth hormone deficiency	Younger	Matches younger age	Can be normal or delayed	Depends on treatment
Genetic syndrome w/ short stature	Approp	Depends on syndrome	Age approp if not affected by syndrome	Short
Chronic disease	Approp	Age approp	Can be normal or delayed	Short

Tall Stature

- Defined as length or height >95th percentile or 2 std dev above the mean for age
- Ddx: Familial tall stature, growth hormone (GH) excess, Klinefelter syndrome, Marfan syndrome, late-onset CAH, can be secondary to obesity, or other genetic syndromes (Beckwith–Wiedemann, Sotos syndrome, Marshall–Smith syndrome)
- Workup:
  - 1st – Physical exam (dysmorphic features, obesity, Tanner stage), midparental height, and height velocity
    - If w/i 5 cm of midparental height, consistent w/ familial tall stature
  - 2nd – Bone age – normal bone age consistent w/ familial tall stature, advanced concerning for precocious puberty (can be assoc w/ late-onset CAH) or GH excess
  - 3rd – Measure body proportions; specifically upper to lower body ratio (normal in childhood 0.89–0.95) & arm span (normally 1 cm shorter than height in childhood and equal to height in adolescence)
    - Klinefelter has ↑ arm span, Marfan has ↓ upper:lower body ratio

Short Stature

- Defined as height <5th percentile or 2 std dev < mean for age
- Ddx: Familial short stature, constitutional growth delay, GH deficiency, genetic syndrome (Turner, Prader-Willi, Noonan), chronic disease, skeletal dysplasia, hypothyroidism, malabsorption (undiagnosed celiac disease, IBD)
- There are growth curves for many conditions, can give hint to cause

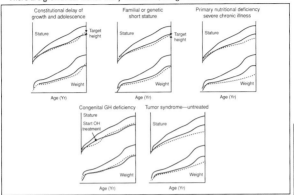

From Rose SR, Vogiatzi MG, Copeland KC. A general pediatric approach to evaluating a short child. Pediatr Rev 2005;26(11):410–420.

- Workup:
  - 1st – Check midparental height, Tanner stage, parental puberty hx, evaluate for chronic disease (renal failure, heart disease, lung disease including cystic fibrosis) or malnutrition
  - 2nd – Bone age, TSH/free T4, IGF-1, IGFBP-3, BMP, celiac panel, ESR, +/– karyotype (Turner syndrome)
  - 3rd – GH stimulation testing if young bone age, ↓ IGF-1, IGFBP-3 (described below)
  - 4th – Consider brain MRI w/ contrast to evaluate for a hypothalamic or pituitary tumor that affects hormone levels (can also assess for ↑ ICP, which can affect hypothalamic or pituitary function)

Constitutional Delay of Growth and Puberty

- Continued growth and pubertal development, but reaches growth spurt and puberty at older age; "late bloomer"
- Workup: Delayed age of parents' pubertal development, delayed Tanner stage, delayed bone age
- No tx necessary

Growth Hormone (GH) Deficiency

- Ddx: Idiopathic, hypopituitarism, pituitary anatomical abnormality, CNS malignancy
- GH stimulation test helps support dx but is not gold standard
  - Use stimulant (insulin, glucagon, clonidine, arginine, or L-dopa) and measure GH elevation every 30 min for 120 min
  - GH level <10 often indicates deficiency, but is lab specific and controversial
- Tx: GH replacement to normalize height until postpubertal or linear growth velocity is <2 cm/yr
  - Limited data on continuing GH therapy after growth plates fuse

Normal Puberty

- Pathway: GnRH (hypothalamus) → FSH & LH (pituitary) → gonadarche (sex hormones) released from gonads → gametogenesis in gonads
- Girls:
  - 8–13 yo (7–13 yo if obese, black, or Hispanic): Starts w/ thelarche
    - Estradiol → breast development (thelarche)
    - Menarche (10–16 yo) occurs 2–2.5 yr after thelarche, during Tanner stage IV
    - Adrenarche (pubic and axillary hair, acne, body odor)
- Boys:
  - 9–14 yo: Starts w/ testicular enlargement (>3 mL)
    - FSH → testicular enlargement
    - LH → testosterone → growth of penis, muscular changes
      - Nocturnal emissions, facial hair, voice deepening are late changes (Tanner V)
    - Adrenarche (pubic hair, axillary hair, acne, and body odor)

GROWTH, PUBERTY 5-3

	Breast	Pubic Hair	Genitals	Pubic Hair
Stage 1	Small nipples. No breast	No pubic hair.	No signs of puberty. Scrotum, testes, and penis as in childhood.	No pubic hair.
Stage 2	Breast and nipples have just started to grow. The areola has become larger. Breast tissue bud feels firm behind the nipple.	Initial growth of long pubic hairs. These are straight, without curls, and of light color.	Initial growth of scrotum and testes. The skin on the scrotum has become redder, thinner, and more wrinkled. The penis may have grown a little in length.	Few hairs around the root of the penis. The hairs are straight, without curls, and of light color.
Stage 3	Breast and nipples have grown additionally. The areola has become darker. The breast tissue bud is larger.	The pubic hair is more widespread. The hair is darker and curls may have appeared.	The penis has now grown in length. Scrotum and testes have grown. The skin of the scrotum has become darker and more wrinkled.	Hairs are darker and curlier and still sparse, mostly located at the penis root.
Stage 4	Nipples and areolas are elevated and form an edge toward the breast. The breast has also grown a little larger.	More dense hair growth with curls and dark hair. Still not entirely as an adult woman.	The penis has grown in both length and width. The head of the penis has become larger. The scrotum and testes have grown.	More dense, curly, and dark hair. The hair growth is reaching the inner thighs.
Stage 5	Fully developed breast. Nipples are protruding, and the edge between areola and breast has disappeared.	Adult hair growth. Dense, curly hair extending toward the inner thighs.	Penis and scrotum as an adult.	Pubic hair extends upward to the umbilicus. It is dense and curly.

Sequence of Puberty in Girls

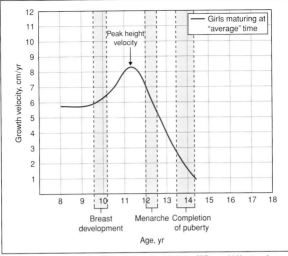

From Rasmussen AR, Wohlfahrt-Veje C, Tefre de Renzy-Martin K, Hagen CP, Tinggaard J, Mouritsen A, Mieritz MG, Main KM. Validity of self-assessment of pubertal maturation. Pediatrics 2015;135(1):86–93.

Sequence of Puberty in Boys

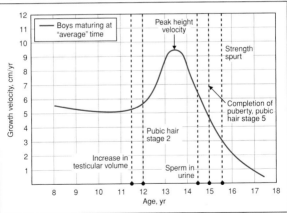

Biro FM, Chan YM. Normal puberty: sequence of puberty in girls. Hoppin AG, ed. UpToDate. Waltham, MA: UpToDate Inc. https://www.uptodate.com (Accessed on February 22, 2018.)

Precocious Puberty

- Definition: Thelarche or testicular enlargement starting before above listed ages
- Workup: LH, FSH, testosterone (male), estradiol (female), bone age
  - Elevated LH may indicate true precocious puberty, as it is unmeasurable before pulsatile GNRH is secreted in the prepubertal period
  - Gold-standard test is a GNRH stimulation test: Positive test for central precocious puberty will be peak levels of LH >9.2 mIU/mL 30–40 min following stimulation by GNRH agonist

- Evaluate for central precocious puberty, if positive
  - Consider brain MRI in all males, any child w/ neurologic sx, or fast progression of puberty
  - CNS abnormalities (including tumors such as hamartomas affecting the hypothalamus and pituitary or other lesions causing ↑ ICP that can disrupt hypothalamic or pituitary function) are the most common cause of central precocious puberty in boys
- Tx (if no CNS lesion is found): GNRH agonist (e.g., leuprolide 0.2–0.3 mg/kg Q1 mo or Q3 mo) prevents LH/FSH secretion -> w/in 6 mo of therapy, will see halting of progression +/– regression of secondary sexual characteristics
- **Benign forms of partial precocious puberty:**
  - Premature adrenarche: Precocious appearance of pubic hair or other signs of adrenarche w/out other signs of virilization
    - Ddx: Consider adrenal tumor especially if fast progression & nonclassical CAH
  - Premature thelarche: Precocious appearance of breast development in girls w/ no other sign of sexual maturation, accelerated growth velocity or bone age advancement
    - Common during first 2 yr of life and in obese 4–8 yo
  - Gynecomastia: Not a form of precocious puberty, but benign breast growth in males (occurs in 50% of males during puberty)
    - Concerning when postpubertal or w/ rapid progression

	Premature Adrenarche	Premature Thelarche	Precocious Puberty
Glandular changes	–	+	+
Areolar changes	–	–	+
Sexual hair	+	–	+
Somatic growth	nl	nl	↑
Bone age	nl or advanced	nl	advanced

Delayed Puberty

Definition: No breast development in girls by age 13 or no testicular development by age 14 in boys
- Ddx: Constitutional delay of growth and puberty (see above), hypogonadotropic hypogonadism (hypothalamic or pituitary tumors, hypopituitarism, malnutrition, chronic illness), or hypergonadotropic hypogonadism (high FSH due to gonadal failure: congenital [Turner and Klinefelter syndromes] or acquired [chemo, surgery, radiation, trauma, torsion, infection, autoimmune])
- Workup: LH/FSH, testosterone, estradiol, bone age, prolactin, IGF1, TFTs, cortisol, karyotype
  - Also should be considered in patients w/ pauses in pubertal progression

Irregular Menstruation
- **Prepubertal vaginal bleeding:**
  - Ddx common: Irritation, urethral prolapse, foreign body, trauma, abuse
  - Ddx rare: Malignancy (rhabdomyosarcoma including sarcoma botryoides and endodermal sinus tumor), especially if <3 yo; McCune–Albright syndrome (triad of peripheral precocious puberty, fibrous dysplasia, café au lait macules)
  - Workup: Noninvasive exam – look for foreign body, consider precocious puberty (above)
- **Amenorrhea:**
  - Primary amenorrhea: The absence of menstruation by the age of 15 yr in girls who have never menstruated
    - Evaluate if: (1) >5 yr since the first evidence of puberty, (2) failure of any pubertal development by 13 yr of age, below
  - Secondary amenorrhea: The absence of menstruation for 3 or more months in women w/ past menses
    - Evaluate if: <9 menses in a 12-mo period (oligomenorrhea), below
  - Ddx: Pregnancy, anovulation, anatomic, ovarian failure
    - Never forget to consider pregnancy even for primary amenorrhea!
  - Workup: Pelvic exam, pelvic ultrasound, bhCG, FSH, TSH; possibly prolactin, testosterone, 17-OHP, DHEA-S
- **Chronic anovulation:**
  - Hypothalamic dysfunction 2/2 eating disorders, exercise, systemic illness, thyroid dysfunction, polycystic ovary syndrome (PCOS), hypothalamic neoplasms, or adrenal hyperplasia
    - Test prolactin – If elevated, evaluate further for pituitary neoplasms or medication effect

- Hypopituitarism
  - Test by measuring other pituitary or downstream hormones (TSH, FSH, LH, IGF-1, IGF-BP3, cortisol)
- **Anatomic causes of amenorrhea:**
  - Imperforate hymen: Consider in females w/ delayed menarche and otherwise normal pubertal development
    - Will often have cyclic abdominal pain
    - On pelvic exam, found to have an obstructing membrane in vaginal opening that often bulges w/ Valsalva
  - Others: Cervical stenosis, intrauterine adhesions (see ultrasound)
- **Ovarian failure:** Elevated FSH level → obtain karyotype
  - Premature ovarian insufficiency (menopause)
  - Gonadal dysgenesis/streak ovaries seen in Turner syndrome (45,X) and other DSDs

Polycystic Ovary Syndrome (PCOS)
- Diagnostic criteria are controversial and PCOS should not be diagnosed until 2–3 yr after menarche
- Rotterdam criteria, 2 of 3 are present:
  - Clinical evidence of hyperandrogenism (such as acne, hirsutism) or elevated free or total testosterone levels
  - Irregular ovulation (defined as cycle duration >35 d or <8 cycles per yr) or anovulation
  - Polycystic ovaries
  - Exclude other disorders w/ elevated androgens: 21-hydroxylase deficient CAH, androgen-secreting tumors, or hyperprolactinemia
- Assoc conditions: Obesity, acanthosis nigricans, and glucose intolerance w/ insulin resistance
  - Patients should be screened for diabetes w/ hemoglobin A1C
- Tx:
  - Lifestyle changes for obesity
  - Progestin or oral contraceptive to reduce endometrial hyperplasia from unopposed estrogen
  - Consider metformin to increase insulin sensitivity
  - Rarely, fertility agents can be used to induce ovulation including clomiphene citrate and letrozole

Disorders of Sexual Development (DSDs) Typically Presenting at Puberty
- **CAH –** Described below
- **Turner syndrome (45, X karyotype):**
  - Have accelerated loss of ovarian follicles, leaving only connective tissue causing the appearance of "streak ovaries"
  - Characteristics present in variable degrees: Short stature, low hairline and webbed neck, shield-like chest, and lymphedema of the ankles
  - Assoc w/: Horseshoe kidneys, autoimmune disorders including Hashimoto thyroiditis, and cardiovascular disease including coarctation of the aorta, bicuspid aortic valve and other vascular abnormalities
- **Klinefelter syndrome (47, XXY karyotype):**
  - Assoc characteristics: Tall stature, small testes, infertility, gynecomastia, ↓IQ, osteoporosis
  - Labs: ↓ testosterone, ↑ estrogen
  - Tx w/ androgen replacement therapy
- **Androgen insensitivity:**
  - Chromosomes 46, XY w/ mutations in the androgen receptor gene making the androgen receptor partially or nonfunctional
  - Normal testicular development and testosterone production but w/ limited-to-no end-organ effect (e.g., masculinization of external genitalia in utero and adrenarche in puberty)
  - Complete androgen insensitivity: Presents as phenotypically female w/ blind vaginal pouch; typically diagnosed at puberty w/ normal onset of breast development (as androgens are converted to estrogens), primary amenorrhea (given lack of uterus) and lack of pubic hair (given androgen resistance)
  - Partial androgen insensitivity: Presents as undervirilization in otherwise phenotypical males
- **5-alpha reductase deficiency:**
  - Chromosomes 46, XY w/ a deficiency of the enzyme 5-alpha reductase, which converts testosterone to dihydrotestosterone (DHT), the hormone that mediates formation of male external genitalia in utero

- As children, have normal male internal genitalia w/ female external genitalia and blind vaginal pouches; but at puberty, patients undergo male puberty w/ deepening of the voice and virilization of external genitalia

Transgender Health

- **Gender nonconformity:** "Extent to which a person's gender identity, role, or expression differs from the cultural norms prescribed for people of a particular sex" (Int J Transgend 2011;13:165–232)
- **Gender dysphoria:** "Discomfort or distress caused by a discrepancy between a person's gender identity and that person's sex assigned at birth (and the assoc gender role and/or primary and secondary sex characteristics)" (Fisk, 1974; Knudson, De Cuypere, & Bockting, 2010b)
- Sexuality is separate from gender identity
- Terminology: Transmale identifies as male, transfemale identifies as female
- Tx is for dysphoria (not for gender nonconformity)
  - There is little data on persistence of gender dysphoria from childhood to adulthood – often resolves or intensifies at start of puberty
  - Estimated 40% of transgender youth attempt suicide (difficult to study)
- 3 categories of tx – customized to patient's dysphoria
  - (1) Psychotherapy; (2) Pharmacological: Pubertal suppression and cross-gender hormones; (3) Surgery
  - Pubertal suppression: GnRH agonist therapy (pauses puberty to allow for more discussion assessment and thoughtful decision making); typically used from Tanner II until age 16 when cross-gender hormones can be considered; stopping GnRH will allow progression of puberty

ADRENAL DISEASE

Adrenal Insufficiency

- Sx: Hypotension, weakness, fatigue, emesis, diarrhea, and hypoglycemia
- Labs: ↓ morning cortisol (ideally at 7 am), elevated renin, ↓ aldosterone
- Ddx:
  - Primary (adrenal gland destruction): Addison disease (autoimmune), tuberculosis in adrenals, CAH, congenital, x-linked adrenoleukodystrophy, Waterhouse–Friderichsen syndrome (adrenal hemorrhage, commonly due to Neisseria meningitidis septicemia)
- Sx: As above +↑ ACTH gives skin hyperpigmentation, elevated K+
  - Secondary (ACTH deficiency): chronic steroid use, hypothalamic disease, pituitary disease, malignancy, radiation
- Tx:
  - W/ steroids, uses body surface area (BSA aka m^2) in dosing rather than weight:
    - BSA = $0.007184 \times W^{0.425} \times H^{0.725}$
  - Physiologic replacement: 8–12 mg/m^2/d hydrocortisone divided BID or TID (monitor growth and skeletal maturation)
  - Stress dose steroids for illness, particularly vomiting and fever
    - Moderate stress dose steroids: 30–50 mg/m^2/d divided q6h IV (or q6–8h PO) (max 10 mg/dose)
    - Severe stress dose steroids (needed for anesthesia or severe sepsis): 100 mg/m^2 once (max 100 mg) then 75–100 mg/m^2/d divided q6h IV (max 20 mg/dose)
  - If primary adrenal insufficiency: 0.1 mg/m^2/d fludrocortisone and access to salt (NaCl supplementation in infants)

Cushing Syndrome

- Caused by excess cortisol
- Characteristics: Weight gain, central obesity, buffalo hump, moon-face, striae (skin thinning), HTN, hyperglycemia, insomnia, psychosis
- Dx: 24-hr urine cortisol, midnight salivary cortisol, ACTH level twice, +/– dexamethasone suppression test

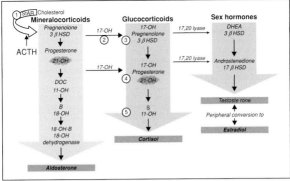

Deficiency	21-OH (4) Classic Complete Enzyme Deficiency	21-OH (4) Non-Classic Partial Enzyme Deficiency	11-βOH (5)	3-βHSD (3)	17-αOH(2)	StAR (1)
Frequency		90%	5%	Very rare	Very rare	Very rare
Adrenal crisis?	1–2 wks of age	When sick	No	1–2 wks of age	no	+
↑ androgens virilization of female/ undervirilization of male	+	+	+	+	–	–
↓ mineralocorticoid	+	+	(HTN)	+	(HTN)	+
Tx	Glucocorticoid Fluorocortisone Salt	Glucocorticoid Fluorocortisone Salt	Glucocorticoid (will ↓DOC)	Glucocorticoid Fluorocortisone Salt supplement		
Labs	↑17OHP ↓glucose, Na, aldosterone ↑K+, renin	↑/nl 17 OHP ACTH stim test →↑17OHP ↓glucose, Na, aldosterone ↑K+, renin	↑DOC, 11-deoxycortisol ↓K+, renin	↑ pregnenolone, DHEA, 17OH -pregnenolone ↓glucose, Na, aldosterone ↑K+, renin	↓K+, renin	

Biro FM, Chan YM. Normal puberty: sequence of puberty in boys. Hoppin AG, ed. UpToDate. Waltham, MA: UpToDate Inc. https://www.uptodate.com (Accessed on February 22, 2018.)

Ddx	ACTH level	Response to high-dose dexamethasone	Further evaluation
Pituitary adenoma (Cushing disease)	High (>20 pg/mL)	Decreased ACTH	Brain MRI
Ectopic ACTH secreting tumor	High	High ACTH remains	Evaluate for neuroendocrine (carcinoid) tumor, rare other tumors
McCune–Albright syndrome	Low (<5 pg/mL)		*
Adrenal adenoma or carcinoma	Low	Not indicated	Adrenal MRI or CT
Chronic steroid use	Not indicated	Not indicated	

*McCune–Albright syndrome: Fibrous dysplasia of bones, café-au-lait skin pigmentation, precocious puberty, other endocrine dysfunction

Congenital Adrenal Hyperplasia (CAH)

- A group of disorders that arise from abnormal steroidogenesis, specifically from a deficiency in any of the 5 enzyme-mediated steps in the production of cortisol (see figure above)
- Each enzyme deficiency leads to deficiency of certain steroid products and elevation of precursors
  - Decreased cortisol leads to ↑ACTH and hyperpigmentation

- Mineralocorticoids: Causes ↑ sodium retention (↑ BP) and ↓ potassium
- Androgens: If ↑ lead to virilization in female (↓ androgen leads to undervirilization of male)
- Infants w/ severe forms will present w/ salt wasting (leading to poor feeding, weight loss, failure to thrive [FTT], vomiting, dehydration, hyponatremia, metabolic acidosis, and hyperkalemia) & adrenal insufficiency (hypotension, adrenal crisis)
  - Males often have more severe presentation as females present w/ virilization and are caught earlier
  - **21-OH deficiency (4):**
    - Depletion of cortisol and aldosterone w/ variable phenotype (variable severity)
    - Leads to accumulation of precursor, **17-OH progesterone (17-OHP)**, which gets shunted to ↑ androstenedione production (measured on newborn screen)
  - **3-β hydroxysteroid dehydrogenase deficiency (3-β HSD) (3):**
    - Similar to 21-OH deficiency CAH, DHEA causes virilization
  - **11-β hydroxylase deficiency (5):**
    - ↑ **deoxycorticosterone (DOC)**, a less potent mineralocorticoid, that leads to salt retention and hypertension
    - Tx: Glucocorticoid → ↓ ACTH → ↓ DOC → ↓ HTN
  - **17-α hydroxylase deficiency (2):**
    - ↑ mineralocorticoids ↓ cortisol ↓ androgen
  - **StAR protein deficiency (1):** Extremely rare form; cholesterol not converted to any adrenal products

Pheochromocytoma
- A catecholamine-secreting tumor (adrenal medulla or paraganglioma in sympathetic chain)
- Sx: Episodes of diaphoresis, HTN, and palpitations; can also have severe refractory HTN
  - Epidemiology: 10% diagnosed in children, causes 1% of pediatric hypertension
- Assoc w/ MEN 2A and 2B, NF1, von Hippel–Lindau, and familial paraganglioma syndrome
- Dx: 24-hr urinary fractionated metanephrines (false + in severe illness, renal disease, and medication effect)
- Tx: DO NOT USE β-blockade, ONLY use α-blockade to mitigate hemodynamic effects until surgical removal of tumor

THYROID DISEASE

Hypothyroidism
- **Congenital:** Large fontanelle, lethargy, constipation, hoarse cry, hypotonia, hypothermia, jaundice; (severe: pale, pot-bellied, puffy face, protruding umbilicus, protuberant tongue)
  - Primary – Defect in thyroid gland development, defect in T4 synthesis, TSH receptor mutation
  - Secondary – ↓ iodine diet of parents
  - Central – ↓ TRH or TSH
    - Note: Newborn screen has high false-positive rate, especially in premature infants →repeat or test blood for TSH, T4
  - Tx: Levothyroxine 10–15 mcg/kg daily, to begin prior to 14 d of life
    - Monitor TSH and free T4 after 1, 2, and 3 wk then every 1–3 mo until age 2, then every 6–12 mo
- **Acquired:** Growth deceleration w/ delayed tooth eruption, fatigue, brittle hair, dry skin, cold intolerance
  - Hashimoto thyroiditis – Often starts as hyperthyroidism due to thyroiditis and TH release
    - Most (97%) have + antithyroglobulin antibodies and antithyroid peroxidase antibodies
  - de Quervain subacute postinfectious thyroiditis – Temporary (most recover, 10% develop permanent hypothyroidism), initially w/ elevated thyroid levels followed by hypothyroid phase
    - Features: + preceding respiratory tract infection, +/- fever & malaise, tender & larger thyroid gland
    - Labs: ↑ ESR, nondetectable thyroid antibodies, ↑ thyroglobulin (due to destruction of thyroid follicles), ↓ radioactive iodine uptake
    - <u>Tx</u>: NSAIDs for pain, levothyroxine as below, β-blocker if severe thyrotoxicosis, +/– prednisone (no clear guidelines in literature)
  - Pseudohypothyroidism – Related to obesity; mildly elevated TSH w/ normal T3, T4
  - Tx: Levothyroxine 1–2 mcg/kg daily
    - Monitor TSH and free T4 after 4–6 wk, then every 6–12 mo

Hyperthyroidism

- Sx child and adolescent: Hyperactivity, irritability, insomnia, heat intolerance, diaphoresis, ↑ appetite, diarrhea, weight loss, palpitations and tachycardia, fatigue, oligomenorrhea, tremor, hyperreflexia
- Sx neonatal and infant: Irritability, insomnia, fever, diaphoresis, poor feeding, diarrhea, weight loss, tachycardia, tremor, hyperreflexia
- Grave disease – Autoimmune, has goiter, can have exophthalmos (peak age 11–15 yo)
  - Workup: ↓ TSH, ↑ T3, T4, + thyroid stimulating immunoglobulin (often >140%), + thyroid peroxidase Ab (TPO) in 95%, + antithyroglobulin Ab in 50%, ↑ radioactive iodine uptake
  - Tx – Methimazole(0.2 mg/kg/d divided TID)
    - If refractory, then radioactive iodine-131 or surgery followed by levothyroxine for resultant hypothyroidism
- Thyroid storm: Life-threatening thyrotoxicosis characterized by hyperthermia, tachycardia, delirium, hemodynamic instability, arrhythmias; rare in children
  - Tx – Per endo consultation due to high morbidity and mortality; propranolol and high-dose potassium iodide to suppress synthesis of T4, short-term PTU (not used long term in children due to hepatotoxicity)
- Neonatal hyperthyroidism: Microcephaly, frontal bossing, IUGR, tachycardia, HTN (SBP > DBP), irritability, FTT, flushing, vomiting, diarrhea, jaundice, thrombocytopenia, heart failure, arrhythmias
  - Mothers have Grave disease and pass antibodies through placenta
  - Tx: Propranolol (0.5–2 mg/kg divided every 6–12 hr), methimazole (0.25–1 mg/kg/d divided every 8–12 hr), digoxin if heart failure

CALCIUM DISORDERS

Hypocalcemia

- Sx: Cramps, ↑ QTc, convulsions, +Chvostek (facial nerve tap causes contraction), + Trousseau (BP cuff causes carpal spasm)
- Tx: IV Ca gluconate (100 mg/kg q6h), calcitriol 0.25–0.75 mcg daily (takes hours to work), ± magnesium

Hypercalcemia

- Sx: Vomiting, abdominal pain, constipation, weakness, paresthesia, polyuria, polydipsia, malaise, nephrolithiasis, rarely pancreatitis
- Hypercalcemic crisis: Ca >13–15 w/ dehydration and AMS
- Tx: NS boluses (for dehydration) and 2–3× mIVF to promote excretion and support hydration; calcitonin (4 units/kg q12h), bisphosphonate

Parathyroid Hormone Effects

- 1) ↑ Ca (by ↑ resorption from bone and GI absorption and ↓ urinary excretion)
- 2) ↓ Phos (↑ GI absorption but ↑ urinary excretion)
- 3) ↑ Vit D (activates production of 1,25-OH vit D in kidney)
- 4) Other labs: Elevated Mg, and ↑/normal alkaline phosphatase

Hypoparathyroidism

↑ Phos, ↓ Ca, ↓ Vit D
- Sx of hypocalcemia
- Ddx: Transient in newborn, DiGeorge, autoimmune, postthyroidectomy
  - Pseudohypoparathyroidism – PTH resistance (same sx, nl to ↑PTH)
- Tx: Ca supplement (20–80 mg/kg elemental Ca daily), calcitriol (0.25–2 mcg daily ≥1 yo), monitor serum and urine Ca and adjust doses
- Sequelae: Skeletal anomalies, short stature, intellectual disability

Hyperparathyroidism

↑ Ca, ↓ Phos
- Sx: Bone pain (from bone reabsorption) and sx from hypercalcemia
- Ddx:
  - Primary disease – Parathyroid gland abnormalities, Ca-sensing receptor or CASR mutation, adenoma, MEN (see below)
  - Secondary disease – Hypocalcemia from rickets or renal failure
- Epidemiology: Rare in childhood prevalence of 2–5 per 100,000 (J Chin Med Assoc. 2012;75:425–434)
- Tx: Hydration, furosemide (0.5–1 mg/kg), hydrocortisone to ↓ GI absorption of Ca (1 mg/kg q6h); less common – calcitonin, bisphosphonates, surgery (if Ca↑1 mg/dL, CrCl <60, or osteoporosis)

Benign Familial Hypocalciuric Hypocalcemia (FFH or BFFH)

- Autosomal dominant – G-coupled protein receptor (Ca-sensing receptor or CASR)
- Sx: Mild ↑ or normal Ca (often asymptomatic), mild ↑ or normal PTH, relapsing pancreatitis may be slightly ↑ (not clear there is a causative relationship), ↑ incidence of chondrocalcinosis and premature vascular calcification (no increase in cardiovascular events compared to general population)
- Labs: 24-hr urine excretion of Ca <200 mg or CaCl/CrCl <0.01
- Can be assoc w/ severe hyperparathyroidism in neonates if homozygous mutation in CASR gene → severe hypercalcemia (Ca >13.5 mg/dL); life threatening and may require urgent parathyroidectomy
- Tx: None needed, total parathyroidectomy only beneficial in neonatal severe primary hyperparathyroidism, relapsing pancreatitis, or persistently elevated serum Ca levels (>14 mg/dL) but can fail (if subtotal resection, hypercalcemia will continue); if give birth should check neonate's Ca levels during 1st few days of life (no tx needed unless symptomatic)

Vitamin D Metabolism

- Produced in the skin from 7-deoxyhydrocholesterol -> w/ UV irradiation makes D_3 -> metabolized in liver and other tissues to 25-OHD (principal circulating form) -> metabolized further to 1, 25(OH)$_2$D (activated form) in the kidney
- 1,25(OH)$_2$D effects: ↑ intestinal Ca and Phos absorption, ↑ bone formation, ↑ Ca resorption in kidney, ↓ Phos resorption in kidney
- Nutritional vit D intake: 400 IU/d for infants, 600 IU/d for children

Rickets

- Low concentration of Ca and/or Phos -> defective bone mineralization
- Sx: Weakness, bone pain, bone deformity, fractures
  - Signs: Widened cranial sutures (enlarged fontanelle), frontal bossing, widening of wrists, rachitic rosary, dental eruption delayed, bow legs, short stature
  - X-ray findings: Best seen in metaphyses of long bones (tibia/fibula, femur), will be widened, cupped/scalloped, frayed, irregular, +/− fractures
- 2 types:
  - Calcipenic: Most commonly 2/2 severe prolonged vit D deficiency nutritionally, can also be nonfunctional vit D enzymes or receptors
  - Phosphopenic:

	Ca	Phos	PTH	Alkaline Phos
Calcipenic	↓	↓	↑	↑
Phosphopenic	Normal	↓	Normal	↑

- Tx of vit D–deficient calcipenic rickets: Vit D (600–6,000 IU/d depending on severity on diagnosis) and Ca supplementation, +/− calcitriol (1,25(OH)D$_2$)
  - Can get hungry bone syndrome in beginning of treatment of severe vit D–deficient rickets: When starting supplementing w/ vit D and Ca, gets depleted quickly due to significant Ca demands w/ osteoid mineralization

PITUITARY DISEASE

Syndrome of Inappropriate Antidiuretic Hormone (SIADH)

- Findings: Hyponatremia w/ concentrated urine; euvolemia or mild hypervolemia
- Etiology: CNS trauma, meningitis, neurosurgery, tonsillectomy and adenoidectomy, pneumonia, pain
- See nephrology chapter for further information

Diabetes Insipidus (DI)

- Sx: Polyuria, polydipsia, FTT, vomiting
- Types:
- Central – CNS trauma, postop, congenital
  - Tx: Vasopressin drip, desmopressin (via rhinal tube, nasal spray, pill), or thiazide diuretics w/ low-solute formula/diet
- Nephrogenic – Congenital or acquired renal tubule resistance to vasopressin
  - Tx: Access to free water and low-salt diet
- Test: Water deprivation test to demonstrate lack of ADH rise
  - Distinguishes from psychogenic polydipsia – Common in young children, due to overdrinking of free water, corrects w/ water deprivation

	SIADH	Central DI	Nephrogenic DI	Psychogenic Polydipsia
Plasma ADH	↑	↓	↑	↓
Serum Na	↓	↑	↑	↓/nl
Urine sodium	↑	↓	↓	↓
Urine output	↓	↑	↑	↑

Hypopituitarism
- Etiology: Hypoplastic gland, infection, trauma, radiation, postop pituitary surgery (craniopharyngioma, adenoma)
- Includes a combination of ↓TSH, ACTH, GH, FSH, LH, ADH – See other sections for sx and evaluation hormone deficiencies

ENDOCRINE SYNDROMES

Multiple Endocrine Neoplasia
- **MEN1:** Pituitary adenoma (functional or nonfunctional), pancreatic tumor (gastrin, insulin, VIP, glucagon), primary hyperparathyroidism
- **MEN2A:** Medullary thyroid cancer, pheochromocytoma, parathyroid gland hyperplasia w/ RET oncogene
- **MEN2B:** Medullary thyroid cancer, pheochromocytoma, GI neuroma

Polyglandular Autoimmune Syndromes (PGAs)
- **Type 1:** Mucocutaneous candidiasis, hypoparathyroidism, adrenal insufficiency
- **Type 2:** Adrenal insufficiency, autoimmune thyroid disease, type 1 DM

DIABETES MELLITUS: TYPE 1 VS. TYPE 2

Diagnosis Criteria
- Fasting glucose >126 mg/dL
- 2-hr glucose >200 mg/dL on oral glucose tolerance test
- Random glucose >200 mg/dL AND sx of diabetes
- Hemoglobin A1C >6.5%

Type 1 Diabetes
- Results from autoimmune destruction of the pancreatic β-cells
- Weak heritability risk – 1st degree relative risk 5–10%
- Assoc illnesses: Autoimmune thyroid disease, celiac disease

Type 2 Diabetes
- Results from insulin resistance; progressive β-cell failure and subsequent insulin deficiency
- Stronger heritability – More than 50% of children have a 1st-degree or 2nd-degree relative
- Assoc illnesses: Obesity, hypertension, hypertriglyceridemia, fatty liver disease, PCOS

Insulin Management
- Basal bolus regimen – Most commonly used regimen
  - Long-acting insulin provides basal coverage – typically given at bedtime
  - Rapid-acting insulin given before meals and snacks – provides coverage for carbohydrates eaten and to correct for ↑ blood glucose
- NPH or mixed regimens (70/30) – Uses peaks to take place of bolus
  - Fixed doses of intermediate-acting insulin is given 2–3 times per day
  - Easiest regimen, but less tightly controlled blood glucose
- Insulin pump
  - Rapid-acting insulin is delivered via SQ catheter continuously at various rates during the day (mimics basal)
  - Bolus doses delivered for meals and snacks and to correct for elevated blood glucose
- Dosing: Typically start at 0.5–1.0 units/kg (higher end of range during puberty) w/ advice from endocrinologist
  - Give half as basal and half divided for boluses

Types of Insulin

Type/Name	Onset	Peak	Duration	Use
Rapid acting NovoLog (aspart), Humalog (lispro), Apidra (glulisine)	10–15 min	60–90 min	2–3 hr	Meal coverage, correct high blood sugars, clear ketones
Short acting Regular	1 hr	2–4 hr	6–8 hr	Used IV for DKA, in TPN. Very short half-life when given IV
Intermediate NPH	1–2 hr	4–8 hr	12–14 hr	Can be used as basal insulin when dosed twice daily. Risk of hypoglycemia, given peak
Long acting Lantus, Basaglar (glargine) Levemir (detemir)	1–4 hr	None	12–24 hr	Used as basal insulin
Mixed 70/30 (NPH/ regular) or 75/25 (NPH/aspart)	30 min	As above	18–24 hr	Used for type 1 or type 2 diabetics only willing to take 2 shots a day

Other Management
- Metformin
  - Mechanism of action: Suppresses hepatic glucose production
  - Side effects: Most common include GI disturbances (usually resolve in 1–2 wk), rarely can cause lactic acidosis if renal function is poor
- Other oral diabetes medications not routinely used in pediatric patients

DIABETIC KETOACIDOSIS (DKA)

Pathophysiology
- Triggered by inadequate insulin/increased insulin need (stress from infection, steroids, etc.)
- ↓ insulin → glycogenolysis + gluconeogenesis + lipolysis
- ↑ glucose → polyuria → dehydration
- ↑ lipolysis leads to creation of ketone bodies, if ↑↑ → ↓pH → electrolyte abnormalities
- Most commonly in type 1 diabetes, can also occur in type 2 diabetes

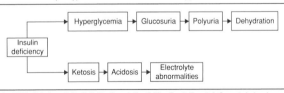

New M, Yau M, Lekarev O, Lin-Su K, Alan Parsa A, Pina C, Yuen T, and Khattab A. Congenital adrenal hyperplasia. In: De Groot LJ, Chrousos G, Dungan K, et al., eds. Endotext [Internet]. South Dartmouth (MA): MDText.com, Inc.; 2000–2019.

Diagnosis
- Glucose >200 mg/dL
- Moderate–large ketones in urine, betahydroxybutyrate in blood
- pH<7.3 or bicarbonate <15 mmol/L
  - Will have elevated anion gap: $[Na^+] - ([Cl^-] + [HCO_3^-])$; nl 6–12 mEq/L

Clinical Manifestations
- Dehydration: Dry mucous membranes, tachycardia
- Ketone breath
- Polyuria, polydipsia, polyphagia
- Abdominal pain & vomiting
- Abnormal respirations (Kussmaul breathing, respiratory compensation for metabolic acidosis)
- Altered mental status, lethargy

Electrolyte Abnormalities
- Hypernatremia secondary to dehydration
  - Often ↓ at presentation as pseudohyponatremia secondary to hyperosmolarity
  - Corrected sodium: Na = Serum sodium + 0.016 × (serum glucose − 100)
- Hypokalemia & hypophosphatemia
  - Whole-body stores are depleted due to osmotic diuresis and vomiting
  - Serum labs show normal–high levels -> K+ and PO_4- efflux out of cells w/ acidosis and insulin deficiency

Management
Principles: Treat dehydration, insulin deficiency, electrolyte abnormalities
- Fluids first! (think ABC's circulation)
  - 1st start w/ a NS bolus 10 mg/kg (DO NOT USE HYPOTONIC FLUIDS – cerebral edema risk)
  - 2nd continuous IV fluids at 1.5–2× maintenance (to rehydrate and avoid dehydration)
  - Use 2-bag system of fluids: one w/ D10 and one w/o dextrose
    - ↑ dextrose-containing fluids once blood glucose <300 and ↓ nondextrose fluids
    - Keep total rate 1.5–2× maintenance
- Get ECG and put on cardiac monitor – Watch for abnormal T-waves w/ abnormal K+ values
  - Monitor potassium q4h and replace if normal and dropping or if ↓
- Insulin infusion – Regular insulin (0.1 u/kg/hr) – start 1 hr after initial NS bolus
  - Goal to ↓ glucose by 50–100 mg/dL/hr
  - Frequent glucose (~q1h), potassium, sodium, and anion gap monitoring (~q4h)
- Transition to SQ insulin when ketoacidosis resolves
  - Give bolus insulin at least 20 min before turning off insulin drip and give long-acting insulin
  - Can start long-acting insulin ~2 hr before stopping drip if no bolus planned

Complications
- Cerebral edema
  - Signs/Sx: Headache, incontinence, altered mental status, emesis, hypertension, bradycardia, irregular respirations
  - Risk factors Include: age <3 yo, severe acidosis (pH <7.1, bicarb <5), severe dehydration (elevated BUN), severe hyperosmolarity (corrected Na >155, glucose >1,000), longer duration of sx, new-onset diabetes
  - Management: Mannitol 0.5–1 g/kg intravenously over 20 min or hypertonic saline (3% NS) 5–10 mL/kg over 30 min
- Respiratory compromise – Rare respiratory failure
- Electrolyte abnormalities:
  - Cardiac dysrhythmias
  - Rapid correction has risk for CNS fluid shifts

HYPOGLYCEMIA

Clinical Definition
- In adults and older children, dx of hypoglycemia made when blood glucose level low enough to cause sx of Whipple triad (sx or signs of hypoglycemia, confirmation of ↓ blood glucose, and resolution of sx w/ restoring of normal blood glucose level)
- Neonates and young children that cannot express sx can have hypoglycemia signs including lethargy, irritability, poor feeding, seizures, hypotonia, sweating, hypothermia, and respiratory distress
- Levels: Brain glucose utilization limited at <55–65 mg/dL, cognitive function impaired at <50 mg/dL; goal to keep BG >70 premeal

Protections Against Hypoglycemia
- Suppression of insulin secretion when blood glucose falls below 85 mg/dL
- Glucagon secretion and ↑ epinephrine release begins when blood glucose is 65–70 mg/dL -> causes glucose release from liver glycogen and subsequently gluconeogenesis
- W/ longer fasting and insulin suppression, ketogenesis occurs (betahydroxybutyrate [BOHB] is the predominant ketoacid and one that is measured in plasma tests; other is acetoacetate)
- In neonates, blood glucose concentrations ↓ more rapidly and ketogenesis occurs sooner due to ↑ energy needs for their relatively larger brains

DDX

- Hypoglycemia can be transient and normal in first 2–3 d of life
  - Risk factors: Prematurity, perinatal stress, maternal diabetes, sepsis, SGA, LGA, polycythemia
  - Recommend waiting to evaluate for other cause of hypoglycemia until >48 hr of life
- Includes: Congenital hyperinsulinism (HI), genetic syndromes (Beckwith–Wiedemann, Turner, Kabuki), hormone deficiencies (adrenal insufficiency, GH deficiency, panhypo-pituitarism), glycogen storage diseases, fatty acid oxidation disorders (defects in fatty acid oxidation and ketone production), liver failure
- HI: Dysregulated insulin secretion, can be congenital, toxic ingestion (sulfonylurea), or stress-induced (assoc w/ perinatal stress)
- Insulinoma: Insulin-producing tumors

Workup of Persistent Hypoglycemia

- Lab tests should be obtained after fasting to provoke blood glucose level <50 mg/dL
  - Labs: BOHB, free fatty acids, insulin, C-peptide, lactate, ammonia, free and total car-nitine and acyl-carnitine profile (to assess for fatty acid oxidation disorder AKA difficulty producing ketones), cortisol, GH
  - Can also stop fast earlier if BOHB >2.5 mmol/L or signs or sx of distress
- To evaluate for HI, a glucagon stimulation test should be performed at end of fast (administer 1-mg glucagon IV/SQ/IM and follow up BG measurements every 10 min for 30 min)
  - A rise of blood glucose >30 mg/dL is diagnostic of HI

Treatments

- Acute hypoglycemia:
  - 2-mL/kg D10W IV
  - Glucagon: 1-mg IV/IM
  - Dextrose infusion, goal to keep glucose infusion rate (GIR) to maintain blood glucose >70 mg/dL
    - GIR = (%dextrose × rate in mL/hr)/(6 × weight in kg)
- Chronic:
  - Dextrose infusion IV or enteral
  - Medications for congenital HI: Diazoxide, continuous glucagon infusion, octreotide (deferred until after infancy due to risk of necrotizing enterocolitis in infancy)

LIPID DISORDERS

Lipid Disorders

- Screening (total cholesterol, LDL, HDL, non-HDL, TG) recommended by NIHANES and AAP once age 9–11 (before puberty) and again 17–21 to identify familial hyper-lipidemia; USPSTF does not recommend citing insufficient data
  - Familial hyperlipidemia – Elevated LDL-C from birth usually due to LDL-receptor gene mutation
    - Sequelae: Xanthomata, early onset CAD
- If lipid levels elevated → Lifestyle counseling and evaluation for secondary causes (includ-ing DM, PCOS, renal disease, alcohol, liver disease, metabolic storage disease, medication)
- Consider referral to lipid specialist if sustained elevation of lipid levels for longer than 6 mo of lifestyle modifications or if LDL level >170

MAINTENANCE FLUIDS

Maintenance Fluids and Calculation (Pediatr Rev 20011;22:380)
- Basal state maintenance fluid needs determined by basal metabolic rate and amount of fluid needed to dissipate heat via respiratory tract and skin
- Holliday–Segar formula equates kcal with mL (1:1) of fluid needed for dissipation

Weight (kg)	kcal/hr or cc/hr (1:1)
0–10 kg	4 cc/kg/hr
11–20 kg	40 cc + 2 cc/kg/hr (for each kg >10 kg)
>20 kg	60 cc + 1 cc/kg/hr (for each kg >20 kg) or wt + 40 cc/hr

(Pediatrics 1957;19:823)

Composition of IV Solutions

Fluid	[Na⁺]	[Cl⁻]	[K⁺]	[Ca²⁺]	[Lactate⁻]
NS (0.9% NaCl)	154	154	–	–	–
½ NS (0.45% NaCl)	77	77	–	–	–
¼ NS (0.2% NaCl)	34	34	–	–	–
Lactated ringers	130	109	4	3	28

(Nelson Textbook of Pediatrics. 20th ed. 2016:384)

- Expect increased losses in fevers (10% for every 1° >37)
- Hospitalized children often in a stressed state leading to excess ADH secretion, stimulating water retention (Nat Clin Pract Nephrol 2007;3:376)
- Some experts have suggested **isotonic fluid (NS)** to decrease risk of hyponatremia. Pts with infection, pulm or CNS disease, and postop have ↑ risk due to ↑ ADH (Pediatrics 2014;133:105)
- D5 provides 17 calories/100 mL and nearly 20% of daily caloric needs. Prevents ketone production and helps minimize protein catabolism (Nelson Textbook of Pediatrics. 20th ed. 2016:384)

HYPOVOLEMIA

- Definition = ↓ in intravascular volume due to: (1) insufficient fluid intake; (2) increased insensible losses (e.g., sweating with exercise, fever); (3) fluid losses from vomiting, diarrhea, excessive urination; (4) fluid shifts

Common Etiologies (Nelson Textbook of Pediatrics. 20th ed. 2016:388)

Vomiting	Pyloric stenosis, SBO or ileus, intussusception, appendicitis, pancreatitis, cholecystitis, pyelonephritis
Poor oral intake	Pharyngitis, stomatitis, peritonsillar abscess
Excessive fluid loss from skin	Burns, Stevens–Johnson, TEN
Excessive urinary losses	Diabetes insipidus, DKA (can have concomitant vomiting)
Third spacing	Nephrotic syndromes, burns, pancreatitis, sepsis, etc.
Hemorrhage	GI bleeds, trauma

Clinical Assessment (Pediatr Rev 2001;36:277)

Clinical Signs	Degree of Dehydration	EWL (mL/kg) for Infants	EWL (mL/kg) for Adolescents
• Tacky mucous membranes • ↓ UOP • Normal cap refill + VS	Mild	5% (50)	3% (30)
• Irritable, UOP <1 mL/kg/hr • Sunken fontanelle, dry membranes • ↑ HR, ↓ or normal BP, deep respirations	Moderate	10% (100)	5–6% (50–60)
• Lethargic, ↓ BP, ↓ / ↑ HR • Oliguric/anuric • Poor perfusion • Deep respirations	Severe	15% (150)	7–9% (70–90)

EWL, estimated weight loss

- Serum [Na] affects clinical manifestations of dehydration such as skin turgor and mucous membranes. The % dehydration is often underestimated by exam in hypernatremia

Deficit Repletion
- Water deficit (L) = preillness wt (kg) − illness wt (kg)
- % dehydration = (preillness wt − illness wt)/preillness wt × 100%

Diagnostic Studies (Pediatr Rev 2001;36:277)
- Electrolytes and acid/base balance typically normal in mild dehydration
- Check serum bicarb, BUN, electrolytes, urine Na (<20 mEq/L if appropriate renal response), urine osmolality and specific gravity (should be elevated), FE_{Na} (<1% if prerenal acute kidney injury)

Management
- **Mild/mod. dehydration:** Trial oral rehydration, 50 mL/kg over 2–4 hr
- **Mod./severe dehydration:** Consider 20 mL/kg bolus × 1 to stop ketone production, than replete remaining deficit + maintenance via IV over 24–48 hr until tolerating PO
- **Clinically unstable** (hypotensive, tachycardic, etc.): Repeat 20 mL/kg NS boluses until resolved; consider pressors for shock if 60 mL/kg given without improvement

HYPONATREMIA

(Pediatr Rev 2013;34:417)

- Defined as Na <135

Clinical Manifestations
- **Nonspecific:** Nausea, headache, lethargy, ataxia, disorientation, seizure, coma (due to cerebral edema)
- Sx more likely if [Na] Δ is rapid (vs. abs level of [Na]). Usually don't see until [Na] <125

Workup
- (1) Acute vs. chronic (>48 hr); (2) neuro status; (3) check BMP, plasma Osm, Uosm, UNa, can check lipids and protein (r/o pseudohypoNa)

Fluid Status
- **Hypovolemic:** Net loss of Na in excess of the net loss of free water
- Intravascular volume depletion: stimulates ADH synthesis → renal water retention
- **Euvolemic:** Gain of free water
- **Hypervolemic:** Greater gain of free water relative to sodium with overall positive balance of both
  - Often a decrease in *effective* blood volume due to third space fluid loss, vasodilation, or poor cardiac output → **ADH** and **aldosterone** production
  - **See algorithm for hyponatremia on next page**

Basic Treatment
- **Hypovolemic:** Isotonic fluid replacement
- **Euvolemic:** Fluid restriction
- **Hypervolemic:** Fluid + Na restriction
  - *Loop diuretics* to increase water excretion for more rapid response
  - *Vasopressin antagonists* block action of ADH causing a water diuresis, helpful in pts with heart failure or cirrhosis (*Nelson Textbook of Pediatrics.* 20th ed. 2016:346–384)
- **Rate of Na correction** in chronic hypoNa should not exceed 12 mEq/L/24 hr to avoid osmotic demyelination

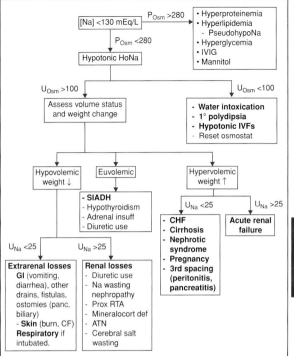

HYPERNATREMIA

(Pediatr Rev 2009;30:412)

- Defined as Na >145
- Deficiency of total body water relative to total body solute. Caused by: (1) water losses, including GI, insensible, or renal; (2) inadequate H_2O intake (i.e., due to impaired thirst or lack of access to H_2O); and (3) excessive Na intake, either oral or parenteral, or mineralocorticoid excess
- Hypertonicity causes water to shift out of cells, leading to contracted intracellular fluid volume

Clinical Manifestations

- **Nonspecific:** Irritability, hyperpnea, muscle weakness, high-pitched cry (infants), insomnia, lethargy, coma (NEJM 2000;342:1493)
- Exam: Increased tone in extremities with brisk reflexes, "doughy" skin turgor, decreased cap refill, nuchal rigidity, myoclonus, asterixis, chorea, seizures (Pediatr Rev 2009;30:412)

Workup

- Determine acute vs. chronic (>48 hr), volume status (vital signs, orthostatics, skin turgor)
- Electrolytes, serum osmolality, urine osmolality (function of ADH secretion), urine sodium

Causes

Extrarenal H_2O loss: Urine$_{Osm}$ >800
- **GI H_2O loss:** Diarrhea (most common) vomiting, NGT drainage, fistula
- **Insensible loss:** Fever, exercise, ventilation, burns

Renal H₂O loss (Best Pract Res Clin Endocrin & Metab 2016;30:189)
- **Diuresis:** Osmotic (glucose, mannitol, urea), loop diuretics
- **Diabetes insipidus:** U_{Osm} <300 mOsm/kg/H₂O ← ADH deficiency (central) or resistance (nephrogenic)
  - **Central:** TBI, space-occupying lesions, infections. Responds to DDAVP
  - **Nephrogenic:** Renal dysfunction, hypercalcemia, severe hypokalemia, **drugs** (lithium, amphotericin, foscarnet, demeclocycline), hereditary (V2 vasopressin receptor or aquaporin-2 gene mutation). DDAVP will not affect urine osmolality

Other: Urine_{Osm} >800
- **Na overload:** Hypertonic saline, sodium bicarb infusion, poorly breastfeeding infants or improperly mixed formula, mineralocorticoid excess

Treatment
- **Restore access to H₂O**
- **Replace free H₂O deficit** (and volume deficit if appropriate). Isotonic bolus(es) indicated in initial resuscitative treatment phase to restore euvolemia
  Free H₂O deficit (mL) = 4 mL × actual body wt (kg) × desired change in serum Na mEq/L
- **Provide maintenance fluids to match ongoing losses**
- **Rate of Na reduction** should not exceed 1 mEq/L/hr and 10–12 mEq/L/24 hr to avoid cerebral edema. Replace deficit over 48-hr period
- **Monitor** serum Na q2–4h in the first 24–48 hr

HYPERKALEMIA

- Defined as K >5.5 in children and >6 in newborns

Etiology (BMJ 2009;339:1019)
- **Extracellular shift:** Acidemia, rhabdo, severe burns, TLS, insulin def., drugs, hyperkalemic periodic paralysis
- **Excessive ingestion** (rare if renal excretion of K normal): Blood transfusions, TPN, or fluids w/ high K
- **Decreased renal excretion:** Renal failure or CKD (most common), adrenal insufficiency, drugs (ACEIs, ARBs, NSAIDs, antifungals, K-sparing diuretics, trimethoprim, pentamidine) sickle cell dx, severe volume contraction (need distal tubule Na delivery to secrete K), genetic disorders, RTA IV, aldosterone deficiency, or resistance

Clinical Manifestations (usually when >7)
- **Sx:** Palpitations, lethargy, weakness, confusion
- **Signs:** Bradycardia, hypotonicity, paralysis

Workup
- Rule out pseudohyperkalemia (hemolyzed sample, WBC >100,000, severe thrombocytosis) with repeat blood draw with heparinized sample
- **Labs:** Initially repeat BMP, Ca, Mag, BG, assess urine output. ABG (if suspecting acidosis). Can consider electrolytes and pH (to r/o RTA), CK (rhabdo), AM cortisol (adrenal insufficiency)
  - **ECG changes** (poor Se): Starts with peaked T-waves → ↑ PR, ↓ P-waves → ↑ QRS, AV blocks/BBBs → VFib/PEA (Arch Dis Child 2012;97:376)
  - Cardiac toxicity enhanced by hypocalcemia, hyponatremia, metabolic acidosis

Management (Arch Dis Child 2012;97:376; Cochrane Database 2005;2:CD003235)
- If **ECG changes** → **stabilize myocardium** → 0.5 mL/kg of calcium gluconate 10% over 5–10 min. Repeat in 5 min if ECG changes persist
- **Drive K intracellularly** (only transient)
  - **IV insulin:** 0.1 U/kg (max 10 U) with dextrose (5 mL/kg D10 <5 yo or D25 2 mL/kg for >5 yo) over 30 min (effect within 20 min, lasts ~4 hr)
  - **β2 agonists:** Albuterol nebs (neonates: 0.4 mg; children <25 kg: 2.5 mg; children 25–50 kg: 5 mg; children >50 kg: 10–20 mg) (effect within 5 min, lasts 1–4 hr)
  - **Na bicarbonate** (if acidotic): 1 mEq/kg (max 50 mEq) over 10–15 min. Effectiveness controversial
- **Excrete K** (↓ total body K)
  - **Loop diuretics:** Furosemide 1 mg/kg IV (↑ urinary excretion)
  - **Cation exchange resins (Kayexalate):** Binds K in gut. Dose 1 g/kg (max 30 g). Risk of electrolyte abnormalities, esp in neonates, and bowel necrosis (don't use if bowel obstructed)
  - **Dialysis:** Use when conservative methods fail or severely hyperK (consider if >7)

- **Discontinue offending drugs** (e.g., ACE inhibitors, K-sparing diuretics, NSAIDs)
- **Low potassium diet:** Avoid many fresh and dried fruits, nuts, seeds, salt substitutes, potatoes

HYPOCALCEMIA

(Pediatr Rev 2009;30:190)

- Defined as Ca <8.4 or iCa^{2+} <4.15

Etiologies of Acute Hypocalcemia by Age	
Early-onset neonate (<5 d)	Stress 2/2 asphyxia, sepsis; IDMs
Late onset neonate (>5 d)	Parathyroid gland immaturity, genetics (absence of parathyroid gland, CaSR mutations, abnl response to PTH)
Infants & children	Sepsis, cardiac surgery, rhabdo, pancreatitis, hepatitis, TLS

Etiologies of Hypocalcemia		
Category	Labs	Etiologies
Hypoparathyroidism	↓PTH	HypoMg, surgery, autoimmune, infiltrative, genetic (e.g., DiGeorge)
Pseudohypoparathyroidism	↑PTH	HypoMg, Albright hereditary osteodystrophy
Vit D def. or resistance	↓PO_4, ↑ALP, ↑PTH	Nutritional/sunlight def (e.g., breastfed infants), fat malabs, liver disease, CKD, genetic
Renal failure	↓1,25-$(OH)_2$D ↑PO_4, ↑PTH	Congenital, glomerular disease (e.g., FSGS), HUS, genetic (e.g., Alports)
Chelation	Variable	Pancreatitis, early rhabdo, TLS, citrate excess (after blood transfusions)

(BMJ 2014;346:f2213; Seldin and Giebisch's The Kidney. 5th ed. 2013:2273)

Clinical Manifestations (Pediatr Rev 2009;30:190)
- Paresthesias, muscle cramps and tetany, ⊕ Chvostek (tap facial nerve → contraction of ipsilateral corner of mouth), ⊕ Trousseau (inflation of BP cuff → carpal spasm), seizures
- Neonates: Apnea, tachycardia, lethargy, poor feeding, vomiting, abd distension
- Chronic: Neuropsychiatric symptoms, cataracts, ↑ ICP
- Rickets: Genu varum or valgum, "rachitic rosary," frontal bossing
- ECG: ↑ QT (torsades), ↓ QRS, flattened T-waves

Workup
- Labs – Ca, albumin, iCa, phos, creat, ALP, PTH, LFTs, vit D metabolites, Mg, UCa
- ECG

Treatment (BMJ 2008:336:1298)
- Symptomatic → 10% Ca gluconate 2 mL/kg or 10% CaCl 0.7 mL/kg
- Asymptomatic: Oral Ca; ergocalciferol (vit D2) or cholecalciferol (vit D3) if vit D def
- PTH deficient or nonfunctional: Calcitriol (active vit D metabolite), consider thiazide. Goal low-nl Ca to avoid hypercalciuria and nephrocalcinosis
- Correct hypomagnesemia (<1.0 mg/dL) if present

HYPERCALCEMIA

(Goldman-Cecil Med e3 2016:1649)

- Defined as Ca >10.5 or iCa >5.25
- Causes – (1) ↑ bone resorption, (2) ↑GI absorption, and/or (3) ↓renal excretion

Category	Etiologies
Parathyroid mediated	1° (adenoma, hyperplasia, carcinoma): Nonfamilial or familial (e.g., MEN syndromes)
	3° (hyperplasia or adenoma in CKD)
Malignancy	PTHrP, excess 1,25$(OH)_2$D production (lymphoma), local osteolysis, cytokines

Vit-D related	Granulomas (sarcoid, TB, histo, IBD), infantile hypercalcemia, vit D intox, Williams syndrome
Endocrine disorders	Thyrotoxicosis, adrenal insufficiency, pheochromocytoma
Drugs	Thiazide, lithium, milk-alkali (Ca & antacids), vit A, TPN
Miscellaneous	Immobilization, fractures

(BMJ 2015;350:h2723; *Goldman-Cecil Medicine*. 3rd ed. 2016:1649)

Clinical Manifestations (BMJ 2015;350:h2723)
- **Renal:** Stones (nephrolithiasis), polyuria, polydipsia
- **MSK:** Bone pain, osteomalacia, fractures, proximal muscle weakness
- **Neuro:** Fatigue, poor concentration, depression
- **GI:** Anorexia, N/V, constipation, abd pain, pancreatitis
- **Cardiac:** Bradycardia, HTN
  - ECG: $\downarrow$ QT, $\uparrow$ PR, $\uparrow$ QRS, BBB, bradycardia, arrhythmias, tall T-waves

Workup
- Labs: Ca, alb, iCa, PO_4, BUN and Creat, ALP, LFTs, PTH, vit D
  - Initial – Repeat Ca, iCa, albumin, phos, Cr/BUN, ALP, PTH, vit D (1,25), Mg
  - Consider – TSH, PTHrP, 24-hr urine Ca, Mg
- ECG; consider renal US and KUB if concern for nephrolithiasis

Treatment (*Goldman-Cecil Medicine*. 3rd ed. 2016:1649)
- Asymptomatic $\rightarrow$ IVF, mobilization, treat underlying etiology
- Severe and/or symptomatic $\rightarrow$ aggressive IVF $\pm$ furosemide (no clear evidence to effectiveness)

Additional Treatment Options for Severe HyperCa		
Treatment	**Onset**	**Comments**
Calcitonin	Within 12 hr	Inhibits osteoclast bone resorption, lowers renal Ca reabsorption. Tachyphylaxis within 24–48 hr
IV bisphosphonates	2–4 d	Inhibit osteoclasts. Risk of renal toxicity
RANKL inhibitor	2–4 d	Denosumab (mAb). Inhibits osteoclasts
Glucocorticoids	2–5 d	Useful in some malignancies, granulomatous disorders
Hemodialysis	Immediate	For comatose pts with ECG Δs, severe renal failure, or cannot receive aggressive IVF

(*Seldin and Giebisch's The Kidney*. 5th ed. 2015:2273)

MAGNESIUM DISTURBANCES

- Dependent on dietary intake, intestinal absorption, and urinary elimination

Hypomagnesemia (<1.7 mg/dL) (*Henry's Clin Diag and Manag by Lab Methods*. 2nd ed. 2017:188)
- **Causes:** Decreased intake/absorption (refeeding, malabsorption, neonatal gut immaturity), renal losses (diuretics, ATN, RTA, Bartter and Gitelman syndromes), misc. (acute pancreatitis, hyperthyroidism, DKA, hyperaldosteronism, cisplatin, cyclosporine, gentamicin, tacrolimus, amphotericin B, chronic PPI)
- **Clinical manifestations:** Sxs when Mg <1 mEq/L. Largely due to associated hypocalcemia (tetany, hyperreflexia, tremors, seizures, muscle weakness, depression, delirium, cardiac arrhythmias)
- **Workup:** BMP, phos, vit D, FE Mg; consider ECG
- **Treatment** (*Williams Textbook of Endocrinology*. 13th ed. 2016:12553)
  - **Mild, asymptomatic:** Oral Mg 20–80 mEq/d in divided doses. MgCl and MgLactate better absorbed than MgOx (can cause diarrhea)
  - **Severe:** Slow infusion of IV Mg sulfate 25–50 mg/kg (max 2 g). Serial Mg levels in pts with compromised renal function
  - Treat concurrent electrolyte abnormalities (Ca, K, PO_4), vit D

Hypermagnesemia (≥2.5 mg/dL) (*Brenner & Rector's The Kidney*. 10th ed. 2016:601)
- **Causes:** Renal insufficiency, excessive intake (Mg-containing antacids & cathartics, Epsom salts, administration for pre-eclampsia), $\uparrow$absorption (IBD, obstruction, GI perforation)

- **Clinical manifestations**
  - Mg >4–6 mg/dL → **Hypotension**, N/V, facial flushing, urinary retention, ileus
  - Mg >8–10 mg/dL → Flaccid paralysis, hyporeflexia, bradycardia & arrhythmias, respiratory depression, coma, cardiac arrest (*Williams Textbook of Endocrinology*. 13th ed. 2016:1253)
- **Workup:** BMP, Mg, review med list (lithium, antacids, laxatives), ECG (↑ QRS)
- **Treatment:**
  - **Mild, asymptomatic:** No treatment needed if renal function intact
  - **Severe:** IV hydration + furosemide; dialysis in renal failure or refractory cases

PHOSPHORUS DISTURBANCES

(Brenner & Rector's The Kidney. 10th ed. 2016:2365)

- Normal values between 3–5 mg/dL; higher range (4–6 mg/dL) in neonatal period and infancy

Hypophosphatemia (<1.5 mg/dL; <4 mg/dL in 1st 6 mo)
- **Causes**
  - **Decreased intake:** Chronic diarrhea, premature infant–fed human milk or term formula, chronic Al or Ca based antacid use
  - **Increased loss:** 1° and 2° hyperparathyroidism, hypoMag, X-linked and AD hypophosphatemia, McCune–Albright, malabsorption, vit D def or resistance, burns, Fanconi syndrome
  - **Internal redistribution:** DKA, **refeeding**, hungry bone, resp alkalosis, sepsis
  - **Miscellaneous:** Hyperaldosteronism, high-dose steroids, estrogens, drugs (ifosfamide, bisphosphonate, cisplatin, diuretics)
- **Clinical manifestations** (*Seldin & Giebisch's The Kidney*. 5th ed. 2013:2369): Heme dysfunction (thrombocytopenia, hemolysis, impaired phagocytosis, prox muscle weakness, rhabdo, CNS Δs (tremor, paresthesias, confusion, seizures), resp depression, rickets
- **Workup:** BMP, Ca, Alb, Mag, PTH, FE phosphate (nl 5–15%), vit D
- Treatment
  - **Moderate/Chronic:** Risk of progression to severe during refeeding
    - Low-fat milk, fleet enema or neutra-Phos (1–3 g/d divided qid), calcitriol (30–70 mg/kg/d)
  - **Severe:** 0.08–0.24 mmol/kg IV over 6 hr (contraindicated in renal failure, hypoCa, HyperCa)

Hyperphosphatemia (>5 in children >2 yr; >7 in neonates)
- **Causes:**
  - **Impaired renal excretion:** Renal insufficiency, pseudo-/hypoparathyroidism, transient PTH resistance of infancy, familial tumoral calcinosis, acromegaly, hyperthyroidism, juvenile hypogonadism, heparin
  - **↑ intake:** Exogenous (laxatives & enemas, vit-D intox, blood transfusion, liposomal ampho B, fosphenytoin); Redistribution (crush injury, rhabdo, tumor lysis, hemolysis, malignant hyperthermia, lactic acidosis)
  - **Internal redistribution:** DKA, metabolic or respiratory acidosis
  - **Miscellaneous:** Hyperostosis; spurious (hemolyzed blood sample, TPA)
- **Clinical manifestations:** Symptoms of hypocalcemia (paresthesias, tetany, seizures, etc.). Can lead to CaPhos deposition in tissues
- **Workup:** Ca, alb, PTH, K, creat, vit D
- **Treatment:** ↑ fluids to promote diuresis, phosphate restriction ± phosphate binders
- Hemodialysis in severe cases/renal failure

ACID/BASE DISORDERS

(Pediatr Rev 2004;25:350)

- Acid–base regulation involves: (1) buffering by extra- and intracellular buffers, (2) controlling the partial pressure of CO_2 via RR, (3) controlling plasma HCO_3 via renal excretion
- **Acidemia:** pH < 7.35; **acidosis:** process in which the $[H^+]$ is increased
- **Alkalemia:** pH >7.45; **alkalosis:** process in which the $[H^+]$ is decreased

Workup
- Determine primary disorder: Check pH, $PaCO_2$, HCO_3
- **ABG** (gold standard) vs. **VBG** (slight increase in PCO_2 and decrease in pH, unreliable P_{O2} – ideally central venous blood) vs. **CBG** (PCO_2 and pH between arterial and venous values) (Pediatr Rev 2016;37:361)

Primary Disorders				
Primary Disorder	**Problem**	**pH**	**HCO$_3$**	**PaCO$_2$**
Met acidosis	Gain of H^+ or loss of HCO_3	↓	↓°	↓$_c$
Met alkalosis	Gain of HCO_3 or loss of H^+	↑	↑°	↑$_c$
Resp acidosis	Hypoventilation	↓	↑$_c$	↑°
Resp alkalosis	Hyperventilation	↑	↓$_c$	↓°

°, primary disorder; c, compensatory mechanism

- Determine if degree of compensation is appropriate

Compensation for Acid/Base Disorders		
Primary Disorder	**Expected Compensation**	**Time Frame**
Met acidosis*	$PaCO_2 = 1.5 \times [HCO_3] + 8 \pm 2$ mmHg or $PaCO_2 =$ $[HCO_3] + 15$ or $PaCO_2$ –2nd two digits of pH	12–24 hr
Met alkalosis	$PaCO_2 = 0.7 \times ([HCO_3] - 24) + 40 \pm 2$ mmHg	24–36 hr
Acute resp acidosis	↑ $[HCO_3]$ by 1 for each ↑ in $PaCO_2$ of 10 mmHg above 40 mmHg	Hr
Chronic resp acidosis	↑ $[HCO_3]$ by 4–5 for each ↑ in $PaCO_2$ of 10 mmHg above 40 mmHg	2–5 d
Acute resp alkalosis	↓$[HCO_3]$ by 2 for each ↓ in $PaCO_2$ of 10 mmHg below 40 mmHg	Hr
Chronic resp alkalosis	↓$[HCO_3]$ by 4–5 for each ↓ in $PaCO_2$ of 10 mmHg below 40 mmHg	2–5 d

*$PaCO_2$ cannot fall <8–12 no matter how severe the acidosis (NEJM 2014;371:1434)

Mixed Disorders (Nelson Textbook of Pediatrics. 20th ed. 2016:346)
- Presence of more than 1 primary acid–base disturbance. Identified if child does not have appropriate compensation
- **pH can be normal** in chronic respiratory processes

METABOLIC ACIDOSIS
(Pediatr Rev 2004;25:350; Pediatr Rev 2011;32:240)

- Divided into anion gap (AGMA) and nonanion gap metabolic acidosis (NAGMA)
  - Formula: $AG = [Na^+] - ([Cl^-] + [HCO_3^-])$; Nl $\sim 16 \pm 4$ mEq/L though ref range varies by lab
  - Correct for hypoalbuminemia if present: Adjusted AG = Obs AG + (2.5 × [nl alb – obs alb])
- **AGMA:** ↑organic acid production or ingestion, inborn errors of metabolism, ↓renal acid excretion from renal failure
- **NAGMA:** Loss of HCO_3 from the GI or urinary tracts or inability of kidney to secrete H+

Clinical Manifestations (Pediatr Rev 2004;25:350)

Adverse Effects of Severe Acidemia (Serum pH <7.2)	
System	**Effects**
CV	↓Contractility, vasodilation, ↑PVR, ↑risk of arrhythmias/Vfib
Resp	Hyperventilation, ↓resp muscle strength, dyspnea
Metabolic	FTT, ↑Met demands, insulin resistance, ↓ATP, hyperK
Cerebral	Inhibition of metabolism, obtundation & coma

Initial Workup
- BMP, Glu, UA, consider VBG (assess acidosis)

Etiologies (NEJM 2014;371:1434; Pediatr Rev 2011;32:241)
Inborn errors of metabolism can present as AGMA (ketones, lactate, other) or NAGMA

Etiologies of AG Metabolic Acidosis

Acid overproduction	Ketoacidosis	DKA, alcoholism, starvation
	L-lactic acidosis	**Type A:** Hypoxic (septic or hypovolemic shock, mesenteric ischemia, hypoxemia, carbon monoxide, cyanide) **Type B:** Nonhypoxic (seizure, meds [e.g., NRTIs, metformin, propofol, intox with salicylates])
	D-lactic acidosis	Short bowel syndrome
Underexcretion	Advanced renal failure: Accumulation of organic anions such as phosphates, sulfates, urate, etc.	
Cell lysis	Massive rhabdo	
Ingestions	Methanol, ethylene glycol, salicylates, paraldehyde	

Etiologies of Non-AG Metabolic Acidosis

Loss of Bicarb	GI	Diarrhea (most common), biliary or pancreatic fistulas, bladder augment using sigmoid colon
	Renal	Type 2 (proximal) RTA, meds (ifosfamide, tenofovir, topiramate, carbonic anhydrase inhibitors)
↓ Renal acid excretion	Early uremic acidosis	
	Type 1 RTA	E.g., ampho, lithium, Sjögren
	Type 4 RTA	Hypoaldosteronism, pseudohypoaldosteronism
Other	Fluid resuscitation with saline, hyperalimentation	

Workup for Non-AG Metabolic Acidosis (Clin J Am Soc Nephrol 2012;7:671)
- **Urine anion gap** (UAG) = $(U_{Na} + U_K) - U_{Cl}$; surrogate measure for renal NH_4^+ excretion; can help differentiate between GI and renal HCO_3 losses
  - Pos UAG → Renal NH_4^+ excretion impaired (Ddx: renal failure, distal RTA, hypoaldo)
  - Neg UAG → Distal NH_4^+ excretion intact (Ddx: diarrhea)
  - UAG unreliable when NH_4^+ excreted with anion other than Cl^- (e.g., β-hydroxybutyrate or acetoacetate), impaired distal Na+ delivery ($U_{Na} <25$ mEq/L). Can't be used in neonates
- **Urine osmolal gap** = measured Uosm − calculated U_{Osm}; measure to assess changes in NH_4^+ concentration irrespective of accompanying anion
  - Calculated $U_{Osm} = 2(Na+K) + urea/2.8 + glu/18$
  - UOG <150 suggests impaired NH_4^+ excretion; >400 suggests intact renal compensation
  - Unreliable in infection with urease+ organism or if ethanol, methanol, or mannitol in urine

Treatment
- Treat underlying disorder
- **If severe (pH <7.2)**
  - Use of IV bicarb therapy controversial. Consider slow infusion in non-AG acidosis to replenish excessive HCO_3^- losses
- **Oral base therapy** for chronic metabolic acidosis (e.g., citrate solutions)

METABOLIC ALKALOSIS

- Net loss of H+ or gain of HCO_3; arterial pH >7.44

Etiologies (Pediatr Rev 2004;25:350)
- Can divide between Cl-responsive and Cl-resistant
- Can only persist if renal HCO_3 excretion is impaired (hypovolemia, ↓effective blood volume, Cl depletion, hypoK, ↓GFR ± ↑aldo)
- With ↓ effective circulating volume, kidneys ↑Na, HCO_3, and Cl absorption → ↓Urine Cl

Etiologies of Metabolic Alkalosis		
Type	U_{Cl} (mEq/L)	Etiologies
Cl responsive	U_{cl} <10	GI (vomiting, NG suction, Cl-wasting diarrhea, laxative abuse); diuretics; posthypercapnia; penicillin; CF
Cl unresponsive	U_{cl} >25	Adrenal disorders (hyperaldosteronism, Cushing); exogenous steroid; alkali ingestion; refeeding alkalosis; Bartter; Gitelman, Liddle, AME

Clinical Manifestations (Pediatr Rev 2004;25:350; Emerg Med Clin North Am 2014;32:453)

Adverse Effects of Severe Alkalemia (pH ≥7.55, HCO_3 >40 mEq/L)	
System	Effects
CV	Arteriolar vasoconstriction, ↓coronary blood flow, ↑risk of arrhythmias
Resp	Hypoventilation
Metabolic	↓K, iCa, Mg, PO_4
Cerebral	↓blood flow, tetany, seizures, delirium

- Sx, if present, often relate to underlying etiology (vol depletion) or hypoK, hypoCa

Workup
- Check **volume status** and U_{cl}, ± renin and aldosterone, cortisol

Treatment (Pediatr Rev 2011;32:241)
- Correct volume depletion, ↓K+, and ↓Cl− (in Cl− responsive cases)
- If volume overload precludes hydration, consider acetazolamide →↑ urinary HCO_3 excretion

RESPIRATORY ACIDOSIS AND ALKALOSIS

- Arterial PCO_2 outside of normal range (39–41 mmHg)

Etiologies of Acute Respiratory Acidosis (Pediatr Rev 2004;25:350)
- **Acute CNS depression:** Drugs (benzo, opiates, barbiturates, propofol); head trauma; CVA; CNS infection
- **Acute neuromuscular disease:** GBS, spinal cord injury, myasthenic crisis, botulism, organophosphate poisoning
- **Acute airway disease:** Status asthmaticus, upper airway obstruction, PNA, ARDS
- **Massive PE**
- **Acute pleural or chest wall disease:** Pneumothorax, hemothorax, flail chest

Etiologies of Respiratory Alkalosis (Pediatr Rev 2004;25:350)
- **Hypoxia**
- **Parenchymal lung disease:** PNA, asthma, diffuse interstitial fibrosis, PE, pulmonary edema
- **Medications:** Salicylate, xanthines (e.g., caffeine), nicotine, catecholamines, analeptics
- **Mechanical ventilation**
- **CNS disorders:** Meningitis, encephalitis, head trauma, space-occupying lesion, anxiety
- **Metabolic disorders:** Sepsis, pyrexia, hepatic disease
- **Hyperventilation syndrome**

Treatment (Pediatr Rev 2016;37:361)
- **Respiratory acidosis:** Enhance CO_2 elimination and treat underlying cause
- Short-term use of positive pressure or mechanical ventilation can improve CO_2 elimination (see 17-7 in PICU for overview of ventilation)
- **Respiratory alkalosis:** Treat underlying cause
  - Acute hyperventilation syndrome often responds to patient breathing into paper bag

ACUTE ABDOMINAL PAIN/VOMITING

(Ped Health 2017;8:83–91)

- Up to 10% of ED visits per year, up to 20% may require surgical evaluation or management
- Initial evaluation should be aimed at differentiating urgent vs. nonurgent etiologies
- Urgent etiologies (by age):
  - <1 yo: Incarcerated inguinal hernia (45%), intussusception (42%)
  - >1 yo: Acute appendicitis (64%), incarcerated hernia (7.5%), trauma (16%), intussusception (6.3%), intestinal obstruction (1.3%), ovarian torsion (1.3%)

Evaluation

- **Red flags:** Bilious emesis (think obstruction), prior history of abdominal surgery (obstruction, incarcerated hernia), pain before vomiting, pain intensifying and well localized, concerning physical exam findings (see below)
- **Physical exam:** Peritoneal signs (involuntary guarding, rebound tenderness, pain with jumping or bed shaking), skin changes (palpable purpura seen in HSP, bruising with pancreatitis), location of pain, general exam (lethargy or ill appearing)
- **Labs:** CMP, CBC, UPT if applicable, consider amylase/lipase, UA, consider ESR or CRP
- **Imaging:** Abd US to start, CT abd if concern for peritonitis, lateral decub or upright KUB if concerned about free air or if previous surgery

Differential by Location of Pain

- **Generalized abdominal pain:** NEC, mesenteric ischemia, perforation; however, often benign
- **RUQ pain:** Hepatitis, cholecystitis/cholelithiasis, referred (i.e., pneumonia, pleural effusion)
- **LUQ/epigastric pain:** Gastric (gastritis, GERD, PUD), pancreatic (radiating to back), splenic (radiating to L shoulder), referred (pulmonary source), ectopic pregnancy
- **RLQ pain:** Appendicitis, ileitis, colitis, mesenteric adenitis, hernia, ovarian (torsion, cyst), ectopic pregnancy, consider *yersinia*
- **Flank:** Acute renal colic, pyelonephritis
- **LLQ pain:** Colitis, constipation, hernia, ovarian pathology (see above)
- **Suprapubic:** Bladder (UTI, cystitis), uterus (pregnancy, PID)

Differential by Type of Emesis

- See diagram on next page

MANAGEMENT OF NAUSEA/VOMITING

(Peds in Review 2013;34[7]:307–321)

Pathophysiology of Nausea

- Main regulator = CNS emesis center @ formatio reticularis in medulla
- Inputs
  - Chemoreceptor trigger zone (area postrema) – influenced by triggers in the blood or CSF – mostly dopamine receptor mediated
  - Vagal afferent system – triggered by GI tract – serotonin mediated
  - Vestibular system – triggered by labyrinthine disorders (i.e., motion sickness) – muscarinic and histamine mediated
  - CNS: triggers not well understood

Antiemetics

- Serotonin receptor antagonists: Ondansetron, granisetron
  - Act @ solitary tract nucleus, vagal afferents, chemoreceptor trigger zone
  - ADRs: Headache, asthenia (lack of energy/weakness), constipation, dizziness
- Dopamine receptor antagonists: Phenothiazines (prochlorperazine, chlorpromazine), butyrophenones (haloperidol), benzamides (metoclopramide, domperidone)
  - Act @ D2 receptors in chemoreceptor trigger zone
  - ADRs: Extrapyramidal sxs (treat with diphenhydramine), drowsiness
- H1 receptor antagonists: Cyclizine, hydroxyzine, promethazine, diphenhydramine
- Muscarinic receptor antagonists: Scopolamine
  - Use: Prophylactic for motion sickness
- Neurokinin receptor antagonists: Aprepitant (PO), fosaprepitant (IV)
  - MOA: Acts on substance P via neurokinin receptors; useful in chemotherapy-related nausea

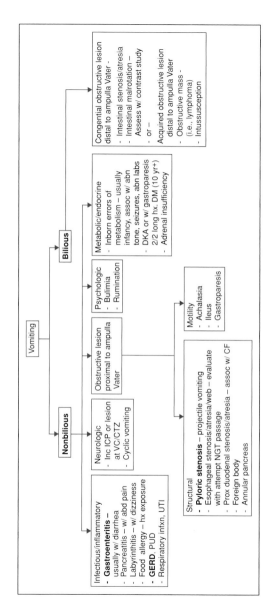

Vomiting

Nonbilious

Bilious

Infectious/inflammatory
- **Gastroenteritis** – usually w/ diarrhea
- Pancreatitis – w/ abd pain
- Labyrinthitis – w/ dizziness
- Food allergy – hx exposure
- **GERD**, PUD
- Respiratory infxn, UTI

Neurologic
- Inc ICP or lesion at VC/CTZ
- Cyclic vomiting

Obstructive lesion proximal to ampulla Vater

Psychologic
- Bulimia
- Rumination

Metabolic/endocrine
- Inborn errors of metabolism – usually infancy, assoc w/ abn tone, seizures, abn labs
- DKA or w/ gastroparesis 2/2 long hx. DM (10 yr+)
- Adrenal insufficiency

Congenital obstructive lesion distal to ampulla Vater
- Intestinal stenosis/atresia
- Intestinal malrotation – Assess w/ contrast study
- or –
Acquired obstructive lesion distal to ampulla Vater
- Obstructive mass (i.e., lymphoma)
- Intussusception

Structural
- **Pyloric stenosis** – projectile vomiting
- Esophageal stenosis/atresia/web – evaluate with attempt NGT passage
- Prox duodenal stenosis/atresia – assoc w/ CF
- Foreign body
- Annular pancreas

Motility
- Achalasia
- Ileus
- Gastroparesis

APPENDICITIS

See page *** in Emergency Department and Infectious Disease

OBSTRUCTION

- Common sxs: Bilious emesis, diffuse abdominal pain, abdominal distention, ↓ stool output

Initial Evaluation
- **Imaging:** Start with KUB or abd US depending on exam; consider upper GI series if significant emesis (Ped Health 2017;8:83–91)
  - CT may be necessary if peritoneal signs present or if other imaging inconclusive
- **Labs:** BMP (assess for metabolic alkalosis), CBC (look for infection) consider FOBT or occult blood on NG output

Etiologies
- **Malrotation (with midgut volvulus):** Most common in infants <1 yo
  - **Dx:** Abd ultrasound or upper GI series
  - **T:** Urgent surgery due to risk of ischemia
- **Intussusception:** Most common age 6–12 mo
  - Telescoping of bowel at lead point (Meckel, Peyer patch, enlarged lymph nodes; found in 25% of cases) (Am J Roentgenol 2016;207[2]:424)
  - **Sxs:** Severe, intermittent abdominal pain; pull knees to chest
  - **Exam:** Palpable sausage-like abd mass, currant jelly stool (late sign ← bowel necrosis)
  - **Dx:** Abd US (97.9% Se, 97.8% Sp, NPV ~100%) (Ped Radiol 2009;39[10]: 1075–1079)
  - **Tx:** Air enema (83% success rate) vs. surgical reduction (more likely required if >3.5 cm) (Academic Radiology 2017;24:521–529)
- **Pyloric stenosis:** 1 in 250–1,000; M 4–8× > F; usually 3 wo–5 mo
  - **Pathophys:** Pyloric hypertrophy → pyloric obstruction → frequent, nonbilious projectile emesis
    - **RFs:** Erythromycin exposure
  - **Exam:** "Olive-like" mass in epigastric region, visible peristaltic waves
  - **Labs:** Hypochloremic metabolic alkalosis (from gastric acid loss)
  - **Dx:** US measuring pylorus length (cutoff depends on weight and age)
  - **Tx:** IVF (for acidosis, dehydration), pyloromyotomy; medical management of pyloric stenosis with atropine is possible, but rarely done in the US (Ped Surg 2016;25[4]:219–224)
- **Meconium Ileus:** 95% of pts have CF, only occurs in 15% of CF pts
  - **Dx:** KUB showing distended loops of bowel
  - **Tx:** Gastrografin enema (40% success rate), potentially operative mgmt

CONSTIPATION

(Peds in Review 2015;36[9]:392)

- **Epi:** 3% of PCP visits, 10–25% of peds GI referrals (Am Fam Phys 2014; 90[2]:82–90)
- **Red Flags:** Fever, FTT, abnormal exam, blood in the stool, delayed passage of meconium
- **Etiologies:**
  - Obstructive: Anal stenosis, anterior displacement of anus, mec ileus, colonic stricture
  - Meds: Opioids, anticholinergic agents, TCAs
  - Neurologic: Hirschprung (below), neuronal dysplasia, anal achalasia, spinal disorders
  - Metabolic: Hypothyroidism, celiac disease, diabetes, CF
  - Dietary: Cow's milk protein allergy, low-fiber diet, ↓ fluid intake for age
  - Functional: Infant dyschezia, functional constipation (below), nonretentive fecal soiling

HIRSCHSPRUNG DISEASE

- Fetal defect of migration of neuroblasts → aganglionic distal colon → impaired relaxation
- **Epi:** 1/5,000; M 3× > F; 10% of pts not dx until >3 yo
  - Assoc w/ trisomy 21 (2%), MEN2, familial dysautonomia, Waardenburg syndrome
- **Sxs:** Failure or delayed passage of meconium, bilious emesis, abdominal distention
- **Eval:** Contrast enema initially, confirmed via rectal suction bx
- **Mgmt:** Surgical resection of affected segment
- See page *** in NICU for more details

FUNCTIONAL CONSTIPATION

- Most common cause of constipation; no underlying pathologic cause
- **Sxs:** Withholding behaviors, abdominal pain, poor appetite
  - **Encopresis:** Repeated passage of feces into inappropriate places (usually underpants)
- **Exam:** Assess for tenderness/masses, external anal inspection for fissures, skin tags, hemorrhoids, consider DRE
- **Diagnosis:**
  - Rome III Criteria, 2 or more of the following: ≤2 defecations in toilet/wk, ≥1 × fecal incontinence/wk, hx of retentive posturing, hx of painful or hard BMs, presence of large fecal mass in rectum, hx of large diameter stools
- **Tx:** Education and reassurance, may require initial disimpaction or clean out, maintenance therapy to maintain goal of 1–2 soft BMs/d
  - Diet: Encourage ↑ dietary fiber, adequate fluid intake
  - Stool softeners, laxatives, osmotic agents

DIARRHEA

ACUTE DIARRHEA

- **Def.:** Abrupt onset ↑ in stool output or change in stool consistency lasting <2 wk
- **Epi:** 10% of admissions <5 yo; average 1–2 episodes/yr in children <5 yo
  - Major cause of pediatric mortality in developing countries

Causes
- **Infectious:** Viruses (25–40% rotavirus), bacteria, parasites
  - **EHEC O157:H7:** Avoid abx as ↑ risk of HUS (2/2 ↑ toxin release), monitor renal function
  - **C. diff:** Consider in patients w/ recent abx use, uncommon in <1 yo
    - Risk of toxic megacolon
    - **Dx:** Stool PCR (>97% Sen)
    - **Tx:** Metronidazole and/or po vancomycin depending on severity and prior hx
- **Postenteritis:** Diarrhea due to loss of intestinal ciliary border
- **Diarrhea secondary to systemic illness:** DKA, UTI

Evaluation
- **Hx:** (recent exposures, travel, antibiotic use, family history, blood in the stool?)
- **Labs:** Stool cx (gold standard) or PCRs, C. diff assay, fecal elastase (steatorrhea), stool-reducing substances (malabsorption), fecal leukocytes, stool for ova and parasites

Management
- Rehydration (oral rehydration preferred over IVF)
- Probiotics: Lactobacillus may shorten duration of symptoms by 1 d (Pediatrics 2010; 126[6]:1217–1231)
- Antibiotics only indicated if C. diff, or if bacterial etiology with severe sxs

CHRONIC DIARRHEA

- ↑ Stool output or loose stools, consistently for >1 mo

Causes
- **Cow's milk/soy protein intolerance:** Common cause of chronic diarrhea in infants
  - **Sxs:** Vomiting, colic, bloody stools
  - **Tx:** Protein hydrolysate formula (elemental formula if ineffective)

- **Lactose intolerance:** Common, 2/2 to impaired ability to break down and absorb lactose → osmotic diarrhea
  - **Dx:** Clinical but can consider lactose hydrogen breath test
  - **Tx:** Lactose avoidance or lactase supplementation
- **Infectious:** Viral, bacterial (*salmonella*), parasitic (*giardia*, cryptosporidium)
- **Immune:** Food allergy, celiac dz (below), IBD (below); immunodeficiencies (will often have diarrhea)
- **Others:** Small Intestinal Bowel Overgrowth (SIBO), short bowel, protein-losing enteropathy
- **See Chronic Diarrhea algorithm for more details**

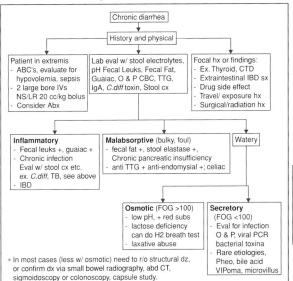

CELIAC DISEASE

- Autoimmune reaction to gliadin (found in dietary gluten) → small bowel inflammation → chronic malabsorptive diarrhea
- **Epi:** ~1% of general population; 1:22 risk in pts with 1st-degree relative
  - Assn w/ T1DM, hypothyroidism, GERD
- **Sxs:** Diarrhea (27%), bloating, bulky/foul-smelling/floating stools, flatulence, malabsorption (growth failure, anemia, etc.), aphthous stomatitis (18%), GERD (12%)
- **Exam:** Dermatitis herpetiformis (classic rash)
- **Dx:** Tissue transglutaminase IgA & serum IgA levels (check both in case of IgA def), antiendomysial ab (>90% Se, high Sp)
  - Gold standard: Endoscopic bx w/ villous atrophy and crypt hyperplasia
- **Complications:** ↑ risk for osteoporosis, enteropathy-associated T-cell lymphoma, small-intestinal adenocarcinoma (risk decreases with adherence to gluten-free diet)
- **Tx:** Gluten-free diet (treats both GI and other sxs)

INFLAMMATORY BOWEL DISEASE

(Peds in Review 2016;37[8])

	Crohn Disease	**Ulcerative Colitis**
Epidemiology	40/100,000, F > M	28/100,000, M > F
Symptoms	Abd pain, diarrhea, weight loss, N/V, oral & perianal dz	Bloody diarrhea, peridefecatory abd pain, tenesmus, n/v

Features	Transmural inflammation; skip lesions	Rectal/colonic mucosal inflammation extending proximally
Pathology	Noncaseating granulomas	Crypt abscesses
Complications	Fistulas, malabsorption, Ca oxalate nephrolithiasis	Pseudopolyps, risk of colon CA (>10 yr)
Associations	AS, sacroiliitis, MPA	PSC, pANCA (+)

- Combination of genetics, microbiome, and environmental factors
- **Sxs:** As above + growth failure ± extraintestinal symptoms (~25% will have)
  - GI: Aphthous stomatitis, PSC, autoimmune hepatitis, Budd–Chiari syndrome
  - CV: Pericarditis, myocarditis, heart block
  - Pulmonary: Bronchitis, pulmonary fibrosis
  - Skin: Erythema nodosum, pyoderma gangrenosum, abscesses, skin tags, hair loss
  - Musculoskeletal: Osteopenia, arthralgias, arthritis
  - Others: Fever, iron deficiency, uveitis
- **Differential**
  - Chronic sxs: IBS, lactose intol, celiac dz, anorexia nervosa, *giardia*, ovarian cyst
  - Acute sxs: Appendicitis, mesenteric adenitis, hemorrhoids, Meckel diverticulum, infectious (*salmonella, shigella, yersinia, giardia*), HSP
- **Evaluation**
  - **Labs:** CBC, CMP, ESR/CRP (nml in 15% of pts, albumin; stool cultures)
  - Endoscopy with bx is gold standard, but can use MRE (>90% Se, better assesses small intestine)
- **Management**
  - Medical management is mainstay: Initially use 5-ASA derivatives & escalate as necessary
    - Monitor nutritional status closely
    - Surveillance for complications (regular colonoscopy starting 8–10 yr after dx)
  - Surgery when needed (can be curative in UC)

Agent (Mechanism)	Clinical Use	Side Effects
Aminosalicylates (sulfasalazine, mesalamine)	Mild to mod UC or colonic CD; distal terminal ileitis	Headache, diarrhea, pancreatitis
Corticosteroids	Induce remission (not long-term med)	Adrenal suppression, hyperglycemia, weight gain, impaired growth, HTN
Immunomodulators (Azathioprine, 6-MP, MTX)	Maintain steroid-free remission, often w/ biologics; 75% response rate; takes 3–6 mo to see effect	BM suppression, hepatotoxicity, pancreatitis, ↑ risk of lymphoma
Biologic agents (anti-TNF-α; Infliximab, Adalimumab)	Severe or steroid-dependent/refractory IBD; 90% response rate	Immunosuppression
Enteral nutrition (elemental diet, polymeric formulas) or TPN	Bowel rest in severe disease, may help induce induction	Adherence challenging

(Peds in Review 2016;37[8])

ESOPHAGEAL DISORDERS

ESOPHAGEAL ATRESIA

- Assn w/ VACTERL (vertebral, anorectal, cardiac, tracheal, esophageal, limb) syndrome
- **Sxs:** Polyhydramnios, excessive oral secretions, aspiration (with feeding or on secretions), inability to pass NG tube into stomach
- **Eval:** KUB (airless abdomen), endoscopy
- **Tx:** Surgical correction

FOREIGN BODY/INGESTIONS

- **Sxs:** Cough, inability to manage secretions, refusal to eat, new-onset stridor
- **Eval:** AP and lateral XR from nose to rectum (will only show radiopaque bodies)

- **Treatment:**
  - Indications for removal: Failure to pass through esophagus in 24 hr, airway compromise, specific objects (sharp, magnet, battery, superabsorbent polymer), fever, abdominal pain, vomiting (Gastrointest Endosc 2002;55[7]:802–806)
  - If none of above indications for removal met and radiopaque object can follow serial XR

EOSINOPHILIC ESOPHAGITIS

(Peds in Review 2015;36[8])

- **Epidemiology:** Up to 40/100,000
  - Risk factors: 3× male predominance, atopic history, Caucasian race
- **Sxs:** Nonspecific feeding issues, food impaction, dysphagia, abd pain (similar to GERD)
- **Dx:** EGD (≥15 eosinophils/hpf on Bx), ↑ IgE level, ↑ peripheral eos (40–50% of cases) (Clinical Gastroenterology and Hepatology 2009;7[12]:1305–1313)
- **Tx:** Food elimination (targeted or complete); topical steroids (swallowed fluticasone – MDI w/o spacer), PPI

GERD

(Peds in Review 2012;33[6]:243)

- **Def.:** Passage of gastric contents into esophagus resulting in sxs
- **Epidemiology:** Common (up to 67% of infants will have some degree) until 12 mo
  - Risk factors: Prematurity, obesity, lung dx, esophageal atresia
- Sxs:
  - Infants: Spitting up, FTT, feeding issues; arching of back or irritability; ALTEs
  - Children: Vomiting, abd pain, chronic cough, dental erosions, epigastric pain
- **Evaluation:**
  - Indications for workup: Bilious emesis, GI bleeding, FTT, forceful emesis, emesis start >6 mo, fever, diarrhea, lethargy, bulging fontanelle, suspicion of metabolic dx
  - Esophageal pH and impedance monitoring ± consider imaging (barium swallow or gastric emptying study)
  - In older children evaluation can start w/ empiric trial of acid suppression × 4 wk
- **Prognosis:** Most infants outgrow by 7–12 mo
- **Tx:** Lifestyle modification (infants: Hold upright, frequent burping, add rice cereal; older children: Avoid high-fat or late meals)
  - Pharmacologic: H2 blockers are first line with addition of PPI if needed
  - Refractory symptoms require surgical correction (Nissen fundoplication)

PEPTIC ULCER DISEASE

- **Sxs:** Recurrent epigastric abdominal pain (may awaken child from sleep), postprandial pain, emesis, may have blood in stool or in emesis
- **Evaluation:**
  - Focused hx: Assess for symptoms above, weight loss, dietary intake, meds
  - Exam: Growth chart, oral exam, abdominal exam
  - **Labs:** CBC, LFTs, ESR, stool for ova and parasites; females → UA and UPT; H. pylori testing (bx ideal, else serology; stool test for recurrent)
  - **Imaging:** Upright KUB if concerned for perforation
  - **Indications for endoscopy:** Negative workup, lack of response to antacids, evidence of GI bleed, abnormalities on imaging
  - **Tx:** H2 blockers (1st line), PPI (if refractory), sucralfate (if evidence of injured mucosa)
  - **H. pylori:** Triple vs. quadruple therapy depending on local resistance patterns
    - Triple: Clarithromycin, amoxicillin (metronidazole if PCN allergic), PPI × 14 d
    - Quadruple: Tetracycline, metronidazole, bismuth, PPI × 14 d

GI BLEEDING

(Peds in Review 2014;35[6]:243)

	Upper GI Bleeding (UGIB)	Lower GI Bleeding (LGIB)
Source	Proximal to ligament of Treitz	Distal to ligament of Treitz
Symptoms	Coffee-ground emesis, hematemesis	Hematochezia (can be seen with rapid UGIB)
Causes	PUD, gastritis, esophagitis, varices, prolapse gastropathy, Mallory–Weiss, swallowed maternal blood (infants – Dx via apt test)	Allergic colitis, enteric infections, juvenile polyps, IBD, volvulus, HUS, angiodysplasia, hamartomas, HSP

- Note: Ingestion of red substances (beets, red food dyes) can cause red-colored emesis/stools, oral iron supplements and bismuth salicylate may cause melanotic appearance to stools
- **Causes**
  - **Anal fissure:** RF – constipation; sxs – bright red blood on outside of stool, pain with defecation
  - **Meckel diverticulum:** Usually ~2 yo, M > F; secondary to ectopic gastric mucosa within 2 ft of the ileocecal junction; dx – technetium-99 scan; tx – surgery
  - **Colonic polyps:** Painless rectal bleeding
  - **Intussusception:** See Obstruction
  - **NEC:** RFs – prematurity, sepsis, LBW, asphyxia; XR shows pneumatosis; tx – ABX, NPO, surgery if indicated
  - **Milk protein intolerance:** Usually w/i 1st 3 mo of life; present with blood in stool; tx – hypoallergenic formula (likely to react to soy as well)
- Eval
  - **Labs:** CBC, LFTs, BMP, fecal occult
  - Gastric lavage via NG (assess UGIB vs. LGIB)
  - **Imaging:** KUB initially; consider additional pending history (i.e., Meckel)
  - **Endoscopy:** Diagnostic and can be therapeutic
- **Tx:** Stabilize initially (2 × large bore IVs, IVF prn, PRBCs if anemic, correct coagulopathies)
  - Depends on etiology; endoscopy can be therapeutic; consider H2 blockers or PPIs

HEPATIC DISORDERS

Patterns of Liver Injury

	AST	ALT	Bili	ALP
Hepatocellular	↑↑	↑↑	+/–	+/–
Cholestatic	+/–	+/–	↑↑	↑
Infiltrative	Nml	Nml	Nml	↑↑

- **Hepatocellular:**
  - >15× nml ← acute viral hep, drug, or toxin mediated, ischemic hepatitis, Budd–Chiari
  - <5× nml ← viral hep, hemochromatosis, NASH, Wilson, autoimmune hepatitis, celiac dx
- **Cholestasis:** Sometimes with jaundice, see below
- **Infiltrative:** Lymphoma, TB, sarcoidosis, histoplasmosis

JAUNDICE

(Peds in Review 2001;22[7]:219)

- **Def.:** T bili >2–3 mg/dL; D bili >2 mg/dL
- **Pathophys:** Due to ↑ production, ↓ conjugation, or impaired excretion
- **Initial eval:** CMP, albumin + PT/INR (assess synthetic function), GGT (more Sp to biliary tract than ALP)

↑ Production → Predominantly Indirect Hyperbili
- **Hemolysis:** Dx via CBC, Coombs, LDH, haptoglobin, smear, hgb electrophoresis
  - Causes – Autoimmune, G6PD, PKD, HS, HE, sickle cell, thalassemia

Impaired Conjugation → Mixed Hyperbili
- **Gilbert:** 5% of ppl; benign; impaired conjugation of bilirubin → episodic jaundice when ill or stressed
- **Rotor:** AR glutathione transferase deficiency → asymptomatic jaundice with hyperbilirubinemia; elevated urinary coproporphyrin III
- **Dubin Johnson:** AR mutation, M > F; primarily indirect hyperbili; dark brown/black liver on gross histology
- **Crigler–Najjar syndromes:** AR mutations in UDP-glucoronosyltransferase; usually present in first few days of life
- Others: Autoimmune hepatitis (see below), A1AT, Wilson dx

Impaired Excretion → Predominantly Direct
- **Extrahepatic cholestasis**
  - **Biliary atresia**
    - **Epi:** F > M, 1/10,000–20,000 (Pediatrics 1997;99[3]:376–382)
    - **Pathophys:** Rapidly progressive destruction of the extrahepatic biliary tree
    - **Sx:** Jaundice and firm hepatomegaly most commonly at 3–6 wk of age
    - **Imaging:** Triangular cord sign on abd US (85% Se, 100% Sp) (J Ped Surg 1997;32[11]:1555–1559)
    - **Tx:** Kasai portoenterostomy (palliative bridge to transplant, more effective if performed earlier)
  - **Cholelithiasis:** Uncommon in children, dx via abd US (check CBD) or HIDA; Tx: ERCP vs. cholecystectomy, ABX if signs of infection
    - RFs: Sickle cell dx, female, obese, OCP use
- **Intrahepatic cholestasis**
  - Primary sclerosing cholangitis (PSC)
    - **Epi:** M > F, usually presents in adolescence. Associated with UC
    - **Sx:** Intermittent abdominal pain, anorexia, weight loss, jaundice, and pruritus. Failure to thrive, delayed puberty
    - **Labs:** ↑ GGT, ↑ ALP; +/– transaminitis; (+) ANCA staining
    - **Imaging:** MRCP (can consider ERCP, liver biopsy)
    - **Tx:** Ursodiol for sxs, immunosuppression (↓ progression); often require transplant; high risk of cholangiocarcinoma (9–15% lifetime risk) (N Engl J Med 1995;332:924–933)
  - Choledochal cysts

Multifactorial
- **Neonatal hyperbilirubinemia:** See page *** in NICU
- **Anatomical causes:** Pancreatic divisum, annular pancreas, choledochal cyst, congenital strictures
- **Other causes:** Idiopathic, drug-induced, postprocedure (ERCP), systemic disease precipitating cholestasis (infection, trauma, metabolic disorder, autoimmune process)

Imaging Types and Indications
- **Abdominal US:** Assess for obstruction, hepatomegaly, abnormal echotexture or masses
- **Abdominal CT:** Not often needed; more detailed anatomical view of liver
- **HIDA scan:** Use radiotracer to assess patency of hepatic ducts; use in direct hyperbili
- **ERCP:** Procedure; visualized extrahepatic biliary tree; can be therapeutic (papillotomy, stent placement). Risk of postprocedure pancreatitis
- **MRCP:** Allows for visualization of intrahepatic and extrahepatic biliary anatomy

HEPATITIS

- **Def:** Elevation of AST and ALT secondary to inflammation

Causes
- **Toxin/drug induced:** Most common cause of acute liver failure in children is APAP overdose. Other causes: EtOH, meds (antiepileptic medications, antibiotics), amanita mushroom. Tx: Supportive, NAC for acetaminophen overdose (see ED)

- **Infectious hepatitis:** Hepatitis A/B/C/D/E, TORCH infections, EBV
  - **HepA:** Fecal oral transmission (contaminated foods). Acute, self-limiting infection presenting with jaundice, fatigue, nausea/vomiting. DDx via (+) IgM. ↑ risk of fulminant liver failure if underlying liver disease. Prevent in high-risk populations with vaccination. Tx primarily supportive
  - **HepB:** Vertical transmission vs. exposure to infected body fluids. Not transmitted through breast milk. Prevent vertical transmission with hep B vaccine and HBID within 12 hr of delivery if mother HBsAG positive or unknown. Isolated positive anti-HBs Ab indicative of prior vaccination. Chronic infection → risk for cirrhosis/hepatocellular carcinoma (monitor annual AFP, hepatic ultrasound)
  - **HepC:** Transmitted through infected body fluids vs. vertical transmission. Not transmitted through breast milk. Can cause acute or chronic infection. Often asymptomatic. Mgmt: Supportive, vaccinate against other hepatitis viruses, genotype guides tx. Chronic infection increases risk for cirrhosis/hepatocellular carcinoma
  - **HepD:** Only infects patients with hep B. Treated supportively
  - **HepE:** Fecal oral transmission. Acute infectious process, increased severity in pregnant patients
- **Genetic disorders:** Alpha-1 antitrypsin deficiency (A1AT), Wilson dx, metabolic disorders (mitochondrial disorders, galactosemia, hereditary hemochromatosis)
  - **A1AT:** Autosomal codominant inheritance (SERPINA1 gene mutation) with incomplete penetrance. Jaundice in first 2–4 mo of life, later develop cirrhosis, COPD/emphysema. Dx: Alpha-1 antitrypsin level (<11 μmol diagnostic), genetic testing. Tx: Supportive until liver transplant (curative)
  - **Wilson dx:** Autosomal recessive inheritance. Copper deposition in the liver, kidney, cornea, and central nervous system → hepatitis, cirrhosis, renal dysfunction, depression, psychosis. Kayser–Fleischer rings on ophthalmologic exam. Labs: Notable for elevated AST/ALT, low/normal alkaline phosphatase, hemolytic anemia, low ceruloplasmin levels (low sensitivity/specificity), elevated urinary copper excretion (penicillamine challenge test)
- **Autoimmune hepatitis:** F > M; usually presents in adolescence
  - **Dx:** Positive antismooth muscle antibody (type I), positive anti-liver–kidney microsome antibody (type II, most common), ANA
  - **Tx:** Ursodiol (helps with sxs); immunosuppression (limit progression)
- **Infiltrative processes:** NASH increasing in prevalence in pediatrics

PANCREATITIS

(Peds in Review 2013;34[2]:79)

- **Epi:** 13.2/100,000/yr
- **Sxs:** Epigastric abd pain with radiation to back, N/V, anorexia, AMS; retroperitoneal hemorrhage if severe; shock
- **Initial eval:** CBC, CMP, amylase, lipase (>3× nml; more Sp than amylase). Imaging: US (assess for gallstones or obstruction)
  - Consider CT if diagnosis unclear, prolonged sxs, or if concerned about hemorrhage or cyst
  - ERCP: If recurrent or prolonged pancreatitis, recent trauma, known gallstones

ACUTE PANCREATITIS

- **Etiologies:** None found in 33% of cases
  - Biliary obstruction (10–30%): Congenital anomalies (divisum, annular pancreas), choledochal cysts, gallstones
  - Drug-induced/toxin-mediated (12–25%): Steroids, valproic acid, antiepileptics, antibiotics, furosemide, immunosuppressants, scorpion stings, alcohol
  - Infection: Can be systemic sepsis or localized (mumps, coxsackie B, VZV, EBV, HBV, flu)
  - Blunt abd trauma
- **Tx:** Bowel rest, IV fluids (usually 2–3× maint), pain control (may require PCA)
- **Complications:** Shock, metabolic derangements, cyst formation or pancreatic necrosis, retroperitoneal hemorrhage, infection, ARDS, pericarditis, DIC

CHRONIC PANCREATITIS

- **Def.:** Process leading to irreversible destruction of pancreatic parenchyma with loss of exocrine function; usually preceded by recurrent acute pancreatitis
- **Etiologies:**
  - Biliary: Macrolithiais, microlithiasis, or sludging
  - Congenital anomalies: Anomalous pancreaticobiliary junction, choledochal cyst, annular pancreas, pancreas divisum, sphincter of Oddi dysfxn
  - Genetic – Hereditary pancreatitis (usually AD) – PRSS-1, SPINK-1 mutation, CFTR
  - Duodenal inflammation: Crohn, celiac, infection
  - Meds: Metabolic (hyperCa, hyperTG)
  - Autoimmune (isolated, Sjögren, PBC)
  - Idiopathic (most common)
- Dx is primarily clinical
- **Sxs:** Chronic epigastric abd pain with radiation to pack; weight loss; fatty stools or diarrhea; potentially can present with jaundice
- **Eval:**
  - BGs (risk of DM), fecal elastase (looking for pancreatic insufficiency, poor Se), 72-hr fecal fat collection (best test for steatorrhea); genetic testing (as above)
  - **Imaging:** MRCP (modality of choice), US can be useful as well; ERCP depending on w/u
- **Tx:**
  - Chronic pain control
  - Pancreatic enzyme replacement therapy (Creon with meals)
  - Pancreatectomy with islet cell autotransplant possible; does not improve pain in 20% pts
    - Particularly in pts with hereditary/genetic causes due to risk of pancreatic CA (by 40 yo)

ANEMIA

(Nathan and Oski's Hematology and Oncology of Infancy and Childhood. 8th ed. 2015:293–307)

Definition
- ↓ in RBC mass: Decrease in Hb/Hct compared to general population, is age and sex dependent

Clinical Manifestations
- Symptoms: Most are asymptomatic, blood loss, fatigue, pallor, irritability, pica (assoc. w/ iron deficiency), glossitis, koilonychias, angular cheilitis
- Signs: Pallor (conjunctival, palmar creases), tachycardia, systolic murmur, jaundice (if hemolytic), high-output heart failure if severe

Etiology
- **RBC loss**
  - Blood loss: GI losses (acute GI bleed, milk protein allergy), menorrhagia, trauma
  - Hemolysis: Autoimmune, hemoglobinopathies, intrinsic RBC defects, mechanical destruction, G6PD deficiency, paroxysmal nocturnal hemoglobinuria (PNH), medication-induced hemolytic anemia
  - Splenic sequestration
- **Decreased production**
  - Marrow failure: Aplastic anemia, pure red cell aplasias (Diamond–Blackfan, transient erythroblastopenia of childhood, parvovirus B19 infection), infiltration (malignancy, myelofibrosis), Fanconi anemia
  - Infectious bone-marrow suppression
  - ↓ EPO production: Renal failure, hypothyroidism, hypopituitarism, chronic inflammation, protein malnutrition
  - Anemia of chronic disease
  - Sideroblastic anemia
  - Lead poisoning
  - Nutritional deficiency: Iron, vit B_{12}, folic acid, copper, zinc

Historical Factors
- Age
  - Nutritional anemia rarely occurs before 6 mo of age
  - Neonatal anemia usually due to blood loss, isoimmunization, congenital anemia, congenital infection
  - Anemia at 3–6 mo of age suggests hemoglobinopathy (HbF ↓ around 6 mo)
  - Premature infants are at higher risk for iron deficiency anemia, exaggerated physiologic nadir
- Jaundice/hyperbilirubinemia suggests hemolysis (membranopathy, enzymopathy)
- Pica suggest iron deficiency

MCV, RDW, and Reticulocytes

Retic	Microcytic	Normocytic	Macrocytic
Low	Iron deficiency Lead poisoning Anemia of chronic disease (normocytic too) Aluminum toxicity Copper deficiency Protein deficiency Aluminum toxicity	Pure RBC aplasias Anemia of chronic disease. Bone marrow failure (e.g., malignancy, myelofibrosis) Anemia of renal failure	Folate deficiency B_{12} deficiency DBA Trisomy 21 Liver disease
Normal	Thalassemia trait Sideroblastic anemia	Acute blood loss (early) Dyserythropoietic anemia II	
High	Thalassemias Hemoglobin C disorders	Hemolysis (MAHA, AIHA, membranopathies, enzymopathies) Hemoglobinopathies	Active hemolysis (reticulocytosis) Dyserythropoietic anemia I, III

(Adapted from Harriet Lane Handbook. 21st ed. 2018:364–394)

Workup
- CBC with differential cell count
  - MCV and RDW are helpful in categorizing anemia
- Reticulocytes: Absolute and reticulocyte index (RI = [%retic] x [HCT/Nml HCT])
  - Evaluates marrow production.

- Evaluation for hemolysis: LDH ↑, uncong bilirubin ↑, potassium ↑, haptoglobin (Hp) ↓
  - Hp is a naturally occurring binder of free hemoglobin, inhibiting oxidative activity
- Direct (Direct antiglobulin test-DAT) and indirect (Indirect antiglobulin test-IAT) Coombs
- Peripheral smear
- Iron, ferritin, transferrin
- Hb electrophoresis

MICROCYTIC ANEMIAS

Iron Deficiency Anemia (Lancet 2016;387(10021); Am Fam Phys 2016;93(4); Nathan and Oski's Hematology and Oncology of Infancy and Childhood. 8th ed. 2015:344–381)
- Most common cause of anemia in children
- Diagnosis:
  - Often incidentally discovered. Most infants are asymptomatic
  - Presents with pica. Iron deficiency raises risk for neurocognitive defects
  - Risk factors include: Maternal iron deficiency, feeding problems, poor growth, consuming >24 oz/d cow's milk, non–iron-fortified formulas, feeding problems, poor growth
- Screening:
  - WHO/AAP: Universal screening at 1 yr
  - USPSTF: Insufficient evidence to recommend for or against
- Etiology:
  - Insufficient supply: Dietary insufficiency, rapid growth (infancy), unfortified formula
  - Poor absorption: Celiac dz, IBD, gastric bypass/short bowel
  - Iron losses: GI bleeding, milk-protein enteropathy, menorrhagia, chronic intravascular hemolysis
  - Inaccessible iron stores: Infection, inflammation-induced hepcidin expression → ↓ iron absorption
- Workup:
  - CBC w/ diff at 9–12 mo: Hb <11 g/dL (se 26%, sp 95%), MCV <71 fL (se 86%, sp 83%). Often concurrent thrombocytosis
  - No further workup if IDA suspected
  - Iron studies reveal low iron, low ferritin, high transferrin and TIBC. Ferritin is first to decrease, may be falsely elevated by inflammation
- Treatment: Oral iron replacement

Hemoglobinopathies (below)

Sideroblastic Anemia (Hematol Oncol Clin North Am 2014;28(4))
- Heterogeneous group of bone marrow d/o, congenital and acquired
- Typified by presence of ringed sideroblasts in marrow aspirate
  - Prussian blue-positive granules = mitochondrial iron deposits, typically perinuclear
- Congenital forms may not present in early childhood
- Ineffective erythropoiesis leads to iron overload, causing significant morbidity. Tx with phlebotomy if mild, chelation therapy if transfusion dependent
- Dx: BM aspirate. Genetic testing
- Tx: Pyridoxine if microcytic (until genetic cause can be defined). Management of iron overload

NORMOCYTIC ANEMIAS

Normal Physiologic Nadir of Infancy (Harriet Lane Handbook. 21st ed. 2018:364–394)
- Gradual decrease in Hb until O_2 needs exceed O_2 delivery → ↑ EPO
- Nadir typically occurs at Hb of 9–11 mg/dL
- Generally occurs at 8–12 wk if full term, 3–6 wk if premature
- Tx: Observation only

Transient Erythroblastopenia of Childhood (Harriet Lane Handbook. 21st ed. 2018:364–394; Nathan and Oski's Hematology and Oncology of Infancy and Childhood. 8th ed. 2015:344–381)
- Characterized as severe anemia at 6 mo-4 y, >80% of cases after 1 y
- Brief interruption of erythropoiesis, likely caused by a viral infection. Low reticulo-cytes, RDW
- Spontaneous recovery in 4–8 wk

Lead Poisoning (Pediatr Rev 2010;31(10))
- Lead inhibits rate-limiting enzymes in heme synthesis, ferrochelatase, delta amino levulinic acid dehydrogenase → accumulation of precursors and hypochromatic, microcytic anemia
- See Primary Care section 1-7 for more information

Anemia of Chronic Inflammation
- Can be microcytic
- AKA anemia of chronic disease. Normocytic or microcytic, normochromic, slightly ↑ RDW
- Upregulation of hepcidin → decreased enteral absorption
- Defective iron recycling in marrow → iron sequestration in reticuloendothelial macrophages
- Decreased EPO levels for degree of anemia
- Iron studies: Low iron, high ferritin, high transferrin and TIBC
- Tx: treat underlying disorder. Does not improve with iron therapy

---

HEMOLYTIC ANEMIAS

(Pediatr Rev 2016;27(6); *Nathan and Oski's Hematology and Oncology of Infancy and Childhood*. 8th ed. 2015:311–430)

- Normocytic with reticulocytosis
- Extravascular vs. intravascular:
  - Extravascular = mediated by reticuloendothelial system: autoimmune hemolytic anemia (AIHA), sickle cell, hereditary spherocytosis
  - Intravascular = RBC membrane damage occurs intravascularly: Mechanical destruction, complement-mediated destruction (e.g., mechanical heart valve), microangiopathic hemolytic anemias, cold AIHA
- Intrinsic/congenital vs. acquired:
  - Intrinsic: Enzymopathies (G6PD deficiency), membranopathies (hereditary spherocytosis & elliptocytosis), PNH, hemoglobinopathies (sickle cell disease)
  - Acquired: Hemolytic disease of newborn, warm AIHA, mechanical heart valve, HUS/MAHA
- Signs and symptoms:
  - Dark urine: Hemoglobinuria (intravascular hemolysis)
  - Jaundice: Unconjugated hyperbilirubinemia. If present at 1st day of life, investigate for hemolysis
  - Splenomegaly: Sequestration of RBCs
  - Pallor, fatigue, light headedness, murmur
- Diagnostic evaluation:
  - Reticulocytosis: Usually >2% with absolute reticulocyte count >$100 \times 10^3/\mu L$
  - Release of RBC contents → ↑ indirect bilirubin, ↑ LDH, ↑ AST
  - Haptoglobin binds free hemoglobin → decreased (not useful in infants <3 mo)
  - Peripheral smear:
    - RBC fragments (schistocytes, helmet cells) → toxin stress, shear stress (e.g., MAHA, mechanical destruction)
    - Microspherocytes → AIHA (structural changes 2/2 membrane bound antibodies)
    - Polychromasia due to reticulocytosis
- Second tier testing:
  - Hemoglobin electrophoresis (sickle cell, β-thalassemias)
  - Antiglobulin (Coombs) testing (once hemolysis is established)
    - DAT:
      1° test: Nonspecific antihuman antibodies added to RBCs, if antibodies present on cell surface → agglutination
      2° test: Human anti-IgG and anticomplement antibodies (implies IgM bound) → Helps differentiate between warm (IgG) and cold (IgM) AIHA
    - IAT: Patient serum is added to donor RBCs. If patient has RBC autoantibodies → binds donor RBC → agglutination with antihuman globulin
- Complications of chronic hemolytic diseases include parvovirus B19 aplasia as well as gallstones

Hemoglobinopathies (below)

Alloimmune Hemolytic Disease of the Fetus and Newborn
- Mediated by maternal IgG against fetal antigens (Rh[D], A, B) and fetal/neonatal RBC destruction
- Ranges from mild neonatal anemia to severe in utero hemolysis and hydrops fetalis

- Prophylactic maternal administration of anti-D IgG and intrauterine transfusions have greatly decreased incidence and severity of disease
  - Maternal prenatal alloimmunization (previous pregnancy, blood products) may lead to severe disease
- In the U.S., neonatal AIHA is now most commonly caused by ABO mismatch
  - Often manifest as hyperbilirubinemia w/o anemia
- Dx: direct and indirect antiglobulin test. Most, but not all cases are positive
  - Prolonged or severe hyperbilirubinemia with negative DAT/IAT should raise suspicion for RBC enzymopathy (G6PD, PK deficiency) or Gilbert's disease
- Tx:
  - Severe fetal disease may require intrauterine transfusions
  - Management of hyperbilirubinemia: Phototherapy and exchange transfusion if indicated
  - Transfusion support
  - Observation: hemolysis ceases in 1–2 months once maternal antibodies have been consumed

G6PD Deficiency
- Most common RBC enzymopathy
- X-linked recessive
  - Likely responsible for 33% of male neonatal jaundice, usually in the 1st day of life, mediated by bilirubin metabolism defects rather than hemolysis
- G6PD critical in defending against RBC oxidative stress (replenishes NADPH via pentose phosphate pathway)
- G6PD deficiency increases risk of intravascular hemolysis with RBC oxidative stress
- Patients usually asymptomatic and unaware of their deficiency
- Hemolytic episodes present with fatigue, back pain, dark urine, jaundice
- Common triggers:
  - Infection: Acute illness, specific triggers include Hep A, Hep B, EBV
  - Fava beans, medications (primaquine, sulfa drugs, nitrofurantoin, naphthalene)
- Dx: Quantitative G6PD activity assay. May be falsely normal in acute phase due to destruction of G6PD-deficient RBCs. Severity of the disorder is related to the quantitative degree of enzyme activity deficiency
- Tx: Episodes generally self-limited, may require RBC transfusion. Education and avoidance of triggers

Paroxysmal Nocturnal Hemoglobinuria
- Incidence of 1–1.5 million cases worldwide
- Complement-mediated hemolysis due to acquired deficiency of complement regulatory proteins (CD55 and CD59)
- Caused by somatic mutations in X-linked *PIGA* gene with subsequent clonal expansion
- Manifestations:
  - Anemia: Intravascular hemolysis (increased reticulocytes, LDH), extravascular hemolysis (phagocytosis of C3-bound RBCs)
  - Bone marrow failure: Not a consequence of gene mutation, cellular autoimmunity to HSCs
  - Thrombosis: Causes severe morbidity and most common cause of mortality. Mechanism poorly understood
  - Smooth muscle dystonia: Abdominal pain, esophageal spasms, dysphagia, erectile dysfunction. Due to free Hb scavenging of free NO
  - Renal tubular damage due to microvascular thrombosis, iron deposits. Mild-to-moderate pulmonary hypertension
- Dx: Confirm clinical diagnosis with peripheral blood flow cytometry to detect deficiency/absence of GIP-anchored proteins
- Tx: Eculizumab (binds C5 and prevents cleavage, thereby inhibiting terminal complement activity/formation of MAC. ↑ median survival ~20 yr, improves outcomes in hemolysis, thrombosis, renal function, pulmonary hypertension, pregnancy. Increases susceptibility to *Neisseria meningitidis*. (N Engl J Med 2006;355:1233–1243)

Hereditary Spherocytosis (Blood Rev 2013;27(4):167–178; Pediatr Rev 2004;25(5): 168–172)
- HS is the most common RBC membrane disorder (incidence ~1/5,000) and manifests usually as chronic mild hemolysis
- Caused by protein deficits in spectrin assembly → unstable RBC membrane → RBC bilayer membrane lipid loss (microvesicles) → ↓ surface area → spherical RBCs
- Spherocytes circulate poorly in small capillaries, thus are phagocytosed → extravascular hemolysis

- Signs and symptoms:
  - Can present soon after birth (suspect with jaundice onset <24 hr of life or lasts >1 wk). Most severe forms can present in utero
  - In older children, HS manifests as a classic triad of pallor (anemia), jaundice, and splenomegaly with varying severity
  - Children may also have poor exercise tolerance, poor growth, academic difficulties
  - Cholelithiasis due to bilirubin stones
- Dx:
  - CBC: ↓ Hb/HCT, ↑ reticulocytes, ↓ MCV, ↑ MCHC (usually >35 g/dL)
    - Degree of anemia and reticulocytosis help classify severity
  - Markers of hemolysis: ↑ unconjugated bilirubin, ↑ LDH, ↓ Hp
  - Peripheral smear: Spherocytes, polychromasia
  - Flow cytometry (Se 92.7%, Sp 99.1%, PPV 97.8%, NPV 97.8%): RBCs labelled with eosin-5' maleimide (binds RBC proteins) to measure surface area loss
  - Osmotic fragility test (Se 68%): Spherocytes have ↓surface area and swell at higher saline concentrations than normal RBCs
  - Glycerol lysis test, Pink test
  - Targeted protein expression analysis with protein electrophoresis

Autoimmune Hemolytic Anemia (Pediatr Rev 2016;37(6):235–246)
- Primary autoimmune hemolytic anemia
  - No clear cause in 30–40% of cases
  - Classified by autoantibody thermal reactivity
  - Warm agglutinins
    - IgG+, bind at 37°C (less commonly involve C')
    - Mostly affects healthy children, occasionally with preceding fever, viral sx
    - Presents with jaundice, splenomegaly, lab evidence of intravascular hemolysis
    - Dx: DAT: +IgG, -C3
    - Tx: Steroids are first line, secondary therapies include rituximab and splenectomy
  - Cold agglutinins
    - IgM+, bind <30°C, maximally at 4°C
    - Presents with acrocyanosis, hemoglobinuria (extravascular hemolysis)
    - Dx: IgM in vitro deposits C' → DAT: -IgG, +C3
    - Tx: Cold avoidance
    - Paroxysmal cold hemoglobinuria: Rare and self-limited 2/2 cold-reactive IgG (Donath–Landsteiner Ab). Typically preceded by viral infection in children (historically caused by syphilis). Dx: DAT -IgG, +C3, DL test. Tx: Supportive care as it is self-limited
  - Some AIHA will be DAT negative (poor antibody binding esp. w/ cold Ab, IgA, NK cell)
- Secondary autoimmune hemolytic anemia
  - Trigger found in 63% of cases in a national cohort study in France
  - Infection: EBV, CMV, mycoplasma, streptococcus, parvovirus
  - Autoimmune disorders: SLE, JIA
  - Malignancy/hematologic disorders: Hodgkin lymphoma, autoimmune lymphoproliferative disorder, CVID
  - Drugs: Cefotetan, ceftriaxone, piperacillin, fludarabine, diclofenac

HEMOGLOBINOPATHIES

Sickle Cell Disease (South Med J 2016;109(9):495–502)
- Occurs in 1/300–400 African American births
- Multiple genotypes lead to a similar disease of RBC sickling, chronic hemolytic anemia, and vaso-occlusive complications marked by painful vaso-occlusive crises and progressive end-organ injury
  - HbSS (60–65% of infants)
  - HbSC
  - HbSβ[0] and HbSβ[+] (coinheritance of hemoglobin S and β-thalassemia mutation)
- HbSS and HbSβ[0] are generally more severe than HbSC and HbSβ[+]
- Complications:

Pulmonary	Acute chest syndrome (ACS)
	• Leading cause of death
	• Second most common reason for hospitalization
	• Children with asthma are at higher risk for ACS
	• Caused by pulmonary infection, intrapulmonary sickling, or fat emboli from infarcted bone marrow
	• Dx: New infiltrate on CXR AND symptoms of fever, cough, tachypnea, dyspnea, chest pain, or hypoxemia

	• Tx: Supplemental oxygen, pain control, parenteral antibiotics (cephalosporin and macrolide). Transfusion or exchange transfusion in deteriorating patients • Use incentive spirometry to decrease the risk ACS in hospitalized children Pulmonary hypertension • Secondary to chronic pulmonary vascular changes and/or chronic thromboembolic disease (left out asthma, OSA)
Gastrointestinal	Cholelithiasis • Secondary to chronic hemolysis • Pigment stones occur in 10–50% of patients with SCD • Tx: Cholecystectomy Sickle hepatopathy • Presents with severe direct hyperbilirubinemia w/o infection or biliary obstruction to fulminant hepatic failure. • Tx: Emergent exchange transfusion

Neurologic	Vaso-occlusive pain crisis
	• Most common reason for admission
	• *Dactylitis*: VOCs in young children that involves mostly hands and feet, manifest as pain with hand/foot swelling
	• No diagnostic tests exist, though CBC w/ diff, CMP, reticulocytes should be measured
	• Tx:
	  • Mild-moderate: Home treatment with heat, oral hydration, ibuprofen, and oral opiates
	  • Severe: Inpatient management with parenteral opioids, IV hydration, NSAIDs
	  • Avoid transfusion for acute painful episodes, unless there is a clear indication
	
	Chronic pain
	• Defined as pain lasting >3 mo, often begins in adolescents and young adults
	• Multifactorial: can be 2/2 joint avascular necrosis, bone infarction, peripheral neuropathy 2/2 soft tissue chronic inflammation and reperfusion injury
	• In advanced cases of AVN, joint replacement may be considered
	
	Stroke (hemorrhagic or ischemic)
	• Prior to current screening interventions, stroke occurred in 11% of children with SCA before the age of 20. Screen with transcranial doppler ultrasound starting at 2 yr for HbSS, HbSβ⁰
	• Dx: Best tests are MRI to detect acute infarct and MRA to evaluate for arterial stenosis or obstruction
	• Tx: Emergent exchange transfusion
	• Secondary prophylaxis with regular transfusion therapy to maintain HbS ≤30%
	• *Moyamoya syndrome*: Occurs in ~40% of children after ischemic stroke and significantly increases stroke risk. Characterized by stenotic large cerebral artery with development of collateral circulation
	• Primary prevention: Screening with transcranial Doppler yearly for patients 2–16 yr. Those with ↑ cerebral blood flow velocity (>200 cm/s) should receive chronic transfusion therapy to decrease HbS to ≤30%, which decreases risk from 30–3% (N Engl J Med. 1998;339:5–11)
	• *Silent cerebral infarct*: Strokes apparent on MRI w/o associated neurologic deficit
	  • Prevalence increases with age
	  • Most common in HbSS, also occurs with HbSC and HbSβ⁺/⁰
	  • Associated with worse neurocognitive outcomes, ↑ risk of stroke
	  • Dx: MRI at 5 yr for all children with poor school performance
	Tx: Chronic transfusions ↓ incidence of additional SCI, ↓ risk of stroke, but did not improve neurocognitive measures

ANEMIA 8-6

Genitourinary	<u>Priapism</u> • Can affect males at any age • Presents as stuttering pattern or prolonged erection (>4 hr) • Home Tx: Exercise, warmth, ejaculation, urination, hydration, and oral analgesics • If >4 hr, should manage in the ED with IV fluids, analgesics, and urgent urologic management (aspiration/irrigation of the corpus cavernosum ± injection of α-adrenergic agonists) • Goal of tx is to prevent penile fibrosis and erectile dysfunction (ultimately develops in 40% of patients with multiple episodes of priapism)
Infectious	<u>Fever</u> • Given risk of pneumococcal sepsis (incidence lower with PCN ppx), requires careful evaluation • Workup: CBC w/ diff, reticulocytes, blood cultures. UA or CXR if indicated • Tx: Parenteral 3rd generation cephalosporin <u>Aplastic crisis</u> • Most commonly associated with parvovirus B19, though may occur with other viral infections • Viral infection and suppression of erythropoietic precursors leads to severe anemia in pt with increased RBC turnover • May present with acutely with severe symptomatic anemia (syncope, hypotension) or with indolent worsening of anemia • Dx: Severe anemia, low reticulocytes • Tx: Small aliquot transfusions to avoid volume overload
Splenic	<u>Splenic dysfunction</u> • Occurs as early as 5 mo and in most w/ HbSS by 4 yr. Pt w/ HbSC and HbSβ⁺ retail splenic tissue longer • Substantially increases risk of bacteremia with encapsulated organisms (*Streptococcus pneumoniae, Haemophilus influenza, Neisierria meningitidus*) • Primary prevention of infection with penicillin prophylaxis and immunization against pneumococcus, meningococcus, HiB <u>Splenic sequestration</u> • Common cause of acute anemia in young children, occurs prior to complete autoinfarction • Presents with rapidly enlarging spleen 2/2 sequestration of sickled RBCs. May present with shock in severe cases • All parents/caregivers should be trained to examine for splenomegaly • Dx: Splenomegaly, abdominal pain, acute on chronic anemia ↓Hb ≥2 g/dL from baseline, thrombocytopenia • Tx: IV fluid volume support and small volume PRBC transfusion may be indicated (avoid large transfusion as spleen will release sequestered RBCs) • Recurrence is common, thus splenectomy is indicated if recurrent or symptomatic
Renal	<u>Nephropathy</u> • Sickle cell vasculopathy affects renal tubules and glomeruli • Hyposthenuria (inability to concentrate urine) manifests as urinary frequency, nocturnal enuresis • Screen yearly for microalbuminuria starting at 10 yr • Evaluation by nephrology recommended if proteinuria detected or elevated serum creatinine • Some data suggest hydroxyurea and ACEi may be protective
Ophthalmologic	<u>Proliferative retinopathy</u> • More often affects patients with HbSC disease (prev 45%) than HbSS (prev 11%) or HbSβ⁺ (prev 17%) • Vascular disease leads to retinal ischemia, neovascularization (proliferative retinopathy), and eventual retinal detachment • Screen with yearly dilated exams starting at 10 yr

- Health maintenance
  - *Penicillin prophylaxis for pneumococcal sepsis:* Recommended from infancy through at least 5 yr. 84% reduction in pneumococcal sepsis (N Engl J Med 1986;314(25): 1593–1599)
  - *Immunization* against encapsulated bacteria—Streptococcus (N Engl J Med 1977; 297:897–900), HiB (Pediatrics 1989;84(3):509–513), N. meningitidis
  - *Stroke:* Yearly transcranial Doppler ultrasound for HbSS, HbSβ⁰ starting at 2 yr
  - *Retinopathy:* Yearly dilated retinal examinations for all genotypes annually, starting at 10 yr
  - *Nephropathy:* Yearly urinalysis with microscopic analysis starting at 10 yr
- Hydroxyurea
  - Mechanism: Increased HbF production and total Hb, decreases neutrophil count as well as intracellular adhesion, increases NO bioavailability
  - In children, improves outcomes for mortality, VOC, ACS, hospitalization, quality of life
  - Treatment indicated in HbSS and HbSβ⁰ disease, but should be considered with HbSC and HbSβ⁺ if severe symptoms. HU should be started at age 9 months
  - Adverse effects: Neutropenia, thrombocytopenia, rash, nail changes
- Role of transfusion
  - Transfusion to an Hb >10 g/dL while HbS >30% → hyperviscosity and ↑ risk of vaso-occlusion, splenic sequestration, ACS, stroke
  - Risks of chronic transfusion include iron overload and alloimmunization

Sickle Cell Trait (Hematology Am Soc Hematol Educ Program 2015;2015(1):160–167)
- Now detected due to high frequency of universal screening in the U.S.
- Provides protective benefit against malaria
- Clinical complications:
  - *Exercise-related injury:* Manifests as sudden death, rhabdomyolysis, heat-associated collapse. Increased risk at high altitude, with high-intensity exertion
  - *Renal disease:* CKD, hematuria, papillary necrosis. Renal medullary carcinoma occurs almost exclusively in SCT
  - *Increased risk of VTE:* Unclear risk of arterial events (i.e., MI, CVA)
  - Risk of pregnancy complications is controversial

Thalassemias (Pediatr Clin North Am 2013;60(6):1383–1391)
- Normal Hb variants
  - α-globin production (chrom 16) begins in utero, remains constant, binds with β, γ, or δ globin from β-globin locus (chrom 11)
  - HbF (α₂/γ₂): Fetal hemoglobin, present in utero and declines with ↓ γ-globin expression in 1st 6 mo of life
  - HbA (α₂/β₂): Begins late in gestation, reaches adult levels at 1 yr. Predominant hemoglobin
  - HbA₂ (α₂/δ₂): Minor adult hemoglobin. Increased in β-thalassemia syndromes
  - ~5% of global population has ≥1 globin allele variant
  - RBCs of thalassemia carriers are less susceptible to *Plasmodium falciparum*
- **α-Thalassemia**
  - 2/2 decreased or absent production of α-globin chains, severity depends on number of alleles affected
  - **Silent carrier** (1 allele mut [αα/α-]): Asymptomatic
  - **α-Thalassemia trait** (2 alleles mut [αα/–] or [α-/α-]): Generally asymptomatic w/ mild hypochromic microcytic anemia
  - **Hemoglobin H disease** (3 alleles mut [α-/-]):
    - Early production of Hb Bart (γ4) w/ later expression of HbH (β4)
    - HbH unstable, precipitates → ineffective erythropoiesis, oxidative damage leading to ↓ RBC lifespan
    - Generally not transfx dependent w/ moderate microcytic anemia, may need transfx in times of stress (e.g., infection)
    - HbH constant spring assoc w/ nondeletion mutation of α allele: usually transfusion dependent
  - **Hydrops fetalis** [4 alleles mut (–/–)]: Severe, usually fatal phenotype, intrauterine anemia
- **β-Thalassemia**
  - Severity depends on degree of α-globin excess
  - Usually presents as anemia in the first 6 mo and HbF expression declines. Severe forms can present earlier with sx of irritability, jaundice, ↓ growth, abdom distension, and hepatosplenomegaly 2/2 extramedullary hematopoiesis

- **β-thalassemia minor (trait)**
  - One defective β-globin gene
  - Significant microcytosis, hypochromia, with mild anemia
  - HbA_2 usually mildly elevated (>3.5%), may have HbF elevation
  - No treatment required
- **β-thalassemia intermedia**
  - Due to a many different β-globin mutations, with less significant disease severity
  - Significant microcytic hypochromic anemia
  - Usually do not require chronic transfusions, only during times of stress
- **β-thalassemia major (Cooley Anemia)**
  - No β-globin chains are produced
  - Generally presents after 6 mo in previously healthy children with ↓ HbF
  - Marked microcytic hypochromic anemia + α-chains precipitate → ineffective erythropoiesis, hemolytic anemia
  - Sx: Irritability, growth failure, extramedullary marrow expansion → maxillary hyperplasia & frontal bossing, jaundice/chronic hemolysis
  - Tx: Chronic transfusion

MACROCYTIC ANEMIAS

(Nathan and Oski's Hematology and Oncology of Infancy and Childhood. 8th ed. 2015:293–307, 344–381, 1555–1613.e30)

Megaloblastic Anemia
- Def: Macrocytic anemia with megaloblastic appearance of nucleated cells, suggests asynchrony of nuclear/cytoplasmic maturation
- Can manifest as anemia (or pancytopenia if severe) with reticulocytopenia
- Primarily caused by folate and vit B_{12} deficiency. Less commonly inborn errors of folate/B_{12} transport or metabolism, hereditary orotic aciduria, or 3-phosphoglyceride dehydrogenase deficiency
- Neutrophils are characteristically hypersegmented (>6 lobes)
- **Folic acid deficiency**
  - Deficiency is rare in children 2/2 mandated folate fortification of food
  - Risk factors: Dietary insufficiency (exclusive goat milk feeding, alcoholism in adults), poor absorption (celiac dz, IBD), ↑ requirements (low stores in premature infants, chronic hemolysis, pregnancy), antifolate medications (e.g., MTX), other medications (anticonvulsants, OCPs)
  - Dx: Serum folic acid level (high Se, low Sp), will ↓ after 2–3 wk of poor intake. Consider RBC folate (more stable, can be falsely ↑ by, B_{12} def, Fe def, hemolysis)
  - Tx: Folic acid supplementation
- **Vit B_{12} deficiency**
  - Normal absorption: Digested vit B_{12} bound by intrinsic factor (IF) → Vit B_{12}: IF absorbed by apical brush border (most abundant in distal ileum)
  - Sx: Symmetric myelopathy of posterior and lateral columns and peripheral neuropathy 2/2 demyelination → axonal degeneration → gliosis (may be irreversible, feet affected first), atrophic glossitis, stomatitis. Infants may have prominent GI sx, recurrent infx if severe
  - Risk factors: ↓ intake (vegan, exclusive breast feeding esp. if B_{12} def mom), ↓ IF:Vit B_{12} formation (acid suppression, pernicious anemia, chronic gastritis, partial/whole gastrectomy), ↓ absorption (ileitis [Crohn dz, bacterial overgrowth], resection/bypass of ileum, parasitic infx)
  - Dx: Serum cobalamin level (falsely ↓ by folate def, pregnancy, OCPs, obesity), elevated methylmalonic acid level (98% Se)
  - Tx: Cobalamin repletion (initial dose usually parenteral)

Chronic Illness
- Renal failure 2/2 ↓ EPO
- Hypothyroidism ↓ RBC mass 2/2 ↓ O_2 req, can be normocytic. ↓ EPO
- Chronic liver disease ± acanthocytes 2/2 ↑ chol in RBC membrane

Myelodysplastic Syndromes
- Heterogeneous group of clonal disorders that are rare in children, leading to ineffective hematopoiesis → cytopenias → hematopoietic cell dysplasia (trilineage). May transform to AML
- Risk factors: Alkylating agents, Fanconi anemia, Diamond–Blackfan anemia, Shwachman–Diamond syndrome and other bone marrow failure syndromes, chromosomal breakage d/o
- Sx of marrow failure: Fatigue, fever, malaise

- **Exam:** Pallor, bruising/petechiae. HSM/lymphadenopathy are rare
- **Labs:** Macrocytic anemia, reticulocytopenia, neutropenia, thrombocytopenia
- **Smear:** Teardrop cells, poikilocytosis, circulating myeloblasts, progranulocytes, Pelger–Huët cell
- **BM Bx:** Nl or ↑ cellularity, trilineage dysplasia. Karyotype ± FISH analysis to detect clonal abnormalities
- **Tx:** Controversial. Primary tx is HSCT ± AML-type chemotherapy prior, depending on risk and burden of disease

Diamond–Blackfan Anemia (Hematol Oncol Clin North Am 2009;23(2):261–282; Pediatr Clin North Am 2013;60(6):1291–1310)
- One of a rare group of genetic bone marrow failure syndromes. Mixed inheritance
- Genetically and clinically heterogeneous, manifest as erythroid failure, congenital abnormalities, and cancer predisposition
- Underlying defect is defective ribosome biogenesis 2/2 mutations in ribosome subunit genes
- Median age of presentation and diagnosis is 8 and 12 wk, respectively. 93% present in 1st yr of life
  - Rarely presents in adulthood
- Presentation:
  - Red cell hypoplasia ± other cytopenias (uncommon)
  - 30–47% p/w congenital anomalies. Dysmorphic facies (classically Cathie facies) and triphalangeal thumbs
  - May have +family hx of DBA
- **Ddx:** Need to rule out TEC, which should resolve. DBA suggested by congenital abnormalities, age <1 yr, +FHx of DBA, ↑ erythrocyte adenosine deaminase activity (eADA) (↑ in 85%, Se 84%, Sp 95% unknown mechanism), macrocytosis (may be seen in stress erythropoiesis w/ TEC recovery), ↑ HbF
- **Dx:**
  - **Labs:** Reticulocytopenia macrocytic anemia, other cytopenias uncommon. ↑ eADA. ↑ HbF
  - **BM Bx:** ↓ or absent erythroid precursors
  - Confirm w/ gene mutational analysis
- **Tx:**
  - **Corticosteroids:** Prednisone 2 mg/kg po daily to goal of Hb >10 g/dL and reticulocytosis (79% will respond)
  - Blood transfusions if steroid refractory or development of toxicity from corticosteroids
    - May need Fe chelation therapy
  - HSCT is controversial
- **Cancer risk:** Unclear mechanism. 25% lifelong risk of AML. OR 5.4 calculated risk of cancer (hematologic malignancy and solid tumors)
- **Prognosis:** ~20% will enter remission and tolerate steroid wean, ~75% by age 10 yr. Pregnancy, OCPs may contribute to relapse

PLATELET DISORDERS

THROMBOCYTOPENIA

Definition
- Plt <150 × 10^9/L

Clinical Manifestations (Pediatr Rev 2005;26(11):401–409)
- Risk of bleeding is proportional to degree of thrombocytopenia
  - Primary hemostasis is maintained with a Plt >75 × 10^9/L
  - Spontaneous bleeding occurs when Plt <50 × 10^9/L. Surgery acceptable if Plt >50 × 10^9/L
  - Significant hemorrhage rarely occurs with Plt >20 × 10^9/L
  - Most life-threatening hemorrhage occurs with Plt <10 × 10^9/L

Platelet Count (×10^9/L)	Signs and Symptoms
>100	None
50–100	Minimal—bleeding after major trauma, surgery
20–50	Mild—cutaneous symptoms
5–20	Moderate—cutaneous symptoms and mucosal bleeding
<5	Severe—↑ risk for spontaneous CNS hemorrhage

(Adapted from: Pediatr Rev 2005;26(11):401–409)

- Sx: Petechiae, purpura, mucosal bleeding (gingival), epistaxis, menorrhagia, GI bleeding, hematuria, CNS hemorrhage

Etiology (Nelson Textbook of Pediatrics, 20th ed. 2016:2400–2408e)
- Decreased production
  - Congenital: Thrombocytopenia-absent radius syndrome, Fanconi anemia (→ aplastic anemia), Amegakaryocytic thrombocytopenia
  - Bone marrow disorders: Aplastic anemia, MDS, bone marrow infiltrative d/o, osteopetrosis, nutritional (Fe, folate, vit B_{12}) deficiencies, drug induced, radiation, neonatal hypoxia, placental insufficiency
- Destruction
  - Immune: ITP, NAIT, SLE, Evan syndrome, antiphospholipid syndrome, drug-induced (heparin), posttransfusion purpura
  - Nonimmune: TMA (DIC, HUS, TTP), infection (HIV, viral infections, bacteremia, fungemia), eclampsia/HELLP syndrome, congenital heart disease
- Sequestration: Hypersplenism (most commonly 2/2 chronic liver dz, storage dz), Kasabach Merritt syndrome, burns, hypothermia
- Pseudothrombocytopenia: In vitro clumping of platelets due to EDTA anticoagulant

Historical Factors (Pediatr Rev 2005;26(11):401–409)
- Neonates
  - Thrombocytopenia manifests as generalized petechiae, ecchymoses, mucosal bleeding
  - Age of onset informs diagnosis in neonatal period (Pediatr Rev 2000;21(3):95–104)
    - **Fetal:** Alloimmune, congenital infx (TORCH), chromosomal d/o, autoimmune, congenital
    - **Early onset (<72 hr):** Placental insufficiency (preeclampsia, IUGR, DM), asphyxia, perinatal infection (E. coli, GBS, H. flu), DIC, alloimmune, autoimmune, thrombosis, Kasabach–Merritt syndrome, metabolic d/o, congenital, bone marrow replacement (congenital leukemia)
    - **Late onset (>72 hr):** Late-onset sepsis, NEC, congenital infections, autoimmune, Kasabach–Merritt syndrome, metabolic d/o, congenital
- Older infants and children thrombocytopenia is most commonly 2/2 ITP
  - Thrombocytopenia typically presents as bruising on torso, arms, and legs (especially pretibial-surface
  - Large soft tissue hematomas, hemarthroses, or muscle hemorrhage are uncommon
  - Thrombocytopenia may be entirely asymptomatic. The presence of symptoms, preceding illnesses, may suggest underlying d/o

Workup
- Initial:
  - CBC w/ diff
  - Peripheral smear
  - PT, PTT, INR
- Secondary:
  - Mean platelet volume (MPV)
  - Platelet function tests (e.g., closure time (PFA-100), aggregation studies)
  - Plt Ab studies, below
- Bone marrow aspirate/biopsy may be needed

Neonatal Alloimmunoe Thrombocytopenia (NAIT) (Pediatr Rev 2005;26(11):401–409; Br J Haematol 2012;156(2):155–162; J Thromb Haemost 2009;7(Suppl 1):253–257; Br J Haematol 2013;161(1):3–14)
- Epi: Frequency of 1/2,000
- Presents as severe thrombocytopenia in the first 24–48 hr of life
- Mediated by transplacental passage of maternal antiplatelet antibodies to paternal human platelet antigens (HPA)
  - HPA-1a is the most common antigen, present on 98% of platelets
  - Anti-HPA-1a and -5b Ab are responsible for 95% of NAIT in Caucasian infants
- Sx: Unexplained bruising, petechia, bleeding. May be asymptomatic
- Feared complication is ICH:
  - Occurs in 10–20% of untreated cases. Most common cause of ICH in term infants
  - Can occur from 20-wk gestation to days of life. ≤80% occur prenatally. Greatest postnatal risk is in 1st 96 hr
  - Associated with severe neurodevelopmental problems (e.g., cerebral palsy)
- Subsequent pregnancies (with same father) are more severe 2/2 maternal alloimmunization

- Dx:
  - Primarily clinical. May send serology for maternal HPA antibodies
  - Obtain head US to screen for ICH (MRI to further define extent, eval post fossa) (Pediatr Blood Cancer 2017;64(12))
- Ddx includes maternal ITP w/ transplacental passage of maternal antiplatelet Abs
  - Mediated by maternal autoantibodies to common platelet Ags
  - Typically less severe thrombocytopenia
  - Postnatal hemorrhage is uncommon. No intrauterine hemorrhage
  - Tx: Observation, IVIG if thrombocytopenia severe
  - High recurrence rate in subsequent pregnancies
- Tx:
  - Random donor platelet transfusion, may only transiently ↑ plt.
    - Prophylactic thresholds vary. Transfusion indicated if bleeding
    - Maternal derived HPA-compatible plt may be obtained via pheresis in resistant or prolonged cases. Must be washed to remove anti-HPA Ab in serum and irradiated
  - IVIG
    - May be used as monotherapy in moderate-severe thrombocytopenia (30–50 × 10^9) without bleeding
  - Typically resolves within 6–12 wk
- Prevention: Mothers at high risk are managed with intrapartum IVIG, prednisone, with elective C-section delivery (↓ birth trauma)

Immune Thrombocytopenic Purpura (Pediatr Rev 2000;21(3):95–104; Blood 2011;117:4190–4207; Hematol Oncol Clin North Am 2010;24(1):249–273; J Pediatr Hematol Oncol 2013;35(1):1–13)

- Caused by markedly ↓ platelet lifespan 2/2 humoral antibody response against platelet Ags → Lifespan ↓ from 8–10 d → hr. Auto-Abs may interfere with production as well
- Epi:
  - Peak incidence 2–6 yr, male = female
  - Incidence 1/10,000 children
- Sx: Acute onset of petechiae, purpura in otherwise well child
  - Often presents in few weeks following a viral infx
  - Bleeding (epistaxis, mucosal bleeding) presents in <1/3 of pt. GI and GU bleeding occur in <10%
  - Fever, ↓ wt, pallor, pain, LAN, HSM, jaundice suggest *against* ITP
- Exam:
  - Widespread petechiae and ecchymoses (bruising in expected distribution, e.g., pretibial)
  - Bruises all in similar stage (acute onset)
  - No lymphadenopathy, hepatosplenomegaly
  - Oral mucosal ("wet") petechiae may suggest need for more aggressive tx.
- Labs:
  - Severe, isolated thrombocytopenia (<20 × 10^9/L in 75% of pt)
  - Nl WBC, Hb/HCT, LDH, uric acid
  - Leukopenia, anemia, ↑ LDH, ↑ uric acid, ↑ PT/PTT suggest against ITP
  - MPV nl or ↑
  - *H. pylori* testing not recommended
  - BM Bx is unnecessary with classic ITP
- Tx
  - Children w/o bleeding or mild bleeding (skin only—bruising and petechia): Observation regardless of plt count
  - Children w/ bleeding: IVIG × 1 or a short course of corticosteroids (IVIG with ↑ plt faster)
    - Not effective: Plt transfusion (rapidly cleared) and pheresis (Abs rapidly reappear)
    - Anti-D Ig tx not advised if ↓ Hb 2/2 bleeding or hemolysis (↑ risk AIHA). May be used in Rh+ nonsplenectomized pt.
  - Splenectomy is not recommended as initial tx for acute ITP, consider for chronic ITP
  - Children with significant bleeding:
    - Rare (ICH incidence 1/1,000), though catastrophic (ICH → ~50% mortality). Massive plt transfx indicated
    - Little data for tx. In addition to above, consider high-dose corticosteroids, plasmapheresis, and splenic artery embolization (prior to splenectomy)

- Children w/ bleeding, not responsive to initial tx:
  - Rituximab
  - Splenectomy
  - High-dose dexamethasone
- Injury prev:
  - "Common sense" approach to injury prevention, e.g., avoid contact sports
  - Avoid NSAIDs, antiplatelet agents
- Chronic ITP
  - Def: Thrombocytopenia 2/2 ITP lasting >6 mo
  - Some may have secondary ITP 2/2 immunologic d/o: Evans syndrome, SLE, autoimm. lymphoproliferative syndrome
  - If other features present consider for alternate dx (e.g., BM Bx, evaluation for SLE)
  - Tx:
    - Observation, may not require tx if no bleeding, acceptable plt
    - Rituximab or high-dose dexamethasone
    - Splenectomy (~60–80% response rate). High risk (↑ risk of thrombosis/infection), consider only after 12 mo or if significant bleeding, intolerance of tx, ↓ QOL
    - Thrombopoietin receptor agonists

Thrombotic Microangiopathies (N Engl J Med 2014;371:654–666; Pediatr Clin North Am 2013;60(6):1513–1526)
- Clinical features: Microangiopathic hemolytic anemia, thrombocytopenia, end-organ injury due to vascular damage 2/2 arteriolar/capillary thrombosis
- **Hemolytic uremic syndrome** (Pediatr Rev 2001;22(11):365–369)
  - Generally preceded by an infection with shiga-like toxin producing *E. coli* in previously healthy children
  - Most common cause of acute renal failure in children
  - Multiple types:
    - Typical (D+) HUS: Usually associated with *E. coli* 0157:H7, preceded by watery/bloody diarrhea. Recurrence rare
    - Atypical (D-) HUS: Associated with *S. pneumoniae*, drugs, primary glomerulopathies, and familial collagen/vascular disorders. Prodrome is rare. Commonly recurs (~50%)
  - Typically presents in a previously healthy child with pallor (anemia) and petechiae (thrombocytopenia) ~5–7 d after onset of abdominal pain and bloody diarrhea followed by progressive renal failure/anuria
  - Dx:
    - Anemia, thrombocytopenia, schistocytes on smear
    - ↑ LDH, ↑ bilirubin, ↓ Haptoglobin
    - DAT negative
    - ↑ BUN and creatinine
    - UA: Hematuria and proteinuria
  - Tx: Supportive care
    - Anemia: RBC transfusion for acute symptomatic anemia
    - Thrombocytopenia: Cautious use of platelets prior to procedures given risk of exacerbating microthrombi
    - HTN: Short-acting hypertensives
    - Renal failure: Fluid management and electrolyte repletion. Hemodialysis or peritoneal dialysis when unable to manage fluid overload or electrolyte imbalances medically
    - Atypical HUS: Eculizumab treatment is associated with improvement in renal function. (N Engl J Med 2013;368:2169–2218)
- **Thrombotic thrombocytopenic purpura** (Curr Opin Pediatr 2013;25(2):216–224)
  - Rare in children
  - Caused by deficiency of ADAMTS13 protein (congenital or acquired)
  - Acquired TTP (antibody-mediated)
    - May be associated with connective tissue disease or preceding infection
    - Often presents with fever, neurologic abnormalities, thrombocytopenia/microangiopathic hemolytic anemia and acute renal failure
    - Dx: Undetectable ADAMTS13 activity only during acute episode, detectable anti-ADAMTS13 IgG
    - Tx: Urgent plasma exchange, corticosteroids. Rituximab may be considered in severe or treatment-resistant cases
  - Congenital TTP (Upshaw–Schulman syndrome)
    - Presents in neonatal period to teenage years
    - Early onset disease associated with increased risk of recurrence (up to 80%)

- Labs: ADAMTS13 undetectable, anti-ADAMTS13 IgG negative, DAT negative, schistocytosis, ↑ LDH, ↑ bilirubin, ↓ haptoglobin
- Confirm dx with genetic testing
- Tx: Plasma infusion to replace ADAMTS13, renal replacement therapy if needed. Neonates may require exchange transfusion for hyperbilirubinemia

Disseminated Intravascular Coagulation (Blood 2018;131:845–854)

- Not a primary disorder, secondary to an underlying condition
- Characterized by systemic coagulation, thrombosis in small/medium vessels. Bleeding occurs due to consumption of clotting factors and consumptive thrombocytopenia
- Triggers:
  - Severe infections (bacteremia, malaria, hemorrhagic fevers)
  - Malignancies (especially APML)
  - Trauma
  - Obstetric diseases (abruptio placentae, amniotic fluid embolism)
  - Vascular malformations
  - Severe immune reactions
- Bleeding occurs in a minority of patients. Lab abnormalities include:
  - Prolonged PT, aPTT, INR
  - Thrombocytopenia
  - ↑ D-dimer or fibrin split products
  - ↓ fibrinogen (may be masked by elevated acute phase reactants)
  - Peripheral smear: Schistocytes, thrombocytopenia
- Tx: Treat the underlying condition
  - If bleeding: Platelet transfusion (thrombocytopenia), FFP (prolonged PT/aPTT), cryoprecipitate (hypofibrinogenemia)
  - If clotting or purpura fulminans: Therapeutic anticoagulation
  - No bleeding/thrombosis: Consideration of prophylactic anticoagulation

PLATELET FUNCTION DISORDERS

(Pediatr Rev 2000;21(3):95–104; Thromb Haemost 2008;99(2):253–263)

Disease	Clinical Features	Platelet Function
Wiskott–Aldrich syndrome	• X-linked inheritance • Eczema • Recurrent infections	• Plt 20–100 • Plt very small on smear • ↓ MPV
Bernard–Soulier syndrome	• Autosomal dominant • Ecchymoses • Gingival/GI bleeding	• ↓ Plt, ↓ Plt adhesion • Large plt on smear (may be > lymphocytes)
May–Hegglin anomaly	• Autosomal dominant • Most asymptomatic	• Giant plt on smear • Inclusion bodies in WBC (Dohle bodies)
Gray platelet syndrome	• Usually mild bleeding • Early myelofibrosis	• Plt enlarged, pale, and oval on smear
Quebec platelet disorder	• Autosomal dominant • ↓ bleeding w/ antifibrinolytic tx • Plt transfx not useful	• ↓ Plt aggregation (↓ w/ epi) • ± thrombocytopenia • Plt w/ ↑ urokinase-type plasminogen activator
X-linked thrombocytopenia	• X-linked inheritance • No immune problems	• ↓ Plt • ↓ MPV
Glanzmann thrombasthenia	• Variable inheritance and severity • Failure of adhesion	• ↓ Plt adhesion

(Adapted from Pediatr Rev 2000;21(3):95–104)

Congenital Thrombocytopenias (Hematol Oncol Clin North Am 2009;23(2):321–331)

- Congenital amegakaryocytic thrombocytopenia
  - Autosomal recessive, 2/2 thrombopoietin (TPO) receptor c-Mpl mutation
  - Presents at birth with severe thrombocytopenia, no congenital abnormalities
  - ↑ risk of myelodysplasia, AML. Progresses to bone marrow failure
  - Dx: ↑ TPO level, BM Bx w/ ↓ or absent megakaryocytes, otherwise nl. Plt w/ nl size and granularity
  - Tx: Supportive care, plt transfx, HSCT
- Thrombocytopenia with absent radii (TAR)
  - Various inheritance patterns, unknown molecular basis. Female > male

- Def: Thrombocytopenia at birth + bilateral radius aplasia w/ present thumbs
  - Additional congenital abnormalities often present
- Plt count often spontaneously recovers to near nl by 1st yr of life. No progression to marrow failure
- Dx: Clinical, ↑ TPO, BM Bx w/ ↓ size and ↓ # of megakaryocytes. Plt w/ nl size and granularity
- Tx: Supportive care while marrow recovers

LEUKOCYTE DISORDERS

LEUKOCYTOSIS

- Pattern in elevation is useful to indicate underlying cause in conjunction w/ clinical context

WBC Lineage	Associated Conditions
Basophils	Allergic conditions, leukemias
Eosinophils	Allergic conditions, dermatologic conditions, eosinophilic esophagitis, idiopathic hypereosinophilic syndrome, malignancy, medication reaction, parasitic infection
Lymphocytes	Acute/chronic leukemias, hypersensitivity reaction, infections (viral, pertussis)
Monocytes	Autoimmune diseases infections (EBV, fungi, protozoan, rickettsia, tuberculosis), splenectomy
Neutrophils	Bone marrow stimulation, chronic inflammation, congenital causes, infection, medication induced (e.g., corticosteroids), reactive, splenectomy

(Adapted from Am Fam Physician 2015;92(11):1004–1011)

NEUTROPENIA

(Pediatr Rev 2003;24(2):52–62; Pediatr Rev 2013;34(4):173–184;
Pediatr Rev 2008;29(1):12–24)

- Def: Decrease in the absolute neutrophil count (ANC) = (%neutrophils + %bands) × WBC count
  - Mild: ANC 1.0–1.5 × 10^9/L, moderate: ANC 0.5–1.0 × 10^9/L, severe ANC <0.5 × 10^9/L
  - Severity predicts risk of pyogenic infection w/ prolonged neutropenia

Clinical Manifestations
- Generally present due to infectious complications. Most commonly skin/soft tissue (cellulitis, abscess, furunculosis), pneumonia, bacteremia
- Recurrent oral ulcers, gingivitis, stomatitis, perirectal inflammation/infection, AOM.
- Most common pathogens: S. aureus, gram-negative organisms (esp. enteric), S. epidermidis, streptococci, enterococci.
- Sx: Fever, erythema, pain, warmth. ↓ neutrophils → ↓ exudate formation, ↓ abscess formation, ↓ LAN

Etiology
- Infection
  - Mechanism: Margination of neutrophils, consumption at site of infection, ± marrow suppression w/ decreased production (esp. preterm pt with ↓ marrow reserves)
  - Viral infx is a common cause of neutropenia in children (RSV, varicella, influenza A&B, measles, rubella)
    - Occurs in the first 24–48 hr of illness, lasts 3–7 d (period of viremia)
  - Also seen w/ bacterial, protozoal, rickettsial, and severe fungal infx
- Drug induced – mediated by multiple mechanisms
  - Immunologic: Induced Ab-mediated destruction
    - Acute (often symptomatic) onset, days to weeks after initiation. +Ab studies
  - Toxic: Direct neutrophil toxicity
    - Insidious (often asymptomatic) onset, weeks to months after initiation
  - Hypersensitivity:
    - Onset weeks to months after initiation, may be w/ systemic sx (fever, rash, LAN) and organ involvement (hepatitis, nephritis, pneumonitis, aplastic anemia)

- Immune mediated (alloimmune, autoimmune)
- Bone marrow failure (aplastic anemia, replacement w/ malignancy).
- Ineffective myelopoiesis, usually 2/2 nutritional deficiency (B_{12}, folate, Cu, Zn)
- Hypersplenism
- Intrinsic disorders (cyclic neutropenia, severe congenital neutropenia, Shwachman–Diamond syndrome, dyskeratosis congenita)

Workup
- Hx: Constitutional sx, current illnesses (viral infx, critical illness), recurrent infection, medication exposures, medical history, FHx
- Exam: Stature, nutrition, any congenital abnormalities of skeleton, skin (albinism, eczema, wars), nails, hair, lymphadenopathy, hepatosplenomegaly
- Labs:
  - Initial: CBC w/ diff to confirm neutropenia, peripheral smear w/ neutrophil morphology and evaluation for blasts/immature neutrophils. Reticulocytes to eval marrow fx
    - Repeat CBC after illness to ensure improvement
    - Weekly CBC w/ diff if cyclic neutropenia is suspected
  - Follow-up investigation depends on suspected d/o
    - *DAT*: Eval for AIHA, present in autoimmune d/o (e.g., Evans, SLE), may see ↑ monos
    - *ANA, anti dsDNA Ab*: If SLE is suspected
    - *IgM, IgG, IgA, lymphocyte subsets*: If underlying immunodeficiency suspected (e.g., SCID, IgA def, CVID, hyper-IgM syndrome)
    - *Antineutrophil Ab*: If autoimmune or autoimmune neutropenia suspected
    - *Vit B_{12}, serum/RBC folate*: If nutritional deficiency suspected
  - Bone marrow examination if severe neutropenia, pancytopenia, or persistent neutropenia to r/o malignancy and BM failure syndromes

Immune Neutropenia

Disorder	Mechanism	Clinical Features	Diagnosis/Treatment
Alloimmune neonatal neutropenia	Transplacental transfer of maternal alloantibodies against child's neutrophils	• Sx w/in 1st 2 wk • Severe neutropenia • Sx: Delayed cord separation, fever, infx (cellulitis, pna)	• + antineutrophil Ab • Tx: supportive care w/ atbx. • Neutrophils usually recover by 7 wk
Autoimmune neutropenia of infancy and childhood	Autoreactive Antineutrophil Ab May be 2/2 "molecular mimicry" after viral infx	• Dx btwn 5–15 mo • Neutropenia may be very severe • 90% w/o recurrent infx	• +antineutrophil Ab (may need to repeat) • Tx: Supportive care w/ atbx, steroids, G-CSF • 95% of infants have remission in 7–30 mo
Secondary immune neutropenia	Autoreactive antineutrophil Ab 2/2 underlying autoimmune d/o	• Assoc w/ Evans syndrome, SLE, RA, systemic sclerosis • May have pancytopenia	• +antineutrophil Ab • Tx: Supportive care w/ atbx, treat underlying disease • May need G-CSF

Cyclic Neutropenia
- Autosomal dominant, incidence 0.6–1/1,000,000
- Caused by mutated neutrophil elastase gene
- Characterized by cyclic episodes of severe neutropenia
  - Mean oscillatory period is 21±4 d, neutropenia lasts 3–6 d
- Sx: Oral ulcers, stomatitis, skin infections (or more severe lung, GI, oral, vagina, rectal infx) when neutropenic
- Dx: 2–3x/wk CBC w/ diff for 2 mo to establish pattern, confirm w/ genetic testing.
  - Monocytes typically cycle in a reciprocal fashion (i.e., ↑ monos when ↓ neutrophils)
  - Periodicity helps differentiate from severe congenital neutropenia
- Tx: G-CSF
  - Changes oscillatory cycle to every 9–11 d w/ 1 d of neutropenia
  - ↓ risk of death from *C. perfringens*, gram-negative infx

Severe Congenital Neutropenia
- Autosomal dominant or recessive (Kostmann disease), incidence of ~1/1,000,000
- Characterized by arrest in myeloid maturation at the promyelocytic state, occurs sporadically. Onset in infancy

- Sx: Symptomatic neutropenia w/ infection. Severe infx (esp. PNA, deep abscesses) common
- Labs: Profound neutropenia (<0.2 × 10⁹/L), ↑ monocytes, ↑ eosinophils, mild thrombocytopenia, mild anemia of chronic inflammation
- Dx: Bone marrow (arrest in promyelocytic stage), genetic testing (may have neutrophil elastase mutations)
- Tx: G-CSF. HSCT if MDS/AML develops
- ~10% ↑ Risk of MDS and AML

COAGULATION DISORDERS

BLEEDING DIATHESES

Clinical Manifestations (Pediatr Rev 2016;37(7):279–291)
- Easy bruising, esp. over bony prominences and btwn ages 1–10 yr
- Defective primary hemostasis (i.e., platelets): easy bruising, petechiae, mucosal bleeding, bleeding after trauma or surgery. Hematomas, hemarthroses uncommon
- Defective secondary hemostasis (i.e., coagulation factors): delayed bleeding (surgery, trauma, deep lacerations), hemarthroses, muscle and soft tissue hematomas
- Neonates: Umbilical stump oozing, oozing from venipuncture/heel stick, bleeding after circumcision, large cephalohematoma or caput succedaneum w/o birth trauma, ICH (if term or near-term)

Workup
- History:
  - Age of onset (expect early in life)
  - Hx, frequency, and severity of previous unprovoked/spontaneous bleeding
  - Hx of bleeding after procedures/surgeries
  - Family hx of bleeding, menorrhagia
- Physical exam: Presence and distribution of bruising (consider nonaccidental trauma), presence of lymphadenopathy, splenomegaly, hematomas, joint swelling
- Labs:
  - Initial: CBC w/ diff, peripheral smear, PT, aPTT, fibrinogen, thrombin time
  - Secondary: von Willebrand antigen and activity, FVIII, VIX. May need further factor testing
  - PT/aPTT can be erroneously prolonged 2/2 erroneous processing (inadequate amount, delay in testing) as well as lupus anticoagulant (often follows viral infx)

Vitamin K Deficiency Bleeding (Blood Rev 2009;23(2):49–59)
- Formerly known as hemorrhagic disease of the newborn
- Classic VKDB: Occurs days 1–7 of life. Sx: Bleeding from GI tract, umbilical stump, epistaxis, circumcision bleeding, skin bleeding. Risk factor: Exclusive breastfeeding
- Early VKDB: 1st 24 hr, associated with maternal drugs that interfere with vit K metabolism (warfarin, anticonvulsants, antituberculous drugs). Sx: Superiosteal, skin, intracranial, intrathoracic, or intra-abdominal bleeding
- Late: Occurs after 1 wk (peak 3–8 wk), 2/2 exclusive breast feeding, cholestasis, underlying disease (e.g., biliary atresia α-1 antitrypsin deficiency, cystic fibrosis), chronic diarrhea, antibiotic therapy
- Primary Tx is prevention with parenteral vit K at birth
- Tx bleeding with vit K if bleeding, add FFP if severe

Hemophilia A and B (Pediatr Rev 2013;34(7):289–295; Pediatr Rev 2016;37(7):279–291)
- X-linked recessive inheritance
- Hemophilia A is a deficiency in FVIII, affects 1/5,000 males, ~1/3 due to spontaneous mutation
- Hemophilia B is a deficiency in FIX, affects 1/30,000 males
- Hemophilia C is a deficiency in FXI
- Disease severity is a function of clotting factor activity
  - Mild (activity >5%): Bleeding w/ trauma or surgery (significant)
  - Moderate (activity 1–5%): Bleeding w/ trauma or surgery (mild)
  - **Severe (activity <1%): Spontaneous bleeding** and bleeding with trauma, surgery
- 90% present in 1st yr of life (esp. when learning to walk)

- Sx: Excessive bruising, intramuscular hematoma, mucosal bleeding, hemarthroses (Knee > elbow > ankle > shoulder > wrists > hips)
  - Sx of intramuscular hematoma: Swelling, warmth, ↓ ROM, pain. May develop "target joints" with recurrent bleeding
  - Mild hemophilia may only present after significant surgeries
- Dx:
  - Labs will initially show ↑ PTT, w/ normal PT, bleeding time, thrombin time
  - Mixing study → PTT normalizes
  - Measurement of factors VIII, IX (and XI if indicated) w/ genetic confirmation
    - FVIII activity is similar btwn adults and infants. FIX activity is ↓ in infants (may only be able to dx after 6 mo if mild hemophilia B)
- Tx:
  - Ppx: lifelong tx with prophylactic factor replacement superior compared to episodic tx ↓ hemarthroses, ↓ joint replacement. Usually 1–4× weekly
  - Bleeding: Factor replacement, based on severity of hemorrhage
    - Mild hemophilia A bleeding: May tx w/ DDAVP if proven responsive (↑ FVIII, ↑ vWF), not all respond
    - Mild mucosal bleeding: Tx w/ antifibrinolytic tx (tranexamic acid, aminocaproic acid)
- Complications:
  - Infections dz have ↓ with advent of factor replacement
  - Inhibitors: IgG against factor replacement, tx w/ prolonged high-dose factor infusion
  - Arthropathy: 2/2 repeated hemarthroses, may need surgical intervention

von Willebrand Disease (N Engl J Med 2016;375:2067–2080)
- Most common bleeding disorder
- Affects 0.6–1.3% of population
- Three types:
  - Type 1: 70–80% of cases, autosomal dominant, quantitative ↓ vW factor
  - Type 2: ~20% of cases, autosomal dominant or recessive, dysfunctional vW factor → Nl/↓ vWF Ag but ↓↓ vWF activity, subdivided:
    - 2A: Defective vWF multimer assembly → absent high molec weight (HMW) multimers → ↓ platelet adhesion. May respond to DDAVP
    - 2B: ↑ affinity of vWF to GPIb → ↑ and spontaneous binding to plt. DDAVP contraindicated. May have thrombocytopenia 2/2 ↑ plt clearance
    - 2M: ↓ vWF platelet adhesion or collagen binding
    - 2N: ↓ vWF to FVIII binding → FVIII (may be misdiagnosed as hemophilia)
  - Type 3: <5% cases, autosomal recessive, complete absence of circulating vWF w/ severe bleeding
- Sx depend on level of vWF activity
  - Most common sx: mucosal bleeding, epistaxis, menorrhagia
  - 60–80% of pt have bleeding after surgeries or dental extractions
  - Menorrhagia (vW dz is dx in 5–20% of women presenting w/ menorrhagia), bleeding after minor wound, GIB, muscle hematomas, postpartum bleeding
  - Hemarthroses are rare (except type 2N)
- Dx: Personal hx of bleeding ± Fhx of bleeding w/ consistent labs
  - Labs: ↓ vWF, vWF activity (level of vWF-dependent plt adhesion by ristocetin assay), FVIII activity (frequently ↓)
    - vWF level affected by age, exercise, inflammation (acute-phase reactant), pregnancy, and menstrual cycle
  - vWD will have abnormal vWF, vWD activity, or both. vWF <5IU/dL indicates type 3 dz
- Tx:
  - Menstrual losses: OCPs, IUD
  - Antifibrinolytics (tranexamic acid or aminocaproic acid)
  - Type 1: Desmopressin
  - vWF-FVIII concentrate or recombinant vWF
  - Type 3: vWF-FVIII concentrate or recombinant vWF

THROMBOTIC DISORDERS

(Pediatr Clin North Am 2013;60(6):1443–1462)
- Thrombosis in children occurs in bimodal distribution: Neonatal and adolescent periods

Clinical Manifestations
- Thrombophilia presents in children w/ multiple manifestations: Venous/arterial thrombosis, pulmonary embolism, arterial ischemic stroke, cerebral sinus venous thrombosis

Etiology
- Acquired risk factors (Virchow triad: Stasis, hypercoagulable state, vascular injury):
  - Stasis:
    - Neonates: CVCs, congenital heart dz
    - Older children: Congenital IVC abnormalities, May–Thurner synd (lt iliac v. compressed by rt common iliac a.), Paget–Schroetter synd (thoracic outlet synd), immobility
  - Vascular injury (neonates and older children): CVCs
  - Hypercoagulable state:
    - Neonates: CVC, cyanotic heart dz, sepsis, dehydration, TPN, maternal antiphospholipid Ab
    - Older children: Antiphospholipid syndrome, malignancy, nephrotic syndrome, TPN, dehydration, sepsis, varicella infx, autoimmune disease
  - **Antiphospholipid syndrome**
    - Due to Ab against phospholipid–protein complexes → ↑ risk stroke, VTE, arterial thrombosis
    - May be primary or secondary (autoimmune dz, infection)
    - Dx: Thrombosis and + antibodies (lupus anticoagulant, anticardiolipin, β2GP), must be + on repeat testing ≥12 wk later
- Inherited thrombophilia syndromes: Protein-C def, protein-S def, ATIII def, Factor V Leiden mut (homo/hetero), prothrombin gene mutation, hyperhomocysteinemia, Lp(a) elevation

Workup
- Testing is strongly indicated in all children with unprovoked, spontaneous thrombosis, less clear when provoked (e.g., catheter-related)
- Labs: Protein C, protein S, antithrombin, factor V Leidin mutation
- Protein C, protein S and AT can be **decreased in the setting of acute thrombosis** → repeat once off of anticoagulation

Inherited Thrombophilia
- **Protein C and S deficiency**
  - Prot C&S are vit K dependent. Activated protein C binds protein S → FVa and FVIIIa degradation
  - Prevalence: Protein C deficiency 0.6%, protein S deficiency 1.2%. ↑ risk of stroke w/ OR 8.76 (protein C deficiency) and 3.2 (protein S deficiency)
  - Can be heterozygous, homozygous. Homozygous dz is life threatening in 1st days of life
    - Homozygous protein C deficiency → purpura fulminans w/ DIC. May have major vessel (renal v., vena cava) thrombosis
    - Heterozygous dz rarely presents in neonatal period
  - Dx: Measure protein C&S activity. May be ↓ by age (check after 6 mo), acute thrombosis (consumptive), and anticoag. Recheck once off of anticoagulation
  - Tx: LMWH, warfarin
- **Antithrombin (AT) deficiency**
  - AT irrev inactivates thrombin, FXa (also IXa, Xia, XIIa, FVIIa)
  - ↑ stroke risk (OR 7.06), venous, arterial thrombosis
  - Dx: AT activity (↓ in newborn esp. preterm, thrombosis, anticoagulation)
  - Tx: Long-term anticoagulation, recombinant antithrombin
- **Activated protein C resistance (factor V Leiden mutation)**
  - Most common congenital thrombophilia d/o. Occurs on 3–8% Caucasians
  - FVL mut → resistant to cleavage by AT, autosomal dominant
  - ↑ risk of VTE (hetero ↑ 3×, homo ↑ 30×), stroke (OR 3.26). OCPs ↑ risk 30–60×.
  - Children usually do not have VTE unless additional risk factor(s) present
  - Dx: Genetic testing
- **Hyperhomocysteinemia:** Assoc. w/ vascular wall injury
- **Lp(a):** Elevated if >30 mg/mL, present in 7–10.3% of population. Competes w/ plasminogen binding on endothelial cells 2/2 (molecular mimicry). ↑ risk 1st VTE (OR 4.49), stroke (OR 6.27)

PANCYTOPENIA

(Pediatr Rev 2016;37(3):101–113)

- Definition: ↓ ≥2 cell lines, may be acute (sepsis, DIC, hemolysis) or chronic (below)
- Sx are dependent on underlying condition and presence of anemia, thrombocytopenia, leukopenia (above)

Etiology
- ↓ marrow function
  - Congenital: Fanconi anemia, dyskeratosis congenita, Schwachman–Diamond syndrome, storage disorders, mitochondrial disorders, other congenital BM failure syndromes
  - Acquired: Leukemia, aplastic anemia, nutritional deficiency, metastatic malignancy/invasion of marrow, MDS, sepsis, congenital TORCH infections
- ↑ cellular destruction
  - Congenital: ALPS, congenital hemophagocytic lymphohistiocytosis (HLH), other congenital immunodeficiencies
  - Acquired: PNH, HLH, macrophage activating syndrome
- Sequestration of cells 2/2 splenomegaly

Workup
- CBC w/ diff, peripheral smear, reticulocytes, AST, ALT, bili, LDH, uric acid
- Bone marrow aspirate/biopsy with cytogenetics indicated to evaluate for leukemia, other dz
- Further testing as indicated by clinical history/context
  - Nutritional deficiency: folic acid, vit B_{12}, copper, ceruloplasmin, zinc
  - Infx: HAV, HBV, HCV, CMV, EBV, parvovirus, HSV, VZV, HHV6, HIV, adenovirus
  - Flow cytometry for PNH if suspected
  - Lymphocyte subsets, immunoglobulins
  - Pregnancy test
  - Autoimmune workup if suspected

Aplastic Anemia (Pediatr Clin North Am 2013;60(6):1311–1336; Pediatr Rev 2016;37(3):101–113)
- Rare (~2/1,000,000 in N Am) though life-threatening dz 2/2 immune-mediated destruction of hematopoietic stem cells
  - Need to r/o infx (viral), nutritional deficiency (Cu, vit B_{12}, folic acid def), drugs (NSAIDs, atbx, anticonvulsants, gold salts, chloramphenicol), chemicals (benzene, insecticides/pesticides), radiation, pregnancy, GVHD, congenital bone marrow failure, PNH, HLH
- Dx:
  - Bone marrow bx w/ decreased cellularity
    - Moderate/nonsevere AA (NSAA): ↓ BM cellularity, peripheral cytopenias
    - Severe AA (SAA): BM cellularity <25% + 2/3 of (neut <500 × 10^6/L, plt <20,000 × 10^6/L, retic <60,000 × 10^6/L)
    - Very severe AA (vSAA): Criteria of SAA + neut <200 × 10^6/L
  - R/o other causes, above
- HLA typing should be obtained early for HSCT donor search
- Tx:
  - Supportive care w/ tx of febrile neutropenia, antimicrobial ppx. Minimize transfx to avoid alloimmunization
  - Early therapeutic tx improves outcomes: immunosuppressive tx (IST) <4 wk, HSCT <12 wk
    - If HLA identical sibling available, progress w/ HSCT (>90% 5-yr survival)
    - IST: ATG + cyclosporine + corticosteroids. Check response at 12th wk. May taper or add tx
    - HSCT: If no response to IST at 12th wk and unrelated donor available

Fanconi Anemia (Pediatr Rev 2016;37(3):101–113; Pediatr Clin N Am 2013;60:1291–1310)
- Rare (1/100,000) multiorgan disease 2/2 mut gene in FA pathway (≥18 genes)
- Signs/Sx: Presentation is variable, FA can affect development of all organs
  - Progressive bone marrow failure, timing varies
  - Congenital abnormalities: Short stature, skeletal abnormalities, VACTERL, café au lait spots, GU malformations
    - ~1/3 of pt have no developmental abnormalities (dx as adolescent, adult)

- Lifetime cancer risk 20% (AML most common)
- Dx: Positive chromosome breakage test, confirm w/ genetic testing
- Tx: Surveillance/supportive care. HSCT once transfusion-dependent BM failure or AML

Shwachman–Diamond Syndrome (Pediatr Rev 2016;37(3):101–113; Pediatr Clin N Am 2013;60:1291–1310)
- Rare (~1/76,000) 2/2 SBDS mutation, pancytopenia assoc. w/ exocrine pancreatic insufficiency, skeletal abnormalities, developmental delay
- Sx: Most common presenting sx are chronic (malabsorptive) diarrhea and FTT
  - Progressive BM failure in early childhood, bone abnormalities vary in severity though w/ metaphyseal dystosis, palate/dental abnormalities
- Dx: Clinical, confirm w/ genetic testing
- Tx: Surveillance and supportive care w/ transfusions, pancreatic enzymes. HSCT when transfusion-dependent or MDS/AML develop

LYMPHADENOPATHY

(Pediatr Rev 2008;29(2):53–60; Pediatr Rev 2013;34(5):216–227)

Definitions
- Lymphadenopathy (LAN) refers to lymph nodes (LN) of abnormal size, number, consistency
- Normal size: Cervical and axillary LN ≤1 cm, inguinal LN ≤1.5 cm
- Generalized LAN defined as ≥2 separate nodal groups/sites

Differential Diagnosis
- After bx, dx are usually: 50% reactive hyperplasia, 30% granulomatous dz (cat scratch dz, scrofula [MTB or NTM]), 13% malignancy (67% of malignancies are Hodgkin dz)
- Infection:
  - Bacterial: LAN can be local (staph, strep, *bartonella*, anaerobes) or generalized (leptospirosis, lymphogranuloma venereum, typhoid fever)
  - Viral infx (generalized LAN): Herpesviruses (EBV, CMV, HSV), HIV, HBV, measles, mumps, rubella, dengue
  - Fungal: Coccidioides, Cryptococcus, histoplasma
  - Protozoa: Toxoplasmosis, leishmaniasis
  - Spirochetes: Lyme dz, syphilis
  - Mycobacterial: Tuberculous and nontuberculous
- Malignancy: Leukemia (ALL, AML), lymphomas, metastatic dz
- Inflammatory/autoimmune dz: ALPS, CGD, dermatomyositis, RA, HLH, Langerhans cell histiocytosis, serum sickness, SLE, angioimmunoblastic LAN with dysproteinemia, Kikuchi dz, Kawasaki dz, sarcoidosis
- Endocrine: Addison dz, hypothyroidism
- Medications (generalized): PCN, cephalosporins, phenytoin, carbamazepine

Workup
- History/Exam
  - Hx of constitutional sx (fever, night sweats, weight loss, anorexia, fatigue), exposures, medications
  - Age: <5 yr more likely infectious, lymphoma more likely in adolescents
  - Duration of LAN (↑ concern if present or no change in 4–6 wk)
  - Palpable LN may be normal (44% of healthy children <5 yr have palpable LN)
  - Tender LN usually indicate infxn (esp if warm, indurated, erythematous, fluctuant). Malignancy may be painful 2/2 intranodal hemorrhage
  - Soft and mobile LN usually benign. Hard, firm, rubbery, immobile LN are assoc w/ cancer
  - Hepatosplenomegaly is less common in infection
- Labs:
  - CBC w/ diff, ESR, LDH
  - Infectious w/u depends on sx: TST (eval for scrofula), monospot/EBV titers, HIV, CMV, *bartonella*
- Imaging:
  - CXR if chronic and generalized or if respiratory sx (cough, dyspnea, CP) to eval for mediastinal LAN
  - US (less Se, more Sp) or CT may help dx abscess. CT helps eval neck deep spaces
- If bacterial lymphadenitis suspected, tx accordingly. If fails tx, obtain TST
- Obtain *excisional biopsy* (FNA has high false −, no architectural detail) if:
  - Supraclavicular LAN
  - Size: >2 cm, ↑ over 2 wk, not ↓ after 4 wk
  - LAN is hard, rubbery, immobile/matted
  - Sx ↑ suspicion for malignancy: Constitutional sx, fever>1 wk, ↓ wt, ↑ ESR, cytopenias, ↑ LDH, mediastinal widening on CXR (LAN), cervical LAN w/o assoc infx, hepatosplenomegaly
- Monitor over time. May need subsequent biopsies to establish dx
- Avoid steroids prior to definitive dx (may mask leukemia, lymphoma, and delay dx)

ACUTE LEUKEMIAS

(Pediatr Rev 2010;31(6):234–241; Nathan and Oski's Hematology and Oncology of Infancy and Childhood. 8th ed. 2015:1527–1613)

Symptoms and Initial Workup
- Difficult to differentiate leukemic subtypes on presentation
- Presentation
  - Sx: Constitutional sx (night sweats, fevers, ↓ wt, anorexia, fatigue) pallor, bleeding, bruising, infxns, bone pain (in 25% 2/2 marrow infiltration). May have respiratory compromise 2/2 mediastinal LAN (~10%, usually w/ T-cell ALL)
    - May have sx of leukocytosis (HA, dyspnea) if ↑↑ WBC
  - Exam: Pallor, petechiae, ecchymoses hepatosplenomegaly, LAN 2/2 leukemic infiltration
    - May have signs/sx of infxn
    - Examine for testicular involvement (sanctuary site)
- Workup:
  - CBC w/ diff, reticulocytes, peripheral smear, LDH, uric acid, BMP, liver function test, coagulation studies
    - CBC, diff, and smear may reveal cytopenias, ↓ retic
    - May present w/ DIC in acute promyelocytic leukemia (APL)
    - ↑ cell turnover → ↑ LDH, ↑ uric acid
    - May have ↑ BUN/Cr 2/2 renal leukemic infiltration and urate-mediated tubular injury
    - Presence of blasts on smear suggests dx, not always observed
  - When leukemia is suspected, a bone marrow biopsy, aspirate, and flow cytometric evaluation of marrow is needed
  - Once diagnosis is established, LP usually performed to assess for CNS disease

Acute Lymphoblastic Leukemia (N Engl J Med 2015;373:1541–1552; Pediatr Clin North Am 2015;62(1):61–73)
- **Epidemiology/risk factors**
  - Yearly incidence 30/1,000,000 in pt <20 yo. Peak incidence at 3–5 yr, M > F (55:45%)
  - Primary genetic risk is trisomy 21, infreq 2/2 radiation, or chemical exposure
  - May be B-cell or T-cell lineage
- **Prognostic factors**
  - Clinical features:
    - Age (1–<10 yr std risk, <1 or >10 high risk), WBC (<50,000/mm^2 std risk, >50,000/mm^2 high risk), sex (female favorable, male averse)
    - Age and WBC risk stratification useful for B-cell ALL, less for T-cell ALL
  - Cell lineage: B-cell w/ more favorable prognosis, T-cell less so (esp w/ early T-cell precursor ALL)
  - Cytogenetics:
    - Favorable: Cryptic t(12;21), high hyperdiploidy
    - Poor: Philadelphia chromosome (Ph) t(9;22), hypoploidy (<44 chrom), 11q23, intrachromosomal amplification of chrom 21
  - Early response to tx: Detected in marrow specimen via PCR and flow cytometry
    - Response after 1 wk of prednisone: Good <1,000 blasts/mm^3, poor >1,000 blasts/mm^3
    - After 1–2 wk of multiagent chemo: Favorable M1
    - Minimal residual dz (MRD) during/end of induction: Low (<0.01%) or undetectable is favorable, MRD ≥0.01% is unfavorable (worse prognosis w/ ↑ MRD)
      - MRD is the most important prognostic factor used for risk stratification
      - MRD ≥0.01% → ↑ risk of tx failure and death by 3–5×
    - MRD at 3–4 mo: Low (<0.01%) or undetectable is favored. Persistent MRD helps select pt for add'l chemotherapy in 1st remission, those appropriate for HSCT
  - Involvement of "sanctuary sites" (hard to penetrate w/ chemotx): CNS or testis
  - Adherence to maintenance therapy: If <90% adherent to tx → ↑ risk of relapse 4×
- **Diagnosis:**
  - Defined as >25% lymphoblasts in bone marrow on biopsy (<25% = stage-IV non-Hodgkin lymphoblastic lymphoma)
  - ~20% of children will have visible blasts in centrifuged CSF, mostly asymptomatic

- **Treatment**
  - Induction (4–6 wk): Steroid (prednisone or dexamethasone), vincristine, asparaginase, ± an anthracycline (doxorubicin or daunorubicin)
    - CNS dz: Intrathecal (IT) chemotherapy (can include methotrexate, cytarabine, hydrocortisone), CNS radiation may be used (↓ in indications 2/2 adverse effects on cognition and secondary neoplasms, used only in highest risk)
    - Almost all enter remission, but universally will relapse w/o consolidation tx
  - Consolidation (6–8 mo): Consolidates remission and prevents CNS leukemia
    - Intensive combination chemotherapy, specific regimens vary w/ protocol
    - Often uses chemotherapy not used in induction therapy. May include MTX, mercaptopurine, thioguanine, cyclophosphamide, etoposide, cytarabine, IT therapy
  - Maintenance (18–30 mo): Lower intensity
    - Usually consists of oral 6-MP (or thioguanine) and oral methotrexate (weekly)
- **Prognosis**
  - Prior to chemotherapeutics, median survival was ~3 mo
  - Current survival is 85% (event free) and 90% (overall survival [OS]) at 5 yr

Acute Myelogenous Leukemia (Hematol Oncol Clin North Am 2010;24(1):35–63)
- **Epidemiology/risk factors**
  - Yearly incidence of 5–7/1,000,000, peak incidence at 2 yr (11/1,000,000)
    - Trimodal incidence: 2 yr, adolescence, adults ~55 yr
  - Only 15–20% of acute leukemia cases, but responsible for 30% of deaths
  - No sex predominance
  - Risk factors: Most children w/ AML have no identifying RF
    - Prior radiation or chemotherapy, esp alkylating agents and intercalating topoisomerase II inhibitors
    - Genetic d/o: Trisomy 21, Fanconi syndrome, severe congenital neutropenia, Shwachman–Diamond syndrome, DBA, NF1, Noonan syndrome, dyskeratosis congenital, familial platelet disorder, congenital amegakaryocytic thrombocytopenia, ataxia-telangiectasia, Klinefelter syndrome, Li–Fraumeni syndrome, Bloom syndrome
    - Acquired BM failure: Aplastic anemia, MDS, PNH
- **Presentation:** Some presenting factors differ from ALL
  - Children w/ APL are more likely to p/w DIC
  - Chloromatous tumors (granulocytic sarcomas, myeloblastomas), tumors of myeloblasts, most common in orbit and epidural space. Can occur anywhere
  - Leukemia cutis: Subcutaneous nodules, "blueberry muffin" spots
  - CNS involvement more common, ~15%
- **Diagnosis and classification**
  - Defined as >20% myeloblasts in bone marrow
  - FAB classification: M0 (AML w/ minimal differentiation), M1 (AML w/o maturation), M2 (AML w/ maturation), M3 (APL), M4 (acute myelomonocytic leukemia), M5 (acute monocytic leukemia), M6 (acute erythrocytic leukemia), M7 (acute megakaryoblastic leukemia)
- **Prognostic factors**
  - Clinical: Age (↑ age assoc. w/ ↓ survival), tumor burden (WBC, hepatosplenomegaly), race and ethnicity (Caucasian children w/ ↑ survival compared to Latino and African American children), overweight and underweight children have worse prognosis
  - FAB classifications are no longer used
  - Cytogenetics:
    - Favorable t(8;21), inv(16), NPM1 and CEBPA mut
    - Poor: Monosomy 5, del(5q), monosomy 7, FLT3-ITD mut
  - MRD: Detectable MRD assoc 2/ ↑ risk of relapse and death
- **Treatment**
  - Induction: Based on high cumulative dose anthracycline and/or cytarabine, multiagent therapy pending protocol
  - Postremission tx: W/o postremission tx, almost all pt will relapse
    - Based on three strategies:
      - Autologous HSCT: No benefit over chemotherapy observed, no current US trials
      - Allogeneic HSCT: ↓ relapse rate, but OS comparable to chemo due to morb/mort of HSCT
      - Continued chemotherapy: Choice of chemotherapeutic agent and number of cycles is controversial
  - APL: Often present w/ DIC. Tx with *all-trans* retinoic acid (ATRA) and intensive chemotherapy
- **Prognosis:** Complete remission obtained in 80–90% with OS of 60%

LYMPHOMA

(Nathan and Oski's Hematology and Oncology of Infancy and Childhood. 8th ed. 1626–1672.e15)

HODGKIN LYMPHOMA

(Mayo Clin Proc 2015;90(11):1574–1583)

Epidemiology/Classification
- Rare, incidence of 9,000/yr in children and adults
- Hodgkin lymphoma should be viewed as 2 discrete clinical entities, classic Hodgkin lymphoma and nodular lymphocyte-predominant Hodgkin lymphoma (NLPHL)

Classic Hodgkin Lymphoma
- **Definition:** Characterized by presence Hodgkin and Reed–Sternberg cells (large, abundant slightly basophilic cytoplasm, ≥2 nucleolar lobes/nuclei, prominent eosinophilic nucleolus)
  - Often malignant cells are a minority in an inflammatory infiltrate (lymph, eosinophils, PMNs, plasma cells) w/ collagen formation and fibroblasts
  - If dx in patient <15 yo, then is childhood Hodgkin lymphoma
- **Classification:** Based on biopsy (characteristics of inflammatory infiltrate)
  - Lymphocyte-rich Hodgkin lymphoma (LRHL): Rare in peds
  - Lymphocyte-depleted Hodgkin lymphoma (NSHL): Rare in peds (assoc w/ old age, AIDS)
  - Mixed-cellularity Hodgkin lymphoma (MCHL): Prevalent in children (or elderly pt) and usually presents in advanced stage, may have poor prognosis
  - Nodular sclerosis Hodgkin lymphoma (NSHL): Usually presents in adolescents and young adults w/ localized dz in mediastinum and supraclavicular or cervical LAN
- **Epidemiology:** 92–95% of pt with HL; bimodal incidence (15–34, >60 yr) w/ peak at 15–20 yr. M > F (2–3:1) in childhood dz, M = F in older pt
- **Risk factors:**
  - Childhood CHL: ↑ family size, ↓ SES
  - CHL in adolescents, adults: ↓ family size, ↑ SES
  - EBV associated in 40%
- **Clinical presentation:**
  - Sx: Persistently enlarged LN (most commonly supraclavicular or cervical), usually painless and firm/rubbery. Fatigue and anorexia are common
    - 30% have constitutional sx in prior 6 mo. Pel–Ebstein fever = evening fever that ↑ w/ time
  - May have severe pruritus (can precede LAN)
  - Pain at sites of dz with alcohol ingestion, unclear mechanism
  - LN may ↑ or ↓ in size, but atbx have no effect
  - Often spreads to contiguous LNs/sites
  - LAN may be incidental finding on physical
  - Of 2/3 pt w/ cervical adenopathy, >2/3 have intrathoracic disease (may cause airway obstruction)
  - Extranodal sites: Spleen, liver, lungs, bone marrow
- **Diagnosis:**
  - Labs: CBC w/ diff, ESR, BMP, ALP, albumin, LDH
    - Nonspecific CBC (may have mild anemia, ↓ lymph, ↑ PMNs, ↑ monos, ↑ eosinophils), ↑ ESR and CRP, ↑ ferritin, ↑ Cu. If bone involvement ↑ ALP. ↑ LDH
  - Initial imaging: CXR (eval for mediastinal LAN, which ↑ risk of general anesthesia)
  - Excisional biopsy (fine needle or core inadequate, they do not maintain architecture)
  - Staging: CT of neck/chest, CT or US or MRI of abdomen and pelvis, PET scan (more Se than conventional imaging)
    - May need repeat biopsies
    - Bone marrow biopsy (may avoid in stages IA, IIA)
- **Ann Arbor staging classification:**
  - Designate: A (No B sx), B (+B Sx, def as fever [T >38°C for ≥3 d], drenching night sweats, ↓ wt by ≥10% in past 6 mo)
  - Stage I: Single LN region (I) or single extralymphatic organ or site (IE)
  - Stage II: ≥2 LN regions on same side of diaphragm (II) or single extralymphatic organ or site and its regional LN on same side of diaphragm (IIE)
  - Stage III: LN regions on both sides of diaphragm (III). If III involves spleen (IIIs), if contiguous involvement of extralymphatic organ or site (IIIE), or involves both (IIISE)
  - Stage IV: Involvement of ≥1 extralymphatic organs or tissues ± LN involvement

- **Treatment:**
  - Poor prognostic indicators: ↑ stage, +B sx, bulky dz, anemia, ↑ ESR, latent EBV infx, males
  - Tx determined by risk stratification using stage ± clinical factors, depending on protocol
    - Low risk: 2–4 cycles multiagent chemotherapy (limits anthracyclines, alkylating agents, etoposide/teniposide to ↓ adverse effects) + low-dose involved-field radiation
    - Intermediate–high risk: 4–6 cycles of multiagent chemotherapy, usually w/ combo of ABVD (doxorubicin, bleomycin, vinblastine, dacarbazine) and MOPP (mustargen, vincristine, procarbazine, prednisone) + increased intensity radiation tx (esp if bulky dz)
    - PET at dx and after 2 cycles of chemotherapy to assess response to therapy. Subsequent therapy may be intensified for patients who do not have a complete metabolic response on PET scan

Nodular Lymphocytic-Predominant Hodgkin Lymphoma

- **Definition:** Monoclonal B-cell neoplasm characterized by small lymphocytic infiltrate with associated follicular dendritic network with lymphocytic and histiocytic cells
- **Epidemiology:** 5–8% of pt with HL, peak incidence at 13 yr. M > F (3:1). Not assoc. w/ EBV
- **Presentation:** Generally more indolent, presents w/ localized peripheral LAN. Mediastinal involvement rare. Often spreads in noncontiguous pattern. 5–12% transform to non-Hodgkin lymphoma (NHL)
- **Diagnosis and staging:** Similar to that for CHL
- **Treatment:**
  - Little data. Pt w/ low-stage disease may be amenable to curative resection w/o chemo
  - Often lower-intensity regimens used give favorable prognosis, low disease burden
  - Current investigation into rituximab ongoing

NON-HODGKIN LYMPHOMA

(J Clin Oncol 2015;33(27):2963–2974)

Definition/Classification
- Lymphoid origin malignant neoplasms that are not classified as Hodgkin lymphoma
- Heterogeneous group of malignancies w/ varying classification systems
- 2008 WHO classification widely used, though others exist (Rappaport, Lukes–Collins, Kiel)

Epidemiology/Risk Factors
- 7% of all cancer in pt <20 yr (4th most common)
- Children have different distribution of subtypes compared to adults. Mostly B-cell, high grade
- Incidence in children varies by age, subtype, location. In the U.S. annual incidence by age is:
  - >5 yr: 5.9/1,000,000; 5–14 yr: ~10/1,000,000; Adol: 15/1,000,000; Adults: 150/1,000,000
  - Incidence higher in Caucasians than African Americans
- Subtype varies with age as well:
  - <3 yr: NHL very rare
  - Young children: Burkitt lymphoma, Burkitt leukemia
  - >15 yr: Diffuse large B-cell lymphoma (DLBCL), anaplastic large-cell lymphoma (ALCL)
- 2× more likely in females (varies by subtype)
- Risk factors:
  - Immunodeficiency (acquired or inherited) is strong RF for NHL
    - Inherited: Ataxia telangiectasia, Wiskott–Aldrich syndrome, SCID, Nijmegen breakage syndrome, X-linked lymphoproliferative dz, ALPS, CVID, X-linked hyperimmunoglobulin M syndrome
    - Acquired: HIV/AIDS, immunosuppressive medications

Presentation
- Most common sx is painless LAN (may be rapidly progressive)
- Most common sites: Cervical LN, abdomen (including liver, spleen), mediastinum, head & neck (e.g., tonsils, sinuses, bony structures). Can affect bones, soft tissues, kidney, skin. CNS involvement not uncommon
- Severity of sx varies widely, depends on size and location
- Signs/sx depend on site:
  - Intraabdominal dz: Bowel obstruction, abdominal distension, N/V, GIB
  - Mediastinal dz: Airway obstruction, cough, SOB, orthopnea
  - CNS dz: Headache, vision changes, CN palsies, paresis, ↑ ICP

Diagnosis
- Labs: CBC w/ diff, LDH, BMP, LFTs, coags
- CXR to evaluate for mediastinal dz
- Excisional biopsy with immunocytochemical and flow cytometric studies
- Evaluation for organ involvement/metastasis:
  - CT chest, CT/MRI of abdomen (pending presenting sx)
  - Craniospinal imaging and LP if any concern for CNS disease
  - PET commonly performed for staging

Staging
- St. Jude staging system
  - Stage I: Single extranodal tumor or 1 anatomic nodal area (excludes mediastinum and abdomen)
  - Stage II: Single extranodal tumor w/ regional LN involvement or ≥2 nodal areas on same side of diaphragm or 2 single extranodal tumors ± regional LN involvement on same side of diaphragm or GI tumor ± LN involvement that is completely resectable
  - Stage III: 2 single extranodal tumors on opposite sides of diaphragm, ≥2 LN areas on both sides of diaphragm, any intrathoracic tumor, extensive intraabdominal disease, any paraspinal or epidural tumor
  - Stage IV: Any of the above + involvement of CNS, bone marrow, or both

Mature B-cell Lymphomas
- **Burkitt lymphoma (BL)** (Lancet 2012;379:1234–1244)
  - Epidemiology: >80% of B-cell NHL in children
  - Most common sites: Abdomen (60–80%), head/neck. Endemic BL most often head & neck
  - Advanced stage (BM and/or CNS dz) in 20–25% of children
    - If >25% blasts in BM = Burkitt leukemia.
  - Fastest growing tumor (doubling time 24–48 hr)
  - WHO classifications: Endemic (90% EBV associated), sporadic, immunodeficiency-related
- **Diffuse large B-cell lymphoma (DLBCL)**
  - DLBCL represents 10–20% of B-cell NHL in children
  - Most commonly present with nodal disease (peripheral, mediastinal, intraabdominal)
  - Commonly presents in an advanced stage
  - BM and CNS involvement rare
- **Prognostic indicators:**
  - Poor: CNS dz (blasts in CSF, CN palsy, IC mass), mediastinal dz, poor response to reduction tx, presence of minimal disseminated dz in BM, unfavorable genetics (+7q, del(13)q)
- **Symptoms:** Depend on site of presentation
  - Rarely BL causes leadpoint → intussusception
- **Treatment:** BL and DLBCL treated similarly
  - Risk stratification: Important for planning. Involves stage, LDH, CNS involvement
  - Localized dz: Surgical resection +2 cycles moderate intensity chemo (e.g., cyclophosphamide, vincristine, prednisolone, doxorubicin)
  - Advanced disease: More intensive tx required
  - Evaluation of role of rituximab currently underway
- **Prognosis:**
  - Generally excellent with event-free survival (EFS) >90% for stages I–III and even IV w/o CNS involvement
  - Pt w/ CNS dz or Burkitt leukemia have worse prognosis
    - Burkitt leukemia: EFS and OS almost 80%
    - CNS dz: EFS 70–75%
- Survival similar btwn BL and DLBCL, except DLBCL may relapse after up to 3 yr
  - Relapse is rare, though with dismal outcomes (cure rate <30%)

Lymphoblastic Lymphoma (LL)
- T- and B-cell subtypes, morphologically indistinguishable
- Distinguished from ALL by <25% BM lymphoblasts (less likely to have cytopenias)
  - Cellular marker: Terminal deoxynucleotidyl transferase (TdT)
- **T-cell LL:**
  - 80–90% of LL
  - Generally presents with mediastinal tumor (90%) in advanced stage (III–IV in >90%)
    - BM involved in ~30%, CNS involved in ~5%

- **B-cell LL:**
  - 10–20% of LL
  - Generally presents with limited stage: Isolated LN, bone, or skin (most commonly scalp)
- Sx depend on site and degree of involvement
- **Treatment:** Usually based on ALL-like protocols w/ ↑ CNS intensity
- **Prognosis:** Low stage >90%, stage III–IV ~80%
  - Relapse, refractory disease in 10–20% (mostly T-cell w/ mediastinal dz), dismal prognosis

Anaplastic Large-Cell Lymphoma (ALCL)
- 10–15% of NHL in peds
- Two forms:
  - Systemic ALCL: LN involvement (peripheral, mediastinal, intraabdominal), usually w/ constitutional sx and extranodal involvement
  - Cutaneous ALCL: Remains confined to skin, excellent prognosis
- **Presentation:**
  - Sx: Almost all w/ LAN, indolent, LN may ↑ and ↓ in size
    - Can be present w/ fevers, B-sx
  - 60% present w/ extranodal dz (skin/soft tissue, bone, lung)
    - Skin/soft tissue (most common): One or multiple skin lesions (bluish nodules, ulcerated lesions, or red-yellow papillomatous lesions) or subcutaneous/muscle soft-tissue tumors
    - Bone: Lesions vary from osteolytic lesions to large bone tumors
  - CNS dz rare (1–4%)
- **Treatment:** No consensus on optimal therapy
  - EFS is 70–76% across many diverse tx protocols
  - Uniquely, ALCL recurrence is sensitive to chemotherapy

CNS TUMORS

(Nathan and Oski's Hematology and Oncology of Infancy and Childhood, Ch 57, 1779–1885.
e42; Pediatr Rev 2013;34(2):63–78; Pediatr Clin North Am 2015;62(1):167–178;
Nelson Textbook of Pediatrics, 20th ed. 2453–2460.e1)

Epidemiology
- 2nd most common malignancy in children (after leukemia), 25% of pediatric malignancies. Most common solid tumor
- Leading cause of cancer-related death in children
- ~4,100 malignant CNS tumors diagnosed each year
- Incidence (malignant and nonmalignant) of ~5/100,000 (~3/100,000 malignant)
  - Peaks 0–4 yr (5.77/100,000), lowest at 10–14 yr (4.78/100,000)
  - Slight male predominance
- Age adjusted mortality rate 0.6/100,000 → 500 deaths/yr
- Tumor location varies with age:
  - <1 yr: Supratentorial (choroid plexus complex tumors, teratomas)
  - 1–10 yr: Infratentorial (juvenile pilocytic astrocytoma, medulloblastoma)
  - >10 yr: Supratentorial (diffuse astrocytoma most common)

Symptoms/Presentation
- Most common sx is headache (1/3 of pt w/ newly diagnosed CNS tumor). 1/3 will also have nausea, vomiting
- Progressive headache, N/V (may be early in the morning), gait imbalance should raise suspicion for ↑ ICP
  - Most common presentation of posterior fossa tumors
  - Young children: Macrocephaly (40%), emesis (30%), irritability (25%), lethargy (20%)
- Sx may indicate tumor location:
  - Supratentorial: Lateralized defects (weakness, sensory), language changes, seizures (40% of cortical tumors). Infants will have premature hand preference
  - Infratentorial and midline: HA, N/V, papilledema
  - Infratentorial: Ataxia, coordination changes, gait changes, blurred vision, diplopia, nystagmus
  - Brainstem: Gaze palsy, CN palsy, upper motor neuron deficits
  - Optic pathway: Visual changes, oculomotor pathway disturbances, nystagmus

- Suprasellar/3rd ventricle: Neuroendocrine deficits (obesity, ↓ growth, DI, galactorrhea, delayed/precocious puberty, hypothyroidism)
- Diencephalic syndrome: FTT and emaciation in spite of normal caloric intake in happy infant
- Pineal region: Parinaud syndrome = upward gaze paresis, pupils react to accommodation not light, nystagmus to convergence or retraction, eyelid retraction

Workup/Diagnosis
- Modality depends on urgency of presentation
- **CT scan:** Faster. If AMS, behavioral changes, ↓ cognition w/ HA, N/V, ataxia. CT w/o contrast should be obtained (contrast rarely needed, unless abscess is in ddx)
  - Sensitive to detect blood, calcification
  - CT can miss brainstem, cerebellar, and suprasellar tumors as well as infiltrative tumors
- **MRI ± gadolinium:** Standard of care, most sensitive modality. Has limitations (sedation required, poor sensitivity to blood, dental braces affect images)

POSTERIOR FOSSA TUMORS

Tumor (Relative Incidence)	Presenting sx	Dx	Prognosis
Medulloblastoma (35–40%)	2–3 mo HA, N/V, truncal ataxia	Hetero- or homogeneously enhancing 4th ventricle mass; may be disseminated	65–85% survival, dependent on stage/type. Poorer in infants (20–70%)
Cerebellar astrocytoma (35–40%)	3–6 mo limb ataxia, HA, N/V	Cerebellar hemisphere mass, usually with cystic & solid components	90–95% survival in totally resected pilocytic type
Brainstem glioma (10–15%)	1–4 mo diplopia, unsteadiness, weakness, CN palsies	80%: Diffusely expanded, minimally or partially enhancing mass. 20%: More focal or cervicomedullary lesion	>90% mortality in diffuse tumors; better in localized
Ependymoma (10–15%)	2–5 mo unsteadiness, HA, diplopia, facial asymmetry	Usually enhancing 4th ventricular mass w/ cerebellopontine predilection	>75% survival in totally resected lesions
Atypical teratoid/rhabdoid (ATRT) (>5%, 10–15% of infant malig. tumors)	As in medulloblastoma, primarily in infants assoc w/ facial weakness, strabismus	As in medulloblastoma, but often more laterally extended	≤20% survival in infants

(Adapted from Pediatr Clin North Am 2008;55:121–145)

MEDULLOBLASTOMA

Epidemiology
- Most common malignant brain tumor. 15% of all pediatric brain tumors, 1/3 of posterior fossa tumors
- Bimodal distribution (peaks at 3–4 and 8–9 yr). Median age of dx is 5–7 yr
- M > F (~2:1)
- ~80% of children cured

Presentation/Diagnosis
- **Symptoms:**
  - Commonly present with sx 2/2 obstructive hydrocephalus (HA, N/V [especially in the morning]) occur in the mo prior to dx
  - Truncal ataxia (50–80%), personality changes/irritability, ↓ grades, lethargy, diplopia, head tilt/torticollis (CNVI palsy 2/2 ↑ ICP, can also be a sign of cerebellar tonsil herniation), truncal ataxia
- **Exam:** Esotropia, papilledema, ataxia, dysmetria, CN palsies
- **Imaging:** Initial w/ CT or rapid-sequence MRI to evaluate for obstructing tumor. Will require full MRI ± gadolinium of brain and spine
  - MR: Solid, midline mass in posterior fossa. Arises from cerebellum, occupies 4th ventricle. Variable and heterogeneous enhancement

- Metastatic dx present in 20–30% of children at diagnosis (visualized on MR or CSF analysis)
- Lumbar puncture should be deferred if possibility of ↑ ICP exists, perform after resection
- Consider BM biopsy, especially if cytopenias present
- **Risk stratification:**
  - Standard (average) risk: Gross total resection or near-total resection (w/ ≤1.5 cm^2 residual) w/o metastases, classic histology
  - High risk: Residual tumor >1.5 cm^2, presence of metastases, anaplastic large-cell histology
  - Infant risk: <3 yr

Treatment
- Increased ICP:
  - May need emergent 3rd ventricular ventriculostomy (preferred over VP shunt)
  - IV corticosteroids
- Initial treatment is surgical resection
  - Total or near-total resection assoc w/ better survival
  - May be c/b posterior fossa syndrome (cerebellar mutism) in 10–20% of children: Inability to speak ± other deficits, occurs ~72 hr postop. Limited recovery
- Radiation therapy: Targeted radiation therapy with craniospinal radiation. ↑ radiation dose as risk increases
- Chemotherapy: Multiagent therapy during and/or after radiation therapy
  - Usually consists of vincristine, cisplatin, etoposide, cyclophosphamide, or CCNU

Prognosis
- Standard risk: 5-yr survival 75–90%
- High risk: 5-yr survival 40–60%
- Tx has long-term sequelae: ↓ IQ 2/2 radiation tx, endocrine abnormalities (GH deficiency, thyroid dysfunction, precocious/delayed puberty), and permanent neurologic deficits

HIGH-GRADE GLIOMAS (HGG)

Epidemiology
- Most common HGGs are glioblastoma, anaplastic astrocytoma, diffuse intrinsic pontine glioma (DIPG)
- Yearly incidence of 0.8/100,000
- Median age at dx: 9–10 yr (HGG), 6–7 yr (DIPG)

Presentation/Diagnosis
- Often present rapidly w/ sx related to location: ↑ ICP, seizures, weakness, gait imbalance
  - DIPG assoc w/ sx of CN palsies, ataxia, dysmetria, dysarthria, long-tract signs (upper motor neuron deficits)
- Imaging strategy with CT and MRI as above
  - HGGs often heterogeneous masses w/ ill-defined margins ± mass effect. Often associated edema, hemorrhage, necrosis

Treatment
- Tx ↑ ICP w/ corticosteroids. May need emergent resection/debulking
- Initial tx w/ surgical resection
  - Goal of GTR, infiltrative nature makes this difficult
  - DIPG is not amenable to surgical resection, though bx may be obtained
- Radiation tx
  - Mainstay of DIPG tx. Chemotherapy has not been shown to improve outcomes
  - Chemotherapy: Role of chemotherapy and ideal regimen is unclear, investigation is underway currently

Prognosis
- Overall prognosis is poor, but better than that in adults
- Anaplastic astrocytoma: 5-yr PFS 44% w/ GTR, 22% w/ other surgery
- Glioblastoma: 5-yr PFS 26% w/ GTR, 4% w/ other surgery
- DIPG: Median OS 6–16 mo

BONE TUMORS

(Pediatr Rev 2010;31(9):355–363)

Epidemiology
- 6th most common neoplasm, 6% of childhood malignancies
- Peak incidence at 15–19 yr
- Most common malignant tumors are osteosarcoma (more common in adolescents) and Ewing sarcoma (more common <10 yr)

Presentation
- Sx: Pain, swelling, ↓ ROM, limp/refusal to use affected limb, swelling/palpable mass (may be tender)
- Pathologic fx occur in 5–10%

Workup
- Initial test is XR of affected site
- Lytic lesions raise concern for malignant tumor
  - If periosteal reaction is present, obtain CT/MRI for possible osteosarcoma vs. Ewing vs. osteomyelitis
  - Benign lesions (osteochondroma, osteoid osteoma, osteoblastoma, fibroma) generally appear radiolucent with sharp margins. May need biopsy unless radiologic findings are classic for the benign lesion

---

OSTEOSARCOMA

(Nathan and Oski's Hematology and Oncology of Infancy and Childhood. 8th ed. 2018–2055.e11; Pediatr Rev 2010;31(9):355–363)

Epidemiology
- Most common malignant bone tumor, 15% of all bone tumors
- Peak incidence after 10 yr (assoc w/ growth spurt)
- Slight predominance in males (1.5:1) and Caucasians
- Most common sites: Knee (distal femur > proximal tibia) > proximal humerus > middle/proximal femur
- Risk factors: Radiation exposure, bone disorders (Paget dz, enchondromatosis, multiple hereditary exostoses, fibrous dysplasia), cancer predisposition syndromes (hereditary retinoblastoma, Li–Fraumeni syndrome)

Diagnosis
- **Sx:** 25% present w/ localized swelling/palpable mass and pain (usually dull, aching). Pain is sole complaint in 70%. May have pathologic fracture (8%). Constitutional symptoms are rare
- **Exam:** May have palpable, painful, soft mass. ↓ ROM, +joint effusion
- **Labs:** ↑ LDH (30%), ↑ ALP (40%), ↑ ESR
- **Imaging:**
  - XR has "sunburst" appearance, usually mixed pattern of bone sclerosis and lysis
  - MRI/CT for local staging, surgery planning
  - Metastases present in 10–20% at initial dx, primarily lung and bone (61% lungs, 16% bone, 14% both)
    - MRI can detect >80% of bone "skip metastases," which are synchronous w/ primary tumor
  - CT chest to detect pulmonary metastases
- **Biopsy:** Open or percutaneous core biopsy
- **Staging** (Enneking staging system) involves tumor grade, tumor site/extent, presence of metastases

Treatment
- Best prognostic indicator: Extent of necrosis with chemotherapy
- Poor prognostic indicators: Age <14, ↑ ALP, ↑ LDH, tumor volume >200 mL, poor response to chemotherapy or inadequate surgical margins, presence of metastases
- Surgical resection and limb reconstruction w/ neoadjuvant and adjuvant chemotherapy
  - Localized dz: Chemo usually includes high-dose MTX, doxorubicin, cisplatin
  - Metastatic dz: Above as well as ifosfamide, etoposide

Prognosis
- Nonmetastatic osteosarcoma: 60–70% long-term survival
- Metastatic osteosarcoma: 25% long-term survival (if limited pulm mets, 50% may be cured with complete resection of all known tumor nodules)

EWING SARCOMA

(Nathan and Oski's Hematology and Oncology of Infancy and Childhood. 8th ed. 1983–2017. e15; Pediatr Rev 2010;31(9):355–363)

Epidemiology
- 2nd most common bone tumor, 2–3% of all pediatric cancers
- ~250 new cases diagnosed/yr
- Median age of dx is 14 yr. Peak incidence in adolescence (15–19 yr incidence 4.6/1,000,000)
- Male predominance (1.3–1.5:1), primarily occurs in Caucasians
- Most common sites: Long bones (30% [metadiaphysis in 59%, diaphysis in 35%]), pelvis (26%), spine (11%)
- Risk factors: Parental exposures to farms
- 90–95% have characteristic translocation t(11;22)(q24;a12)

Diagnosis
- **Sx:** Pain (up to 89%) and palpable mass
  - May have fever (15–20%) and other constitutional sx
  - Other sx depend on site, e.g., cord compression w/ spinal tumor or urinary obstruction w/ pelvic tumor. Pathologic fx occur in 15% of pt
- **Labs:** ↑ ESR, ↑ LDH (30%), ALP typically not elevated. Cytopenias usually indicate BM metastasis if present
- **Imaging:** Initial XR has "onion-skinning" pattern. MR (and/or CT) for further assessment of primary tumor
  - Metastatic present in ~25% at dx primarily in lungs (50–60%), bone (~25%), bone marrow (~25%). <10% have LN involvement
    - CT chest
    - Whole-body PET or bone scan
    - BM aspirate and biopsy
- Biopsy

Treatment
- Poor prognostic factors: Site (pelvic, axial primary), older age at diagnosis, presence of metastases, tumor >200 mL, ↑ LDH, male sex, poor response to chemotherapy
- Tx of nonmetastatic dz: Surgical resection with chemotherapy (usually involves combinations of vincristine, actinomycin-d, cyclophosphamide, doxorubicin, and etoposide)
- Tx of metastatic dz: Tx will involve a combination of systemic chemotherapy with local control (radiation or surgical) as well as radiation tx of metastases. HSCT (high-dose chemo with autologous stem-cell rescue) may be an option

Prognosis
- Nonmetastatic disease: >70% survival
- Metastatic disease: Long-term survival in up to 30%

SOLID TUMORS

WILMS TUMOR (NEPHROBLASTOMA)

(Pediatr Rev 2013;34(7):328–330; Nathan and Oski's Hematology and Oncology of Infancy and Childhood. 8th ed. 1714–1746.e8)

Epidemiology
- 5% of pediatric malignant tumors, ~500 new cases/yr. Most common renal tumor
- Yearly incidence 7.5/1,000,000 for pt <15 yr
- Average age at dx is 3 yr (sporadic) and 2 yr (hereditary)
- Assoc w/ several genetic syndromes:
  - WAGR: Wilms tumor, aniridia, GU anomalies, intellectual disability
  - Beckwith–Wiedemann syndrome: Overgrowth d/o w/ enlargement of tongue, liver, kidney, other internal organs, neonatal hypoglycemia; some have hemihypertrophy
- 5% of children present w/ bilateral Wilms tumor

Presentation
- Often diagnosed by pediatrician or caregiver detecting abdominal mass
- Most common signs/sx: Abdominal mass (75%), abdominal pain (28%), HTN (26%), gross or microscopic hematuria (18%, 24%), fever (22%)
  - HTN (may be severe) 2/2 renal artery compression → ↑ renin, ectopic renin production, ectopic ACTH production
  - Hematuria 2/2 invasion of renal pelvis
- May have metastases (local or hematogenous spread): Abdominal LN > lungs > liver

Diagnosis
- Ddx for abdominal mass in a toddler: Neuroblastoma, hepatoblastoma, sarcoma, lymphoma, germ cell tumors. Initial imaging w/ abdominal U/S
- Aniridia may suggest underlying susceptibility or Wilms tumor
- Diagnostic imaging/staging:
  - Formal radiologic evaluation: MRI or CT of abdomen/pelvis
  - US w/ doppler to evaluate for tumor thrombus (renal vein, IVC)
  - Chest CT evaluate for pulmonary metastases

Treatment
- **Surgical tx:** All patients considered for immediate surgery
  - Indications for preoperative chemotherapy: Bilateral WT, IVC tumor thrombus above hepatic veins, tumors invading adjacent organs (except adrenal), morbid surgical procedure, significant respirator dz 2/2 mets
  - En bloc tumor resection (spillage ↑ risk of recurrence)
  - LN sampling
  - Resection (or biopsy) of metastases
- **Radiation:** May be required in stage III, IV disease
- **Chemotherapy:**
  - Stage I and II: Chemotherapy w/ vincristine and actinomycin D
  - Stage III: Above w/ doxorubicin and abdominal radiation added
  - Stage IV: Addition of metastasis-targeted radiation tx. May also have etoposide, cyclophosphamide, or carboplatin added if unfavorable histology

Prognosis
- Stage I–II: Cure rate ~90%
- Stage III: Cure rate ~85%
- Stave IV or unfavorable histology: Cure rate ~66%

NEUROBLASTOMA

(Hematol Oncol Clin North Am 2010;24(1):65–86; Nathan and Oski's Hematology and Oncology of Infancy and Childhood. 8th ed. 1675–1713.e14)

Epidemiology
- Definition: Tumor of sympathetic nervous system
- 7% of all childhood cancers
- Incidence 10.5/1,000,000 per year in pt <15 yr
  - Peak incidence in children <4 yr, median age at dx is 10 mo, 40% who present w/ sx are <1 yr
  - Slight male predominance (1.2:1), no racial predominance
- **Risk factors:**
  - Exposures: Paternal electromagnetic field exposure, prenatal exposure to EtOH, pesticides, phenobarbital
  - Genetic disorders: Some chromosomal abnormalities, Turner syndrome, Noonan syndrome, Beckwith–Wiedemann syndrome

Presentation
- Presentation depends on site of tumor. Neuroblastomas can occur anywhere along the sympathetic chain, in any sympathetic ganglia. May be asymptomatic
  - Most common sites: Abdomen (65%, over half in adrenal gland), chest, neck, pelvis. 1% have no detectable tumor
  - Abdominal tumor: Painless mass, abdominal pain/fullness. HTN 2/2 renal vein compression
    - Abdominal and pelvic tumors can cause lower extremity edema 2/2 venous/lymphatic compression and obstruction
  - Thoracic tumor: May cause SVC syndrome, Horner syndrome
  - Parasympathetic ganglia tumor: Can cause spinal cord compression
- 40% present with localized dz, metastasis is via lymphatics and/or hematogenous
- Most common sites of metastasis: Bone, BM, liver. Rarely lungs, brain

- **Paraneoplastic syndromes:**
  - Opsoclonus–myoclonus syndrome (OMS): Rapid random eye movements, myoclonic jerks, ataxia, behavioral problems. Occurs in 2–3% children w/ neuroblastoma
  - Vasoactive intestinal peptide syndrome: Chronic intractable watery diarrhea, FTT

Diagnosis
- Tumor may be incidentally diagnosed on abdominal exam or CXR
- Labs: ↑ urine or serum catecholamines or catecholamine metabolites (dopamine, vanillylmandelic acid, homovanillic acid)
- Bone marrow biopsy and aspirate to evaluate for metastasis
- Imaging:
  - CT/MRI to evaluate tumor extent and evaluate for metastases
  - Metaiodobenzylguanidine (MIBG) scintigraphy, using MIBG (concentrates in sympathetic nervous system) labelled with radioactive iodine is essential for initial staging (and treatment follow-up)
  - Consider bone scan to detect cortical bone disease (especially if MIBG is negative)
- Multiple staging systems that incorporate surgical findings, imaging findings, extent/ location of metastasis, age

Treatment
- Risk stratification determines treatment strategy
  - Patients categorized into low-, intermediate-, or high-risk groups
  - Based on age at dx (younger unfavorable), tumor histology, ploidy, MYCN amplification status
  - Stage IV-S (infants <1 yr, localized primary w/ mets limited to skin, liver, or bone marrow) may be observed as majority undergo spontaneously regression
- **Low risk:** Surgical resection; chemotherapy may be omitted in some patients
- **Intermediate risk:** Surgical resection + moderate-dose multiagent chemotherapy (generally includes cyclophosphamide, doxorubicin, cisplatin, etoposide)
- **High risk:** Induction, local control, consolidation, MRD management w/ biologic agents
  - Induction tx: Intensive chemotherapy (including cyclophosphamide, vincristine, doxorubicin, cisplatin, etoposide) and radiation therapy
  - Local Control: May include surgery and radiation therapy as large primary tumor is difficult to tx w/ chemotherapy alone
  - Consolidation therapy: Myeloablative chemotherapy w/ autologous HSCT
  - MRD treatment: Uses 13-cis retinoic acid

Prognosis
- Low risk: >95% long-term survival
- Intermediate risk: >90% long-term survival
- High risk: 30–40% long-term survival

HEPATOBLASTOMA

(Nathan and Oski's Hematology and Oncology of Infancy and Childhood. 8th ed. 1886–1905.e7; Nelson Textbook of Pediatrics, Ch 504, 2479–2480.e1)

Epidemiology
- Liver tumors in all make up 1.1% of childhood malignancies
  - Incidence of all liver tumors: 11/1,0000,000 in pt <1 yr, 6/1,000,000 in pt 1–4 yr
  - 100–150 new cases of liver cancer/yr
- Hepatoblastoma represents ~43% of pediatric liver cancers
- Hepatoblastoma has bimodal incidence, peaks at 0–1 & 16–20 mo
- Median age of dx is 1 yr
- Risk factors:
  - Overgrowth syndromes: Beckwith–Wiedemann syndrome, hemihyperplasia
  - Li–Fraumeni syndrome, primary biliary atresia
  - Prematurity and low birthweight (↑ risk w/ ↓ wt)

Presentation
- Generally presents as an asymptomatic abdominal mass
- Sx: Constitutional sx (fever, wt loss, fatigue, anorexia), emesis, abdominal pain
- Rarely may rupture → hemorrhage spontaneously or 2/2 trauma
- Rarely causes precocious puberty in boys 2/2 ↑ chorionic gonadotropin

Diagnosis
- Initial imaging: Abdominal US
- **Labs:** CBC w/ diff (may have ↑ plt 2/2 ↑ TPO release), BMP, LFTs (usually nml), ↑ AFP (90%), β-hCG (occasionally elevated)

- **Imaging:**
  - CT or MRI of abdomen to assess extent, surgical planning
  - CT chest to evaluate for metastases
- **Biopsy:** Either with total resection or confirm diagnosis w/ biopsy if unable to fully resect

Treatment
- **If amenable to resection by standard lobectomy:** Resection followed by chemotherapy (may be unnecessary if well-differentiated histology)
- **If unable to fully resect:**
  - Neoadjuvant chemotherapy: Based on platinum agents and doxorubicin with other agents incorporated (vincristine, 5-FU, ifosfamide, etoposide, irinotecan)
  - If amenable to resection after chemotherapy: Surgical resection followed by chemotherapy
  - If not amenable for resection: Proceed w/ liver transplant followed by chemotherapy
  - Isolated pulmonary metastases may be resected

Prognosis
- Survival is >90% in low-stage tumors
- If unresectable at diagnosis, survival is ~60%
- Survival decreased with metastatic disease to ~25%

ONCOLOGIC EMERGENCIES

(Hematol Oncol Clin North Am 2017;31(6):959–980; Nathan and Oski's Hematology and Oncology of Infancy and Childhood, Ch 68, 2267–2291.e4)

FEVER AND NEUTROPENIA

(J Clin Oncol 2017;35(18):2082–2094; Clin Infect Dis 2011;15;52(4):e56–e93; Hematol Oncol Clin North Am 2017;31(6):981–993)

Definitions/Epidemiology
- Definitions:
  - Fever: Single oral T ≥38.3°C or oral T ≥38°C for 1-hr period (practically 2 measurements separated by ~1 hr)
  - Neutropenia: ANC <500/mm³ or expected to decrease <500/mm³
- Avoid rectal temperatures, as can seed tissue/blood stream with rectal flora
- Common complication of cancer treatment and HSCT
- Fever may herald serious bacterial infxn
- Common pathogens:
  - Gram positives: CONS, MRSA/MSSA, Enterococcus spp., Viridans group strep, S. pneumoniae, S. pyogenes
  - Gram negatives: E. coli, Klebsiella spp., Enterobacter spp., Pseudomonas aeruginosa, Citrobacter spp., Acinetobacter spp., Stenotrophomonas maltophilia
  - Less commonly caused by fungi (e.g., Candida and Aspergillus spp.) or mold
  - Viruses

Diagnosis/Workup
- **History & physical:**
  - Hx: Cancer hx, treatment hx, exposures, sick contacts
  - Exam: Vital signs, oxygenation, source-specific exam
  - Evaluation of potential sources: Oropharyngeal (sore throat, erythema), respiratory (cough, dyspnea, wheeze, crackles, rhonchi), GI (abdominal pain, tenderness; may not have peritonitic signs), skin/soft tissue (pain, erythema, induration, ± fluctuance, including perineal area), GU (dysuria, lower abdominal tenderness, CVA tenderness), neurologic (HA, mental status changes; may not have meningismus)
- **Labs/cultures:** Blood cultures from all CVC lumens and peripherally. CBC w/ diff. BMP (determine renal function), LFTs (evaluate for hepatitis, cholestatic dz), coags if toxic
  - Consider UA and urine cx if urinary sx, hx of prior UTI, or hx of GU tract instrumentation
  - Consider C. difficile if diarrhea (stool bacterial cx and O/P exam less valuable)
  - Perform LP and obtain CSF if meningitis/encephalitis is suspected
  - Obtain sputum cultures and respiratory viral PCR if respiratory symptoms present

- **Imaging:**
  - CXR if respiratory sx
  - If significant abdominal pain/tenderness (especially RLQ) obtain CT abdomen to evaluate for typhlitis (also known as neutropenic enterocolitis)

Treatment
- High-risk characteristics: AML, high-risk ALL, relapsed acute leukemia, allogeneic HSCT, prolonged neutropenia, high-dose steroids, ANC <100/mm^3
- Rapid administration of broad-spectrum antibiotics, ideally after blood cx. Do not delay for ancillary studies (e.g., urine culture)
  - Initial tx w/ antipseudomonal coverage (antipseudomonal β-lactam, 4th generation cephalosporin, or carbapenem). Cefepime is commonly used
  - Add additional gram-negative coverage (e.g., aminoglycoside) and/or glycopeptide tx (e.g., vancomycin) if clinically unstable, resistant infxn suspected, or high rates of local resistance
  - Consider discontinuation once blood cx negative for 48 hr AND afebrile 24 hr + marrow recovery
- Low risk may be managed outpatient with oral antibiotics

TUMOR LYSIS SYNDROME

Background/Pathophysiology
- Definition: Syndrome of metabolic derangements (↑ K, ↑ urate, ↑ phos, ↓ Ca, ↑ BUN/Cr) 2/2 breakdown of tumor cells
- Most common pediatric emergency. Mortality in clinical TLS of 17.5%
- Malignancies occur w/ ↑ turnover and high tumor burden. Most commonly ALL and high-grade NHL (e.g., BL)
- Commonly seen with introduction of therapy, but can occur spontaneously
  - Highest risk 12–72 hr after initiation. Can occur up to 7 d later
- Predictors of TLS: Bulky disease, LAN, HSM, ↑ WBC
- Mechanism: ↑ WBC breakdown → release of purines, potassium, phosphorus
  - Purines → uric acid by xanthine oxidase → hyperuricemia → uric acid precipitation
  - Hyperphosphatemia → calcium phosphate precipitation → hypocalcemia → cramps/spasm, cardiac arrhythmias, hypotension, tetany, seizures
  - Uric acid and calcium phosphate precipitation in renal tubules → renal insufficiency
  - Cellular lysis + renal insufficiency → hyperkalemia → cardiac arrhythmias

Diagnosis
- Sx: Nausea, anorexia, cramps, oliguria, AMS, arrhythmias, seizures, oliguria/anuria
- Hande–Garrow definition of lab TLS: 25% ↑ in phos, K, uric acid, BUN, or 25% ↓ in Ca from pretreatment values
- Hande–Garrow definition of clinical TLS: >2.5 mg/dL ↑ Cr, K >6 mmol/L, Ca <6 mg/dL, life-threatening arrhythmia, death
- Cairo-Bishop Grading System more clinically relevant, incorporates degree of ↑ Cr, type of arrhythmia, presence of seizures

Prevention and Treatment
- **Prevention:** Aggressive hydration (2–4× maintenance) ± diuresis to maintain brisk UOP, monitoring (labs q6–8h)
- **Electrolyte abnormalities:** See "FEN"
- **Hyperuricemia:**
  - Urine alkalization (promotes urate excretion) is controversial
    - May consider w/ allopurinol, do not use w/ rasburicase
  - Allopurinol 300 mg/m^2/d PO q8h (max 800 mg/d) or 200–400 mg/m^2/d IV one-to-three times daily (max 600 mg/d)
    - Inhibits xanthine oxidase, thus blocks uric acid formation
    - Will take 2–3 d to decrease uric acid levels
  - Rasburicase 0.15–0.2 mg/kg IV as needed daily up to 5 d
    - Recombinant urate oxidase, directly and rapidly breaks down uric acid
    - Contraindicated in G6PD deficiency
- **Renal insufficiency/failure:** Monitor I/Os, avoid nephrotoxins, may need renal replacement therapy

HYPERLEUKOCYTOSIS AND LEUKOSTASIS

Definition/Epidemiology
- Definition: WBC = 100×10^9/L
- Occurs in 5–20% of childhood leukemia. Assoc w/ ALL, AML, childhood CML
- Mortality is 20–40%
- Pathophysiology: Stasis of leukemic cells and migration of blasts into tissues → aggregation/thrombi formation → obstruct circulation. Any small vessel organ can be affected

Presentation
- Sx depend on involved organ(s)
- **Lungs:** Dyspnea, tachypnea. May have hypoxia, ARDS, respiratory failure
- **CNS:** HA, confusion, ataxia, stroke/focal neurologic deficits, ataxia, intracranial hemorrhage
- **GU:** Priapism
- **Renal:** Renal insufficiency or failure
- **Cardiac:** Ischemia, acute myocardial infarction, heart failure
- **Eyes:** Blurred vision, papilledema, distension of retinal artery or vein
- **Skin:** Plethora, cyanosis

Treatment
- Acute tx: Aggressive IV hydration with TLS ppx
- Leukapheresis or exchange transfusion may be used
  - Coagulopathy and ↑ risk of bleeding 2/2 proteases released from blasts and coagulation factor consumption may limit ability to perform leukapheresis
- Avoid PRBCs, which ↑ viscosity. Plt transfusion may be used
- Definitive treatment is induction chemotherapy

SUPERIOR MEDIASTINAL SYNDROME

Definition/Etiology
- Anterior mediastinal mass causing SVC obstruction (SVC syndrome) or tracheobronchial compression
- Anterior mediastinal masses assoc w/ SMS in children: NHL, ALL, HL. Less commonly neuroblastoma paraganglioma, germ cell tumors, thymoma

Presentation
- May have gradual or sudden onset
- Sx: Facial edema, plethora, venous engorgement (face, neck, upper extremities), dyspnea, cough, wheeze, stridor, cyanosis, orthopnea, AMS, syncope, and shock
- Respiratory sx occur in 40–60% of children w/ anterior mediastinal masses
- May have associated pleural effusion
- Sx often worse in supine position

Diagnosis
- CXR
- CT may be considered (only if pt can tolerate supine position). May attempt in supine or decubitus positioning
- Initiate least-invasive workup of underlying malignancy: CBC w/ diff, peripheral smear, BM aspirate/biopsy, pleurocentesis, LN biopsy, percutaneous biopsy of mass

Treatment
- Pt with respiratory sx have ↑ risk of anesthesia risk. CT scan (tracheal cross area <50% = high risk) and spirometry (<50% predicted expiratory flow rate = high risk) can help assess risk
- Sedation/anesthesia can precipitate airway obstruction, should be avoided if possible
- If severe, diagnostic procedures may be too risky. Empiric tx w/ IV steroids, radiation, combination chemotherapy
- Definitive tx depends on underlying malignancy

SPINAL CORD COMPRESSION

Definition/Epidemiology
- Definition: Neurologic deficit 2/2 external compression from a tumor
- Occurs in up to 5% of children with cancer. Most cases (67%) occur in initial presentation of cancer
- Majority of SCC caused by extradural tumors (71%)
- >50% caused by neuroblastoma, soft tissue sarcomas (including Ewing sarcoma and rhabdomyosarcoma)

Presentation
- **Hx:** Back pain is most common sx (94%), weakness, gait disturbance, urinary retention, constipation
- **Exam:** Tenderness to palpation and percussion. Depends on level of compression w/ ↓ strength, ↑ and ↓ reflexes, ↓ sensation
- **Localization:**
  - Spinal cord: Rapid progression of symmetric profound weakness, reflexes ↑ or absent, extensor Babinski, symmetric sensory loss, sphincter function preserved early
  - Conus medullaris: Variable on set (can be rapid), reflexes: ↑ knee and ↓ ankle, extensor Babinski symmetric saddle anesthesia, sphincter function lost early
  - Cauda equina: Variable (may be slow) onset of asymmetric weakness and sensory deficit, asymmetric ↓ reflexes, plantar Babinski, sphincter function may be spared

Diagnosis
- **CXR:** Se only 30%, but can provide useful information (lytic/sclerotic lesions, interpeduncular widening, neural foramina widening, intratumor calcification)
- **Emergent MRI:** Best test to aid in diagnosis, evaluation extent of tumor, and surgical planning. MRI can also visualize cord compression and displacement as well as edema

Treatment
- Urgent dx and tx important, as *SCC can lead to permanent deficits if treatment delayed*
- Combination of steroids, surgery, chemotherapy, and radiation
  - Laminectomy, surgical removal of vertebral lamina (± biopsy and debulking)
    - Benefits: Rapid decompression to stabilize/improve neurologic function, tissue diagnosis
    - Cons: ↑ risk of kyphosis or scoliosis (osteoplastic laminotomy may have ↓ adverse effects)
  - Steroids: Rapid administration of IV dexamethasone 1–2 mg/kg recommended when there is high suspicion for tumor-induced SCC with any neurologic compromise
    - Do not delay for imaging, diagnostic certainty
    - May interfere with dx of lymphoproliferative malignancy
  - Radiation therapy will shrink most pediatric tumors causing SCC, sometime with rapid response. May interfere with diagnosis
  - Chemotherapy depends on having established dx

HEMATOPOIETIC STEM CELL TRANSPLANTATION

(Ped Rev 2016;37(4):135–145)

Definitions
- **HSCT:** The infusion of donor blood stem cells into a recipient
- HSC donor types:
  - Autologous: Recipient and donor are the same person
  - Allogeneic: Recipient and donor are different people
  - Syngeneic: Recipient and donor are identical twins
  - Haploidentical: Donor is first-degree relative, shares one haplotype
- HSC sources: Peripheral blood, bone marrow, umbilical cord blood (UCB)
- Conditioning: Regimen of chemotherapy, immunotherapy, and/or radiotherapy given prior to HSCT. May be:
  - Myeloablative: Intensive tx sufficient to cause bone marrow aplasia w/o HSCT
  - Reduced intensity: Nonmyeloablative and less intense
- Graft vs. host dz (GVHD): Donor T-cell–induced inflammation in recipient
- Graft vs. tumor: Desired effect of donor cells attacking host malignant cells

Indications for Allogeneic HSCT
- **Malignancy:** Very high risk or relapsed ALL, AML with high-risk features or relapsed AML, MDS, relapsed or refractory NHL, certain subtypes of NHL, HL that has relapsed after autologous HSCT or refractory HL
- **Nonmalignant:** Severe immune deficiencies, severe hemoglobinopathies (thalassemia major, sickle-cell dz), inherited BM failure syndromes (aplastic anemia, Fanconi anemia, Shwachman–Diamond, DBA, dyskeratosis congenita, amegakaryocytic thrombocytopenia), infantile osteopetrosis, certain mucopolysaccharidoses, certain leukodystrophies, and others

Hematopoietic Stem Cells

- **Donor selection**
  - Allogeneic HSCs are matched according to 10 major histocompatibility loci, better matches decrease risk of GVHD
  - Minor histocompatibility antigens also influence GVHD risk
  - Preference of donor: Matched sibling donor > matched related donor > matched unrelated donor > mismatched donors
- **HSC sources**
  - BM: High engraftment rate, low rate of chronic GVHD (cGVHD). Difficult to harvest
  - Peripheral blood: High engraftment rates, higher HSC yield. Higher rates of GVHD, thus rarely used in children
  - UCB: Can be obtained quickly. Low rate of GVHD (permissive of HLA mismatch). High rate of graft failure, delayed engraftment, and viral infxns (delayed recovery of immune function)

Conditioning

- Generally administered over 4–7 d prior to HSC infusion. Necessary to prevent rejection
- Consists of combinations of chemotherapy (may be disease directed) ± immunotherapy (antithymocyte globulin or alemtuzumab [anti CD52]) ± radiation
- **Myeloablative:** Goal is to replace all cell lines w/ donor cells. Standard of care for malignant disease
- **Reduced intensity:** Increasingly used to tx nonmalignant dz, where mixed BM chimerism is tolerable. Has greater safety profile, though higher risk of graft failure → replacement by recovery of recipient HSCs
- **GVHD ppx:** Calcineurin inhibitors (e.g., tracrolimus) started 1 d prior to HSC infusion. Short course, low dose methotrexate also commonly added in the first 10 d after HSC infusion

Complications/Risks

- **Infection:**
  - Bacterial infxns/bacteremia are common. At risk for opportunistic fungal infxn, respiratory viral infxn
  - May have primary infxn or reactivation of EBV or CMV (can affect engraftment). Warrants surveillance w/ PCR
  - BK viremia can cause hemorrhagic cystitis, renal dysfunction
- **Mucositis:** Occurs in almost all w/ myeloablative conditioning. Occurs w/ neutropenia, resolves with reconstitution. Tx w/ opiate pain control. ↑ risk of bacterial translocation
- **Cytopenias:** Transfusion support needed prior to engraftment
- **Sinusoidal obstructive syndrome:** Seen in 1–10% of HSCT pt, ↑ risk w/ preexisting liver disease, allogeneic HSCT, high-risk neuroblastoma, busulfan, cyclophosphamide, TBI
  - Pathophysiology: Microthrombi obstruct sinusoidal venules → hepatic swelling, pain, fluid retention, hepatorenal syndrome
  - Labs: Cholestasis w/ variable liver enzyme elevation
- **Pulmonary:** Infxn, radiation- or chemotherapy-induced pneumonitis, cGVHD. Intubation/mechanical ventilation assoc w/ high mortality
- **GVHD**
  - Acute: Affects skin, GI tract, liver. May have graft vs. tumor effect
  - Chronic: Mimics autoimmune dz. Involves skin, GI tract, liver, lungs, and muscles/joints

TRANSFUSION THERAPY

(Hematol Oncol Clin N Am 2017:1159–1170)

Blood Products

Blood Product	Dosing	Notes
PRBC	10 mL/kg	Washed, irradiated, leukoreduced
Platelets	5–10 mL/kg	Single (pheresis) or pooled donors
FFP	10–15 mL/kg	Stable clotting factors, albumin, immunoglobulins
Cryoprecipitate	1 unit/5 kg → ↑ fibrinogen by 100 mg/dL	Is the precipitate of FFP. ↑ content of factor VIII, vWF, fibrinogen

(Adapted from Hematol Oncol Clin N Am 2017;31:1159–1170)

Blood Product Transfusion Reactions (Hematol Oncol Clin N Am 2017:1159–1170)
- **Febrile nonhemolytic transfusion reaction**
  - Definition: ↑ temp by ≥1°C w/ chills, rigors, discomfort
  - Mediated by host reaction to leukocyte Ag in transfusion and cytokines in transfusion
  - Sx similar to more severe reactions, thus transfusion stopped
  - Tx w/ premedication with acetaminophen and Benadryl
- **Allergic transfusion reactions**
  - Occur in 1–3% of transfusions. Mediated by type-I hypersensitivity reaction
  - Occur within 1st 2 hr after transfusion
  - Sx: Urticaria and pruritus. May be severe w/ anaphylaxis (bronchospasm, angioedema, hypotension)
  - Tx: Stop transfusion, tx allergic rxn
  - May prevent w/ saline-washed RBCs can premedicate w/ diphenhydramine
- **Hemolytic transfusion reactions**
  - Rare (1/1.5–1.8 million transfusions) but potentially fatal. Can be acute or delayed
    - Acute: Occurs w/i 24 hr 2/2 destruction of incompatible RBCs by preexisting Abs. Responsible for the majority of fatal cases
    - Delayed: Occurs ~7–10 d after transfusion 2/2 destruction of incompatible RBCs by immune response against an Ag the recipient has been previously exposed to
  - Sx: Fevers, chills/rigors, back or flank pain, hypotension
  - Labs: Renal failure, hemolysis
    - Urinalysis w/ hemoglobinuria. Red discoloration of plasma
    - Direct antiglobulin test +
    - Retype and screen donor and recipient blood
  - Severity depends on Ag (ABO mismatch most severe)
- **Transfusion-associated circulatory overload (TACO) and transfusion-related acute lung injury (TRALI)**
  - TRALI and TACO are the more severe adverse reactions
  - Sx generally occur in the first 6 hr with dyspnea and hypoxia
  - TACO is transfusion-related volume overload (usually in pt w/ ↓ cardiac function) → ↑ hydrostatic pressures → pulmonary edema → respiratory distress
    - Dx: New onset respiratory distress, hypoxia (SpO_2 <90%, PaO_2/FiO_2 ≤300 mmHg), CXR w/ bilat infiltrates, evidence of elevated LA pressures
    - Tx: Diuresis, noninvasive and invasive ventilation
  - TRALI is transfusion-related noncardiogenic edema
    - Dx: Onset of new acute lung injury (CXR w/ bilateral infiltrates + SpO_2 <90% or PaO_2/FiO_2 ≤300 mmHg) w/in 6 hr from transfusion. Pulmonary artery pressure ≤18 mmHg
    - Tx: Noninvasive and invasive ventilation, supportive care. Fluids may be helpful
    - Most cases resolve in 96 hr

CHEMOTHERAPY

NAUSEA AND VOMITING

(Nathan and Oski's Hematology and Oncology of Infancy and Childhood. 8th ed. 2349–2396.e14)

Chemotherapy-Induced N/V (CINV)
- Acute (aka posttreatment) CINV: N/V in 1st 24 hr after chemotherapy
- Delayed CINV: N/V 24 hr after chemotherapy, lasts up to 5 d
- Risk factors: Prior CINV, prechemotherapy nausea or anxiety, female, hx motion sickness, low performance status, low social function
- Prophylaxis:
  - Prevention of acute CINV → reduce delayed CINV
  - High-risk acute CINV: 5-HT receptor agonist (ondansetron or granisetron), dexamethasone, aprepitant (if >12 yr), lorazepam. Can add scopolamine, metoclopramide, dronabinol if needed
  - Low- to moderate-risk CINV: 5-HT receptor agonist, dexamethasone ± lorazepam. Can add scopolamine, metoclopramide, dronabinol if needed
  - Delayed CINV: Ondansetron, aprepitant, dexamethasone. Can add metoclopramide cannabinoid as needed
  - Anticipatory CINV: Lorazepam, nonpharmacologic measures
- Treatment of breakthrough N/V: Use same medications as for ppx. May have to administer scheduled antiemetics if persistent

LATE EFFECTS OF CHEMOTHERAPY

(Pediatr Rev 2006;27(7):257–263)

System	Agent	Potential Effects	Monitoring
Central and peripheral nervous	IT chemotherapy	Cognitive dysfunction	Neurocognitive evaluation
	High doses of methotrexate or cytosine arabinoside	Leukoencephalopathy, seizures, hemiplegia, neuropsychiatric changes	Neurologic evaluation
	Cisplatin	Peripheral neuropathy, hearing loss	Physical exam, audiogram
	Corticosteroids	Cataracts	Eye exams
Respiratory	Bleomycin, BCNU, and CCNU	Pulmonary fibrosis	Pulmonary function tests with DL_{CO}, chest radiography
Cardiac	Daunomycin, doxorubicin, idarubicin	Cardiomyopathy, congestive heart failure, arrhythmias	Echocardiography, electrocardiography
Renal	Cisplatin, carboplatin, ifosfamide	Glomerular or tubular injury, insufficiency	BUN, creatinine, blood pressure, urinalysis
Genitourinary	Cyclophosphamide, ifosfamide	Bladder fibrosis if tx for hemorrhagic cystitis, dysfunctional voiding, bladder malignancy	History, urinalysis
Reproductive	Cyclophosphamide, ifosfamide, carboplatin, cisplatin	Hypogonadism, infertility, early menopause	History of pubertal development, menstrual cycles, and sexual function; LH, FSH, estradiol, testosterone
Skeletal	Methotrexate, corticosteroids	Osteopenia, osteoporosis	Bone density evaluation
	Corticosteroids	Avascular necrosis	History, physical exam, radiographs if indicated
Psychosocial	Any cancer experience	Depression, anxiety, posttraumatic stress, social withdrawal, isolation, limitations in health care and insurance	Clinical interview
Hematologic	Cyclophosphamide, ifosfamide, cisplatin, carboplatin, etoposide	Secondary AML	Complete blood count

(Adapted from Pediatrics in Review 2006;27(7):257–263)

ACUTE TOXICITIES

(Harriet Lane Handbook, 21st ed. 607–627)

Chemotherapeutic Agents	Toxicities
Asparaginase	Hypersensitivity reaction, pancreatitis, coagulopathy, hyperammonemia, PEG-asparaginase may have prolonged toxicities
Bleomycin	Hypersensitivity, pneumonitis, pulmonary fibrosis
Busulfan	Significant myelosuppression, seizures, acute lung injury, fibrosis w/ high cumulative dose
Carboplatin	Myelosuppression, thrombocytopenia. Less N/V, neuropathy, renal injury, ototoxicity than cisplatin
Cyclophosphamide	Severe N/V, hemorrhagic cystitis, SIADH, cardiotoxicity w/ high doses

Cisplatin	Acute and delayed N/V, neuropathy, renal toxicity (glomerular and tubular), ototoxicity, ↓ Mg, ↓ phos
Clofarabine	N/V, capillary leak syndrome, fever, rash, tachycardia, hepatotoxicity, nephrotoxicity, prolonged myelosuppression
Corticosteroids	Na retention, hyperglycemia, HTN, gastritis, mood changes
Cytarabine (ara-C)	Fever and rash, N/V, conjunctivitis, prolonged myelosuppression, mucositis, CNS toxicity
Dactinomycin	N/V, stomatitis, rash, radiation recall
Daunorubicin and Doxorubicin	N/V, mucositis, hepatotoxicity, cumulative doses w/ late cardiotoxicity (CHF, cardiomyopathy), turns bodily secretions red
Etoposide	N/V, hypotension, transient cortical blindness
Ifosfamide	Same as cyclophosphamide, also rarely CNS toxicity (seizures, somnolence, can progress to death)
Irinotecan	Diarrhea
Melphalan	N/V, hypersensitivity reaction, prolonged leukopenia, mucositis, cataracts
Mercaptopurine	N/V, hepatotoxicity, nephrotoxicity, headache
Methotrexate	N/V, mucositis, hepatotoxicity, nephrotoxicity, neurotoxicity (encephalopathy, seizures, HA, ventriculitis), diarrhea
Mitoxantrone	N/V, fever, hepatotoxicity, myelosuppression w/ severe mucositis, blue-green urine
Temozolomide	N/V, headache, myelosuppression, constipation, seizures
Thiotepa	Neurotoxicity (cognitive impairment), skin breakdown, myelosuppression
Thioguanine	Hepatotoxicity, mucositis
Topotecan	Diarrhea
Vincristine	Constipation (and paralytic ileus), peripheral neuropathy, jaw pain, hepatotoxicity

CARRIER SCREENING

(Obstet Gynecol 2017;129:e41–55)

- Can be performed at any point during pregnancy, ideally done prior to conception
  - Only needs to be assessed once during lifetime
- Screens offered to all parents: Spinal muscular atrophy (SMN1 gene deletion), cystic fibrosis (CTFR mutation panel), hemoglobinopathies (via CBC with RBC indices)
- Fragile X carrier screening: recommended for women with (+) FH and unexplained ovarian insufficiency or failure before 40 yo
  - Evaluate for premutation by number of trinucleotide repeats of FMR1 gene
- Tay–Sachs disease screening: offered when either parents is of Ashkenazi Jewish, French–Canadian, or Cajun descent
  - Evaluate for autosomal recessive gene mutations or measurement of enzymatic activity of hexosaminidase
- If a patient has a family history of one of the above conditions, then caution must be used when interpreting the results since carrier testing only tests for select mutations and is not exhaustive

SCREENING FOR FETAL ANEUPLOIDY

(Obstet Gynecol 2016;127:e123–137; Genet Med 2016;18(10):1056–1065)

First Trimester Screening
- Offered to all women – can be done at 10 0/7–13 6/7 wk of gestation
- Includes: Nuchal translucency measurement, serum free β-hCG, or total hCG + pregnancy-associated plasma protein A analyte levels
- Specific risk estimates for trisomy 13, 18, and 21 is calculated using these results as well as maternal factors such as maternal age, prior history of aneuploidy, weight, race, and number of fetuses

Quadruple Screen
- Can be performed at 15 0/7–22 6/7 wk of gestation – in additional aneuploidy risk, offered information regarding risk of open fetal defects
- Includes: (1) hCG; (2) α-fetoprotein (AFP); (3) dimeric inhibin A; and (4) unconjugated estriol in combination with maternal factors such as age, weight, race, the presence of diabetes, and plurality to calculate risk assessment

Second Trimester "Genetic Ultrasonogram"
- Used to screen for Down syndrome using specific ultrasonographic findings – combination of ultrasound and serum screening improve detection rates

Cell-free DNA Screening
- Screening can be performed as early as 10 wk until term – evaluates short segments of DNA in maternal blood that are released by placental cells undergoing apoptosis
- Typically offered to mothers at risk for aneuploidy (i.e., due to positive screening test, AMA) but can be performed electively
- Can detect fetal aneuploidy and fetal sex, Rh (+) fetus in an Rh (−) mother, and some paternally derived autosomal dominant genetic abnormalities
- Because cell-free DNA is a screening test with potential for false-positive and false-negative test results, such testing should not be used as a substitute for diagnostic testing
  - Se and false-positive rates (FPR)
    - Trisomy 21 (99.5% Se, 0.05% FPR), trisomy 18 (97.7% Se, 0.04% FPR), trisomy 13 (96.1% Se, 0.06% FPR)
- Because the test cannot distinguish fetal from maternal DNA, a positive screening test result can represent confined placental mosaicism, a resorbing twin or, in rare, instances, a maternal malignancy or maternal aneuploidy

Preimplantation Genetic Screening
- In individuals undergoing IVF, screening for fetal aneuploidy prior to implantation of the embryo is an option; however, screening for aneuploidy is still offered during pregnancy because false-negative tests results can occur with preimplantation genetic screening

(Obstet Gynecol 2016;127:e108–e122)

Chorionic Villus Sampling
- Generally performed b/w 10–13 wk of gestation
- Placental villus samples can be sent for a variety of testing options depending on the clinical scenario including karyotype, FISH analysis, and/or microarray

Amniocentesis
- Amniotic fluid sample is obtained. This contains fetal cells from various sources including skin and hair
- Usually performed b/w 15–20-wk gestation, but it can be performed at any later gestation
- Fluid samples can be sent for a variety of testing options depending on the clinical scenario. These include karyotype, FISH analysis, and/or microarray

GENETIC DISORDERS

ANEUPLOIDY DISORDERS

(Nelson Textbook of Pediatrics. 20th ed. Ch 81; Lancet 2003;361:1281)

Trisomy 21 (Down Syndrome)
- Most common genetic syndrome; incidence ~1:800 live births
- ~95% 2/2 nondisjunction of chr 21; 1% are mosaic; 4% 2/2 Robertsonian translocation
- **Signs/Sxs by system:**
  - Neuro: Hypotonia, developmental delay, seizures
  - HEENT: Epicanthal folds, palpebral fissures slant upward, small ears, flat nasal bridge, midface hypoplasia (→ impaired Eustachian drainage (→ recurrent otitis/sinusitis/pharyngitis))
  - CV: Endocardial cushion defects, (AVSD), VSD, ASD, PDA, aberrant subclavian, pHTN, ToF
    - CHD present in ~50% of patients
  - MSK: Joint hyperflexibility, short 5th digit, single transverse palmar crease, pelvic dysplasia, atlantoaxial instability (misalignment of C1 vertebra in 15%)
  - GI: Duodenal atresia, Hirschsprung, imperforate anus, TE fistula, annular pancreas, and others
  - Pulmonary: OSA
  - Endocrine: Hypothyroidism, infertility
- **Diagnosis**
  - At birth: Constellation of features and confirmation by karyotype
  - Prenatal: Quad screen: Maternal AFP & estriol ↓ /β-hCG & inhibin A ↑
    - Presence of cell-free fetal DNA in maternal serum is diagnostic
    - Fetal US for nuchal translucency, short femurs, cardiac anomalies, duodenal atresia
- **Management:** Regular screening indicated for possible complications
  - CV: Referral to pediatric cardiologist at birth for evaluation
  - Ophtho: Referral at birth to pediatric ophthalmologist (risk of cataracts & refractive errors)
  - ENT: Annual hearing screens and evaluation for serous otitis
  - GI: Monitor for evidence of Hirschsprung, screen for celiac dz w/ anti-TTG & IgA at 2 yr
  - Heme: ↑↑ risk of leukemia, monitor closely for signs/sxs
  - Endocrine: Annual screening for thyroid dz
  - Neuro: Referral to early intervention, wide range of meeting milestones but most expected to be slightly delayed & may be severely delayed
  - MSK: Low threshold for neck films with neurologic sxs or neck/back pain

Trisomy 13 (Patau Syndrome)
- 0.85:10,000 live births, large percentage terminated before birth
- 5% survival > 6 mo
- **Signs/Sxs:** Cleft lip, polydactyly, overlapping fingers, holoprosencephaly, low-set ears, microphthalmia, cardiac defects (~70%), absent ribs, visceral, and genital anomalies

Trisomy 18 (Edward Syndrome)
- 1.29:10,000 live births, large percentage terminated before birth
- 5% survival to 1 yr
- **Signs/Sxs:** Closed fists w/ overlapping digits, rocker-bottom feet, cleft lip/palate, microcephaly, micrognathia, inguinal/abdominal hernia, cardiac/renal anomalies

Turner Syndrome
- X chromosome monosomy (45, X karyotype) or sex chromosome mosaicism; 1/5,000 live female births
  - **Signs/Sxs:** Misshapen or rotated ears, low posterior hairline, webbed neck, broad chest w/ wide-spaced nipples and cubitus valgus, shortened 4th metacarpal, patella dislocation
  - Associated w/ congenital lymphedema, renal anomalies (60%, horseshoe kidney), hearing loss, osteoporosis, hypothyroidism, diabetes, colorblindness, IBD, celiac dz, CHD (~40%)
    - CHD typically coarctation of the aorta or bicuspid aortic valve (can be more severe such as HLHS) → risk of progressive aortic root dilation or dissection
  - Normal IQ, although may have difficulty w/ nonverbal, social, and psychomotor skills
  - Almost all are infertile
- **Diagnosis** (Nat Clin Pract Endocrinol Metab 2005;1:41)
  - Consider in girls w/ short stature (2 SD below mean height for age), primary amenorrhea, lack of breast development, delayed puberty
  - Consider in fetus w/ hydrops, ↑ nuchal translucency, cystic hygroma, or lymphedema
  - Dx made with karyotyping → chromosomal analysis of 30 peripheral lymphocytes
  - 50% w/ missing X chromosome in all cells studied, others w/ 45, X/46, XX mosaic
- **Management** (Endocrine 2012;41(2):200–219)
  - Treat short stature with GH therapy through bone age of 14 yo
  - Estrogen in adolescence for pubertal development and prevention of osteoporosis with Ca + vit D. Continue throughout life
  - Hearing tests, ophthalmology referral for hyperopia/strabismus, regular dental visits
  - Echocardiogram to evaluate CHD risk, 4 extremity BP for coarctation
  - Renal ultrasound for renal malformations
  - Celiac screen should be done in childhood
  - Annual TFTs, LFTs, fasting lipids, and glucose
  - If Y chromosome is present, 12% risk of gonadoblastoma; refer for removal

Klinefelter Syndrome (Int J Endocrinol 2012;2012:324835)
- 80% w/ male phenotype (47,XXY genotype), remainder may be mosaic or variety of multiple sex chromosome aneuploidies (i.e., 48,XXYY; 49,XXXXY)
- Signs/Sxs:
  - Many unnoticed until puberty or young adulthood
  - Almost all men are infertile (3% of all male infertility)
  - Testosterone def, small testes, ↓ facial hair, gynecomastia, ↓ pubic hair, small penis
  - Tall and slender with long legs and short torso
  - May develop osteoporosis
  - Mild neurodevelopmental disorders (can be more severe)
- **Diagnosis**
  - Late or incomplete puberty should prompt a workup
    - FSH and LH ↑ starting in midpuberty w/ ↓ testosterone
  - Karyotype for diagnosis (assess 50+ cells given possible mosaicism)
- **Management**
  - Neurodevelopmental evaluation at diagnosis
  - Hormone therapy for low testosterone levels or if hypergonadotropism is present
  - Gynecomastia predisposes men to breast cancer; 20–50× ↑ risk

---

FRAGILE X SYNDROME

(Nelson Textbook of Pediatrics. 20th ed. Ch 81; Curr Genomics 2011;12:216; Clin Pediatr (Phila) 2005;44:371)

- Fragility refers to chromosome sites w/ propensity to become damaged
  - Fragile X syndrome: Long arm of Xq27.3
- Most common cause of inherited intellectual disability (~3% of male intellectual disability)

- **Signs/Sxs**
  - Classic triad: Macroorchidism, large cupped ears, long narrow face; also associated w/ high arched palate, joint laxity, scoliosis, seizures, strabismus, MV prolapse
  - Intellectual disabilities have wide range from severe ID to autism spectrum disorder
    - 20–30% w/ autism spectrum, 80% with ADHD, 70–100% w/ anxiety disorder
    - Suspect in any infant or toddler w/ developmental delays (particularly speech) or maternal FH of intellectual disability
- **Diagnosis**
  - DNA testing showing trinucleotide repeat inside *FMR1* gene >200 copies
  - ↑ repeats → ↑ intellectual disability
- **Management**
  - Management of neuropsychiatric manifestations as appropriate (i.e., stimulants for ADHD, AEDs for seizures)
  - Monitoring for possible cardiac valve dz, in adulthood should be monitored for progressive neurodegenerative disorder (fragile X-associated tremor/ataxia syndrome)
  - Normal life expectancy

DELETION SYNDROMES

(Nelson Textbook of Pediatrics. 20th ed. Ch 81)

- Loss of chromosomal material, classified by area of deletion (*p* = short arm, *q* = long arm)
- Diagnosis made by routine chromosome preparation, high-resolution banding techniques (FISH), molecular studies (aCGH)
- **More common deletion syndromes + signs/sxs**
  - 5p, Cri-du-chat syndrome: Hypotonia, shrill cry, microcephaly, prominent metopic suture, hypertelorism, intellectual disability
  - 4p, Wolf–Hirschhorn syndrome: Prominent glabella, frontal bossing, hypertelorism ("helmet" facies), ocular anomalies, beaked nose, cardiac/GU anomalies
  - 22q11.2 microdeletion, DiGeorge syndrome: Cardiac anomalies, cleft palate, parathyroid hypoplasia (hypocalcemia), thymic hypoplasia (immunodeficiency)
  - 20p12 microdeletion, Alagille syndrome: Bile duct hypoplasia, pulm artery stenosis, butterfly vertebrae, eye abnormalities
  - 15q11-q13 microdeletion, Prader–Willi if paternal/Angelman if maternal:
    - Prader–Willi: Profound hypotonia, ↑ appetite → obesity, small hands/feet, hypogonadism, intellectual disability, ↓ height (can treat w/ GH supplementation)
    - Angelman: Severe intellectual disability, hypotonia, seizures, fair skin/hair, laughter
  - 11p13 microdeletion, WAGR syndrome: Wilms tumor, aniridia, GU anomalies, intellectual disability

AUTOSOMAL DISORDERS

Ehlers–Danlos Syndrome (Eur J Hum Genet 2007;15:724; J Med Genet 2010;47:476)
- **Def:** Heterogeneous connective tissue disorders involving skin, organs, and joints
- Autosomal dominant, recessive, or X-linked inheritance
- Affects males and females of all racial and ethnic backgrounds
- Villefranche classification w/ 6 subtypes; many rare, uncommon forms
  - **Classical EDS:** AD mutations of collagen type 1 α-1
    - Dx confirmed by FH and clinical features
    - Signs/sxs: Skin hyperextensibility, IUGR, premature birth, joint hypermobility, redundant skin folds, muscle scarring, congenital diverticula of the bladder, inguinal hernias (males), muscle hypotonia, delayed gross motor development
    - Assn w/ MVP and regurgitation
  - **Hypermobility**
    - AD, most common type
    - No known genes and diagnosis is by clinical exam and confirmed by FH
    - Signs/sxs: Smooth, velvety skin; easy bruising, joint hypermobility with unusual ROM, inguinal hernias (males), recurrent joint dislocation, chronic joint/limb pain
    - Assn w/ MVP and regurgitation
  - **Vascular**
    - AD mutations of *COL3A1* with >320 mutation variants; responsible for procollagen, which provides strength in connective tissue
    - Dx confirmed by skin biopsy
    - Signs/sxs: Thin translucent skin over chest and abdomen, acrogeria (loss of subcutaneous fat and collagen of hands and feet), lobeless ears, short stature, extensive bruising, hypermobility of small joints

- **Prognosis:** Based on type; sudden death from vascular rupture or perforation may occur
  - Children with CVA should be evaluated for EDS
- **Tx:**
- Classical and hypermobile types may develop aortic root dilation (up to 28%)
- Root should be measured (echo) at 5 yr of age then every 5 yr thereafter
- Less strenuous activities recommended as to avoid joint strain and damage

Marfan Disease (Heart 2011;97:1206; Eur J Hum Genet 2007;15:724; J Med Genet 2010;47:476)
- **Def:** Connective tissue dz 2/2 to fibrillin mutation (FBN1) affecting heart, eyes, & bones
- Variable autosomal dominance, fibrillin-1 on chromosome 15 in up to 91% of cases
- 1:9,800 births; 27% are from a new mutation
- **Signs/sxs by system:**
  - **CV:** TTE eval of aortic diameter; use pediatric nomogram
    - Progressive aortic dilation, usually at sinus of Valsalva → AV incompetence → aortic dissection and rupture; ↑ risk of aortic dissection in pregnant women
    - LV dilation → cardiac failure
    - Mitral valve prolapse → regurgitation
  - **Ophthalmology:** Myopia, retinal detachment, lens subluxation
  - **Skeletal:** Pectus, wrist and thumb signs, scoliosis (~60%), arm span: Height >1.05
    - Joint hypermobility in 85% <18 yo and 56% of adults
    - Arthralgias, myalgias, and ligamentous injuries
  - Pulmonary: Spontaneous pneumothorax in 4–11% of patients
- **Diagnosis**
  - Suspect if tall, thin, long limbs, arachnodactyly, pectus deformity, and/or scoliosis
  - Family history of aortic aneurysm or familial thoracic aortic aneurysms
  - Original Ghent criteria replaced by new Ghent criteria
- **Tx:** Most common cause of death → aortic dissection (N Engl J Med 2008;358:2787)
  - β-blockers if aorta is dilated; ARBs/ACEIs can slow dilation
  - Follow aortic diameter w/ biannual/annual TTE, and consider surgery when >5 cm
  - Surgery usually involves replacing the valve and aorta (Bentall procedure)
  - Avoidance of high-intensity activity

INBORN ERRORS OF METABOLISM

BASICS OF INBORN ERRORS OF METABOLISM
(Pediatr Rev 2016;37(1):3–15)
- Mutation of enzyme in metabolism → excess or lack of certain metabolites
- When to suspect an IEM (inborn error of metabolism)
  - Overwhelming illness in neonatal period (sepsis without obvious source of infection), vomiting, metabolic acidosis with anion gap, massive ketosis, hypoglycemia, altered mental status, seizures, hypotonia, unusual odor of urine, excessive dermatosis, neutropenia, thrombocytopenia, pancytopenia, developmental delay (especially regression), hepatosplenomegaly, cholestasis, liver failure, cardiomyopathy
  - Most patients will develop symptoms in first 72 hr of life
- IEMs can be broken down into 2 broad categories:
  - Disorders involving breakdown of energy sources
    - Lipids
      - Defects in fatty acid β-oxidation
      - Defects in carnitine shuttle
    - Proteins
      - Amino acidopathies (whole amino acid cannot be metabolized)
      - Organic acidemias (usually due to defects in deamination of amino acids)
      - Urea cycle disorders (depending on degree of defect, can present later in life)
    - Carbohydrates
      - Glycogen storage diseases
      - Galactosemia
  - Organelle dysfunction
    - Lysosomal storage disorders
    - Peroxisomal disorders
    - Mitochondrial disorders

- **Neonatal presentation**
  - Sxs at 24–72 hr of life; prior, mother's metabolism eliminate metabolic intermediates
  - Ill infant w/ nonspecific sxs: Lethargy, diff feeding, vomiting, abn resp, hypotonia and szrs; see acute presentation differential table below
  - Abnormal body or urinary odor
    - MSUD: Urine smells of maple syrup or burnt sugar
    - Isovaleric acidemia and glutaric acidemia type II → pungent, "sweaty feet" odor
- **Late presentation:** >28 d of life; recurrent vomiting, lethargy, or ↓ po intake → coma, liver dysfunction; consider urea cycle disorders
- **Adolescent/adults presentation:** (J Inherit Metab Dis 2007;30:631)
  - Psychiatric d/o, often w/ additional recurrent rhabdo, myoglobinuria, cardiomyopathy
    - Acute cyclic confusion: Urea cycle defect, porphyria, homocysteine defect
    - Chronic psych sxs: Homocystinuria, Wilson dz, adrenoleukodystrophy, lysosomal d/o
  - Intellectual disability & personality Δ: Homocystinuria, nonketotic hyperglycemia
- **Specific triggers of decompensation** (Vademecum Metabolicum 2004:3)
  - Vomiting, fasting, infection, fever, vaccinations, surgery, accident/injury, changes in diet → protein/carbohydrate metabolism disorders
  - High-protein diet and/or catabolic state → aminoacidopathies, organic acidemia, UCDs
  - Fruit, sugar (sucrose), liquid medicines → fructose intolerance
  - Lactose → galactosemia
  - High fat → fatty acid oxidation disorders
  - Drugs → porphyria, glucose-6-phosphate-dehydrogenase deficiency
  - Extensive exercise → disorders of fatty acid oxidation, glycolysis, respiratory chain

Differential Diagnosis of IEMs Based on Lab Findings		
Primary Finding	**Secondary Findings**	**Potential Disorder**
Acidosis	± ↓ BG, ± ↑ lactate, ± ketosis, ± ↑ NH₃, ↑AG	Various organic acid disorders
	Significantly ↑ lactate, normal BG	Mitochondrial d/o, pyruvate dehydrogenase def, α-ketoglutarate dehydrogenase def, pyruvate carboxylase def
	Significantly ↑ lactate, ↓ BG	Glycogen storage d/o type I, fructose 1-6-bisphosphatase def
	Normal AG, ↑ lactate, no ketosis	RTA
Hyperammonemia	Alkalosis or normal pH, normal lactate	Urea cycle disorders
	↓ BG, ↑LFT, normal ketones	Fatty acid oxidation defects
	↓ pH w/ ↑ AG ± ↑ lactate, ± ketosis, ± ↓ BG	Various organic acid disorders
Hypoglycemia	↓ pH w/ ↑ AG ± ketosis, ± ↑ lactate, ± ↑ NH₃	Various organic acid disorders
	Hepatomegaly, ± ↑ lactate	Glycogen storage disorder
	No ketosis or acidosis, normal lactate	Hyperinsulinemia Fatty acid oxidation defects
	↓ Na, ↓ blood pressure	Adrenal insufficiency
	Hepatic failure	Tyrosinemia, glycogen storage disorder type IV, galactosemia, Niemann–Pick type C

(Pediatr Rev 2009;31:131)

METABOLIC EMERGENCIES

(Pediatr Rev 2016;37(1):3–15; *Nelson Textbook of Pediatrics*. 20th ed. Ch 84;
Pediatr Rev 2009;30:131)

- Initial lab workup: Stat D-stick, CBC w/ diff, chem 7, blood gas, NH3, lactate, plasma and urine amino acids, UA, urine reducing substances, urine ketones, urine organic acids, ESR, CRP, CK, ALT, AST, coags
  - Store plasma samples for amino acids, acylcarnitine and filter paper ("Guthrie" card)
- Initial tx prior to dx: Consult metabolic specialist; stop all protein, fat, galactose, fructose

Hyperammonemia

- May result in acute encephalopathy, if untreated can cause permanent brain injury or death
- Causes: Urea cycle defects, organic acidemias (methylmalonic acidemia, propionic acidemia, isovaleric acidemia, and β-ketothiolase deficiency, transient hyperammonemia of newborn)
  - Urea cycle disorders are most common inborn errors of metabolism
  - Others: Lab error due to specimen mishandling (must be placed on ice & processed by lab within 1 hr), liver dz, valproic acid, TPN, perinatal asphyxia
  - Precipitated by either ↑ protein intake → ↑ ammonia production OR poor po intake → catabolism & ↑ proteolysis
  - **Ornithine transcarbamylase deficiency:** Most common urea cycle defect, X-linked
    - Can present from 1 mo of age to childhood w/ significant illness; ↑ urine orotic acid
- **Signs/Sxs:** Severe emesis, tachypnea, cerebral edema, lethargy, stupor, coma, convulsions
  - Severe forms may present hr after birth; less severe forms can present as recurrent episodes of lethargy and vomiting, FTT, acute encephalopathy, protein aversion
- **Diagnosis:**
  - Repeat ammonia with attention to proper specimen handling
  - Blood gas, LFTs, serum electrolytes for anion gap, urine organic acids for orotic acid (↑ in ornithine transcarbamylase & other urea cycle disorders), plasma amino acid analysis
    - ↑ Anion gap suggests organic acidemia, normal suggests urea cycle defect
    - Labs may be overall unremarkable in urea cycle defects (↓ BUN common)
    - Ammonia normally ↑ in neonatal period, true illness usually w/ value >200 μmol/L
- **Tx:**
  - Stop ammonia production
    - Stop protein intake and provide nonprotein energy source w/ D10-NS + IV lipids
    - Will need to provide essential amino acids to prevent catabolism, requires guidance of metabolic dz expert as absolute contraindications exist for each of the following; typical tx includes Arginine-HCl + Na-phenyl acetate + Na-benzoate
  - Remove ammonia
    - Obtain central access, urgent consultation to metabolic dz specialist
    - Monitor for effect of above tx as arginine alone may ↓ ammonia in urea cycle defects
    - Start hemodialysis if coma or ammonia not improving w/ above
  - Avoid hyponatremia (maintain Na >135) due to risk of cerebral edema
  - Time spent in coma correlates with outcome
  - Liver transplantation ↓ episodes of hyperammonemia

Severe Metabolic Acidosis with Elevated Anion Gap

- When 1st episode of severe AGMA presents in infancy, suggests **organic acidemia**
  - **Types:** Propionic acidemia, glutaric acidemia, methylmalonic acidemia, isovaleric acidemia
    - All are autosomal recessive
- **Signs/Sxs:** ↓ po, tachypnea, vomiting, lethargy, coma; may progress to stroke & death
- **Diagnosis:** Urine organic acids, acylcarnitine profile, carnitine analysis
  - Many screened for on newborn screen but initial episode may occur prior to results
- **Treatment:**
  - Stop all protein intake
  - High-dose carnitine supplements
  - Induce anabolic state w/ dextrose-containing fluids, IV lipids, insulin if needed

- Hemodialysis for profound acidosis, severe sxs, hyperammonemia
- IV bicarbonate to correct acidosis
- If dx known, give appropriate cofactors/tailored tx (i.e., B12 for methylmalonic acidemia)
- **Specifics by disorder:**
  - **Propionic acidemia:** Present in newborn period with severe AGMA + ketosis + markedly elevated ammonia. Complications include cardiorespiratory collapse 2/2 acidosis, pancytopenia, pancreatitis, stroke, cardiomyopathy/cardiac dysrhythmias
    - Long-term tx: Dietary avoidance, B12, carnitine, liver/kidney + liver transplant
  - **Methylmalonic acidemia:** Presents similarly to propionic acidemia w/ similar lab findings but with dx based on NBS or UOA & plasma acylcarnitine profile
    - Assn w/ need for kidney transplant
    - Long-term tx: B12, dietary avoidance, liver/kidney + liver transplant
  - **Glutaric acidemia:** Typically does not present as neonate but w/ mild febrile illness in a child → neurologic devastation (subdural hematomas & permanent basal ganglia injury → movement d/os & dystonia); severe injury unlikely after age 6
    - No easily obtainable marker, dx is clinical based on hx/exam (macrocephaly)
      - Tested on NBS but some are "low excretors" w/ normal screen
    - Acute tx w/ high-dose dextrose infusions; long-term w/ dietary avoidance

ANION GAP ACIDOSIS WITH ELEVATED LACTATE

(Neoreviews 2017;18:4)

- **Causes:** Lab error, tissue ischemia, sepsis, 1° metabolic lactic acidosis (rare)
  - Metabolic causes of primary lactic acidosis:
    - Pyruvate metabolism defect: Pyruvate carboxylase def, pyruvate dehydrogenase def
    - Fatty acid oxidation defects
    - Organic acidopathies
    - Electron transport chain defects (mitochondrial dz)
  - Secondary lactic acidosis due to IEM can also occur in ill infants
- Evaluation
  - 1st step: Always repeat lactic acid ensuring good draw and proper specimen handling
  - Check pyruvate:lactate ratio: ↓ in pyruvate defect, ↑ in all other causes of lactic acidosis
  - Acylcarnitine profile: Abnormal in disorders of fatty acid oxidation
  - Urine organic acids: Abnormal in organic acidopathies
  - Molecular testing: Required to make dx of electron transport chain defects
- Associated sxs of various disorders:
  - Pyruvate metabolic defect → presents with illness at ~24 hr of life, structural brain anomalies, fetal alcohol–like facial features
  - Electron transport chain defects → hypertrophic cardiomyopathy, structural anomalies, lens clouding or cataracts, IUGR
- Initial treatment: Correct acidosis regardless of cause
  - Calculate bicarb deficit, replace 50% in 1st hr & rest over 24 hr as HCO_3
    - Calculation: (24-[serum HCO_3]) × (weight in kg) × 0.5 = HCO_3 deficit in mEq
  - Halt catabolism, infuse dextrose to maintain normoglycemia (although expect glycolysis will produce additional lactic acid as byproduct); enteral nutrition preferred if stable
  - With unknown cause of lactic acidosis, can provide cofactors for known defects:
    - Thiamine for pyruvate dehydrogenase def; biotin for pyruvate carboxylase def
  - Cardiac transplant for cardiomyopathy may be necessary, depends on overall stability
- **Prognosis:** For 1° neonatal lactic acidosis prognosis is generally very poor

HYPOGLYCEMIA

(Neoreviews 2017;18:4)

- **Causes:**
  - Disorders of protein intolerance, carbohydrate metabolism, or fatty acid oxidation
  - Hepatic glycogen storage dz (except Pompe); no glycogenolysis (worse with fasting)
  - In neonates must rule out sepsis, SGA, maternal diabetes, slow adaptation
  - With persistent neonatal hypoglycemia, consider hyperinsulinemia or hypopituitarism
- **Diagnosis:**
  - Determine time since last meal, drugs, hepatomegaly, hepatic failure signs, small genitals, hyperpigmentation, short stature

- Labs: Insulin, C-peptide, cortisol, lactate, free fatty acids, 3-OH-butyrate, Ketostix (urine)
  - Acylcarnitine profile for fatty acid oxidation disorder & organic acidurias
  - Urine organic acids

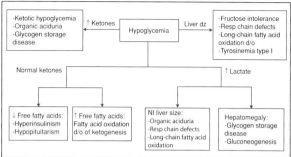

- **Tx:**
  - IV glucose at 7–10 mg/kg/min, for calories and to replace normal liver glucose production → D10% glucose, 110–150 cc/kg/d with electrolytes
    - Maintain BG >100; if glucose needs >10 mg/kg/min → likely hyperinsulinism

Galactosemia (Pediatrics 2006;118;E934)
- **Def:** AR deficiency in enzymes required to break down lactose → glucose + galactose → accumulation of galactose-1-phosphate and galactitol
- **Types:**
  - "Classic galactosemia": Most common with galactose-1-phosphate uridyltransferase (GALT) deficiency
  - Galactokinase (GALK) def
  - Galactose-4'-epimerase (GALE) def – rare
- **Signs/sxs:**
  - Progressive jaundice & liver dysfunction, HSM, food intolerance, hypoglycemia
  - First 2 wk of life: Vomiting, diarrhea, ↓ weight gain, cataracts, ↑ indirect bili (hemolysis)
- **Diagnosis:**
  - Most states screen on NBS; if picked up <5 d can avoid acute morbidity/mortality
  - Galactose (total) 20–30 mg/dL; no rx, outpatient review
    - Repeat screening of dried blood spot, galactose, GALT activity
  - Galactose (total) 30–40 mg/dL; repeat
    - Start lactose-free milk, outpt review, follow-up repeat labs
  - Galactose (total) >40 mg/dL; hospitalization, lactose-free diet
    - Check liver and kidney function, coagulation, and ultrasound
    - Check galactose, galactose-1-phosphate, GALT activity
- **Treatment**
  - Lactose and galactose free diet
  - For acute illness: Supportive care, vit K, FFP, abx for gram-negative sepsis, phototherapy
  - Usually improve w/ removal of galactose; check meds after dx (many contain galactose)
- **Prognosis**
  - Despite dietary therapy, pts develop intellectual disability, verbal dyspraxia, motor abnormalities & hypergonadotropic hypogonadism
  - Many die of *E. coli* sepsis

AMINOACIDOPATHIES
(Pediatr Rev 2016;37(1):3–15)

- Def of enzymes for AA metabolism → toxic products accumulate in brain, liver, and kidneys
- If known disorder of AA metabolism and ill → call metabolic team; often p/w acidosis
- Begin therapy w/ dextrose, stop protein intake, maintain normal [Na] to prevent cerebral edema, HD may be necessary, vitamins and carnitine depending on dx

Phenylketonuria/Phenylalaninemia

- Autosomal recessive; ↑ amino acid phenylalanine in blood
- Deficiency of phenylalanine hydroxylase results in impaired neurotransmitter production
- If >20 mg/dL accumulation of phenylketones → phenylketonuria (PKU), musty body odor
- Spectrum of severity depending on degree of residual enzyme function
  - If untreated: Severe brain damage, MR, seizures, spasticity
- More common in Turkish and Irish populations
- **Diagnosis:** Positive NBS: Check quantitative level of phenylalanine & tyrosine concentrations
- **Treatment**
  - Early dx important, admit to the hospital; inverse relationship b/w time to therapy and IQ
  - Provide protein sources low in phenylalanine; titrate to [Phe] 1–6 mg/dL for 1st 10 yr of life
  - Follow phenylalanine levels; despite therapy pts still have ↑ neuropsych complications

Tyrosinemia

- Accumulation of tyrosine in fluids and tissue
- **Types:**
  - Type I is most severe: Liver failure, neurologic crises, rickets, hepatocarcinoma
    - Deficiency of fumarylacetoacetate hydrolase (FAH)
    - If untreated, death before 2 yo
  - Type II: Deficiency of tyrosine aminotransferase (TAT)
    - Presents with hyperkeratotic plaques on the hands and soles of the feet and photophobia secondary to tyrosine crystals within the cornea
  - Type III: Extremely rare 2/2 deficiency of 4-hydroxyphenylpyruvate dioxygenase
- **Treatment:** Urgent therapy with nitisinone (blocks accumulation of toxic metabolites)
  - Long-term: Phenylalanine and tyrosine-restricted diets

Maple Syrup Urine Disease (Pediatrics 2006;118:e934)

- Deficiency in activity of branched-chain α-oxoacid dehydrogenase complex → accumulation of leucine, isoleucine, and valine
- Autosomal recessive; more common in Mennonite populations
- **Signs/sxs:**
  - Encephalopathy at 4–7 d w/ lethargy, feeding probs, somnolence, cerebral edema, coma
  - Urine w/ maple syrup/burnt sugar smell. If breastfed, see in 2nd wk (↓ protein intake)
- **Diagnosis:** ↑ valine, leucine (plasma >4 mg/dL), & isoleucine in plasma
  - Urine w/ branched-chain oxo-/hydroxy acids
  - Intermittent dz may go undx'd until 5 mo – 2 yr of age; dx'd during a mild illness
  - Intermediate dz: Progressive neurologic decline → intellectual disability; b/w 5 mo–7 yr
- **Treatment:** Glucose & insulin infusion, avoid deficiency of isoleucine & valine
  - Long-term: Follow AAs in the plasma and adjust diet
    - Must have low level of these AAs for growth and development
    - Trial of thiamine supplementation 50–300 mg/d × 3 wk is recommended
  - Best outcomes when treated within first 2 wk of life

FATTY ACID OXIDATION DEFECTS

(Pediatrics 2006;118:E934; Pediatr Rev 2016;37(1):3–15)

- **Def:** Disorder characterized by inability to utilize & break down stored fat during fasting
- Typical presentation is hypoketotic hypoglycemia & metabolic acidosis
  - ↑ transaminases & hyperammonemia ± hepatomegaly

Medium-Chain Acyl-CoA Dehydrogenase Deficiency (MCAD)

- Most common disorder of fatty acid oxidation; autosomal recessive
- Defect in mitochondrial β-oxidation; unable to convert fats to ketones → hypoglycemia
- **Signs/sxs**
  - Vomiting and lethargy after fasting in a 3–15 mo child
  - Most diagnosed <4 yo, undiagnosed mortality ~20–25%
  - Hypoketotic hypoglycemia provoked by fasting (do not present in nonfasting conditions)
    - May develop coma (2/2 hypoglycemia + toxicity of fatty acids & metabolites)
  - Muscle weakness worsens with increased delay in diagnosis

- **Diagnosis:** Detected on NBS
  - Confirm dx with plasma acylcarnitine analysis and urinary organic acids
  - May need skin bx for enzyme eval of fibroblasts to narrow down actual enzymatic defect
- **Treatment:**
  - Avoid fasting or decreased dietary fat intake
  - Supplement with L-carnitine (especially during illnesses)
  - Treat aggressively even during mild illnesses with IV glucose and carnitine

---

LYSOSOMAL STORAGE DISORDERS

(Eur J Pediatr 2004;163:58; Curr Opin Pediatr 2005;17:519)

Gaucher Disease
- AR def glucocerebrosidase activity → accum of glucocerebroside in macrophage lysosome
- Autosomal recessive
- Glucocerebroside accum → hepatosplenomegaly, anemia, thrombocytopenia, growth retardation, skeletal disease
- **Types:**
  - **Nonneuronopathic (Type 1)**
    - Visceral, hematologic, & skeletal involvement
    - Develops in childhood/adulthood; 1:40,000–60,000 (predilection for Ashkenazi Jews)
    - Survival 6–80 yr; early dx and rx with enzyme replacement → better prognosis
  - **Acute neuronopathic (Type 2)**
    - Visceral + heme involvement with a neurodegenerative course
    - Develops in infancy; <1:100,000; survival <2 yr
    - Strabismus, saccadic-initiating defects, opisthotonic posturing (decerebrate w/neck and back arched posteriorly), bulbar palsy/paresis within the first 6 mo of life
    - No data to support enzyme replacement
  - **Subacute neuronopathic (Type 3)**
    - Develops in childhood; <1:100,000; survival 20–40 yr
    - Saccadic initiation defects 1st 3 mo of life; progression of CNS dz occurs in later years
    - No data to support enzyme replacement

Fabry Disease (Pediatr 2004;144:S20)
- Deficiency of α-galactosidase A, which breaks down glycosphingolipids → accumulates in vascular endothelium → ischemia/infarction
- Average age of diagnosis ~29 yo, life span of ~50 yr
- X-linked recessive; female carriers may develop mild manifestations
- Not associated with intellectual disability or physical abnormalities
- Angiokeratomas, hypohidrosis, and acroparesthesia (burning/tingling pain in extremities)
- **Signs/sxs by age**
  - **4–16 yr:**
    - Neuropathic pain (burning/tingling) that usually begins in hands & feet
    - May have fever + elevated ESR, diarrhea, abd pain, N/V, FTT
    - Triggered by stress, heat, fatigue, or exercise (cannot sweat); angiokeratomas (purplish/red nonblanching telangiectasias); ↑ in size and # w/ age
    - Eyes with whorled corneal opacity
  - **Teenage adult:**
    - Renal complications → uremia + HTN → ESRD
    - May have MI, valve abnormality, arrhythmias, LVH, early strokes, and dyspnea
- **Diagnosis:** Deficient or absent α-galactosidase A activity
  - Can dx prenatally with chorionic villi or cultured amniocyte
- **Treatment:** α-galactosidase A replacement (J Inherit Metab Dis 2012;35:227)
  - Avoid pain triggers such as heat, cold, stress, or exertion
  - Some benefit from carbamazepine, gabapentin, diphenylhydantoin, NSAIDs
  - GI symptoms helped with pancrelipase or metoclopramide
  - Check baseline renal, heart, and brain MRI before enzyme rx to follow disease
  - Follow-up: CBC, chemistries, U/A, creatinine: Albumin ratio, CrCl
    - In adolescents: Every other yr echo and ECG to monitor for cardiac abnormality

Pompe Disease (J Pediatr 2004;144:S35)
- Glycogen storage type II disease or acid maltase deficiency; lysosomal storage disorder
- Considered a neuromuscular, metabolic myopathy, & glycogen storage disease
- Muscle d/o caused by deficiency of acid α-glucosidase → lysosomal glycogen accumulation in cardiac, skeletal, and smooth muscle cells
- **Types:**
  - Infantile onset
    - Death within 1st yr of life; present in 1st few mo → floppy baby
    - Hypotonia, muscle weakness, HCM → death from cardiopulmonary failure
  - **Juvenile and adult onset**
    - Less severe cardiac issue; present at any age; survival: Early childhood to late adults
    - Progressive skeletal muscle dysfunction, calf muscle pseudohypertrophy
    - Gower sign → using hands and arms to stand up from a lying position
    - Require wheelchairs and eventual artificial ventilation → respiratory failure
- **Diagnosis:**
  - Clinical syndrome + muscle bx; check acid α-glucosidase activity in skin/muscle fibroblasts
  - Other family members should be tested; genetic counseling recommended
- **Treatment:** Supportive care

Mucopolysaccharide Disorders (MPS) (Pediatr Rev 2009;30:e22; J Pediatr 2004; 144:S27)
- Def of enzyme for degradation of glycosaminoglycans
- Accumulation of glycosaminoglycans in lysosomes → cell, tissue, organ dysfunction
- Autosomal recessive except type II (Hunter syndrome) which is X-linked-recessive
- **Signs/sxs:**
  - Normal at birth, chronic progressive course w/ multisystem involvement
    - Abnormal facies, organomegaly
    - Loss of developmental skills, frequent pneumonias, cardiomyopathy
- **Diagnosis:**
  - Specific enzyme assays for each type
  - 7 types: I–IV, VI, VII, IX; III and IV have subtypes
  - Recommend genetic counseling
- **Hurler syndrome:** Most severe form (MPS I)
  - Deficiency of α-L-iduronidase → dermatan sulfate and heparan sulfate stored
  - Usually normal at birth; death before 10 yo
  - Presents in early infancy or childhood w/ severe somatic & neurologic dz, progressive MR
  - Bone marrow transplantation is helpful, enzyme replacement also available
- **Hunter syndrome** (MPS II)
  - X-linked, seen in males
  - Deficiency of iduronate sulfatase → dermatan sulfate and heparan sulfate stored
  - Supportive therapy

MITOCHONDRIAL DISORDERS
(Pediatr Rev 2016;37(1):3–15)
- Enzyme or enzyme complex disorder involved in ATP production via oxidative phos
  - Enzymes involved include pyruvate dehydrogenase complex, tricarboxylic acid cycle, the respiratory chain, and ATP synthase
- Impacts high-energy-requiring organs → brain, skeletal muscle, heart, kidney, & retina
- Inheritance can be recessive, dominant, X-linked, or maternal w/ variable penetrance
- **Signs/sxs:**
  - Suspected w/ combined neuromuscular and/or nonneuromuscular sxs
    - Progressive course, unrelated organs or tissues involved in disease process
  - Neurologic presentation: Central and/or peripheral sxs, seizures, hypotonia, abnormal movements, resp distress, encephalopathy, coma, poor head control as an infant, cerebellar ataxia, intellectual disability, poor psychomotor development, loss of skills
  - Muscular presentation: Can range from fatal infantile myopathy → progressive muscle weakness; generalized weakness, resp distress, ↑ lactate, exercise intolerance, rhabdo
    - Fatal form, results in death before 1 yo
  - Multisystem disease:
    - Anemia, FTT, liver dysfunction, diarrhea, short stature, DM, cardiomyopathy, FSGS, retinopathy, hearing loss, feeding difficulties

- **Diagnosis:**
  - Full assessment of muscle function, CK, EMG, neuro exam with EEG
  - Lactic acid, CSF lactate, urine organic acids, plasma and CSF amino acids, CSF protein
  - MRI, consider NMR spectroscopy
  - Surgical muscle bx in mitochondrial center → EM for quant mitochondria and morphology, enzyme histo, immunohisto, genetic studies, enzyme studies, and light microscopy
- **Treatment:**
  - Fluids, electrolytes, restrict glucose, avoid drugs that effect the respiratory chain (valproate, tetracyclines, chloramphenicol)
  - Treat acidosis; consider cofactors: Coenzyme q10, biotin, creatine

FEVER IN NEWBORN

- Def: Any infant aged 0–60 d of life with rectal temperature of 38°C/100.4°F requires sepsis evaluation due to a high percentage (10%) of serious bacterial infection in febrile infants (Clin Ped 2000;39:81)
- **All febrile neonates <30 d and ill-appearing febrile infants >30 d** must undergo a full sepsis workup: Blood, urine, and CSF cx and cell count + CBC w/ diff and CRP/pro-calcitonin (Clin Ped 2000;39:81)
  - CXR if focal signs/symptoms
- **Well-appearing febrile infants >30 d** who meet the following criteria below can have the LP deferred, abx withheld, and the patient can be observed while blood and urine cx are pending based on the Rochester criteria:
- Rochester criteria

Clinical	Previously healthy with no underlying illness
	Full term w/o prev hospitalizations or complications
	Well-appearing w/o evidence of bacterial infection on exam or imaging
	No prior abxs including perinatal abxs
Labs	WBC between 5,000–15,000
	Absolute band count <1,500
	Urine WBC <10/hpf
	Stool WBC <5 (if indicated)

- Empiric tx:
  - **<30 d:** Ampicillin 50 mg/kg/dose Q8H + gentamicin 4–5 mg/kg/dose daily or ampicillin 50 mg/kg/dose Q8H + cefotaxime 50 mg/kg/dose Q8H
  - **>30 d & <60 d:** Ceftriaxone 50 mg/kg daily (meningitic dosing 100 mg/kg) daily and ampicillin
  - Acyclovir should be added in any of the above regimen if there is suspicion for HSV infection given maternal risk factors

GROUP B STREPTOCOCCUS IN NEONATES

GBS	Onset of Occurrence	Typical Manifestations	Notes
Early onset	1–6 d of life	Pneumonia, meningitis	More likely to present with shock physiology
Late onset	7 d–3 mo	Bacteremia, meningitis	More likely to have clinically apparent seizures
Late, late onset	>3 mo	Bacteremia, CNS, & MSK focal sites	Common in infants <28-wk gestation

- Lumbar puncture is required in patients presenting with GBS bacteremia infection
- Tx should be penicillin or ampicillin but empiric therapy should include gentamicin to cover possible infectious pathogens such as *E. coli*
- Definitive therapy of GBS bacteremia is ampicillin 150 mg/kg/d for 10 d
- For meningitis, tx duration increases to 14–21 d
- Penicillin G is also an alternative with the same tx duration as ampicillin

MENINGITIS/ENCEPHALITIS

- Meningitis is the inflammation of the leptomeninges, the tough protective layers of tissue surrounding the brain and spinal cord
- Hib and pneumococcal vaccination has resulted in a dramatic reduction in the incidence of bacterial meningitis
- Sx:
  - Generally starts with abnormal vital signs such as tachycardia and fever
  - Irritability, lethargy, refusal to eat, headache, myalgia, photophobia, confusion can also be present
  - Seizures and neurologic signs are late signs
  - Neonates can present with a bulging fontanelle, apnea, or other respiratory signs

- HSV meningitis can lead to encephalitis and can result in cerebral edema and destructive lesions in the brain with a predilection for the temporal lobes. Seizures are common (Pediatrics 2001;2:23)
- **Encephalitis** is an inflammation of the brain parenchyma as opposed to the meninges
  - Signs and symptoms of encephalitis can be similar to meningitis but with alterations in consciousness an earlier sign (*Principles and Practice of Pediatric Infectious Diseases. 5th ed. 2018:305*)
  - Most common causes of infectious encephalitis are viral (HHV, arboviruses, and enterovirus)

Age	Common Organisms of Meningitis
Neonates	*Listeria, E. coli*, GBS, enterics (*Pseudomonas, Serratia*), HSV
1–3 mo	GBS, gram-negative rods, *S. pneumoniae, N. meningitidis*
3 mo–3 yr	*S. pneumoniae, N. meningitidis*, GBS, gram-negative bacilli
3–10 yr	*S. pneumoniae, N. meningitides*
≥10 yr	*N. meningitides*

- Dx: Blood cx, CBC w/ diff, CSF Gram stain and cx, cell count and diff, glucose and total protein

CSF Analysis	Glucose (mg/dL)	Protein (mg/dL)	WBC
Normal	50–80	15–45	0–5
Bacterial	<45	>250	>100 (neutrophil predominant)
Viral	normal	>50, <150	<250 (lymphocyte predominant)

- Empiric tx:
  - Neonates: Ampicillin + cefotaxime in neonates
  - Older children: Ceftriaxone
    - Vancomycin is added if there is concern for resistant *S. pneumoniae* or *MRSA*
  - Consider acyclovir if there is concern for HSV meningitis
- If *Neisseria* meningitis is confirmed, ceftriaxone at 100 mg/kg/d is usually preferred due to ease of administration, although penicillin G can also be used if the pathogen is susceptible. Chemoprophylaxis must also be considered with rifampin 20 mg/kg Q12H ×2 d to others in close contact with patient (Pediatr Rev 2017;38:163)
- Tx for viral encephalitis is mainly supportive and in cases of seizures, antiepileptics would be recommended

ACUTE OTITIS MEDIA AND EXTERNA

Acute Otitis Media
- Dx: Bulging of tympanic membranes or signs of inflammation (erythema, fever, or ear pain) AND middle ear effusion (Acad Pediatr 2012;12:214)
- Common pathogens: *S. pneumoniae*, nontypeable *Haemophilus, Moraxella*, and *S. pyogenes*
- Complications: Mastoiditis +/– intracranial spread, hearing loss, bacteremia, meningitis
- Tx:
  - First line: High-dose amoxicillin 80–90 mg/kg/d BID
  - Recurrent AOM: Amoxicillin–clavulanate 90 mg/kg/d BID
  - PCN allergy: Consider 3rd gen cephalosporin vs. macrolide
  - IM ceftriaxone 50 mg/kg for 1 dose an alternative, esp if recurrent AOM
- Tympanostomy: Indicated if 3 episodes of AOM w/i 6 mo or ≥4 episodes in 1 yr (Pediatrics 2017;139:6)

Acute Otitis Externa
- Def: Infection of the skin of the auditory canal and is classically caused by *Pseudomonas*, (also *Staph* can be a pathogen)
- Dx:
  - Auditory canal narrowing with granulation tissue and edema
  - Pain w/ movement of the tragus/pinna
- Tx:
  - Mild: Otic antimicrobials drops (e.g., ciprofloxacin) +/– steroid drops
  - Severe: Aura lavage
- Complications: Necrotizing otitis externa – osteomyelitis of the skull due. Tx w/ parenteral abx +/– surgical debridement

PHARYNGITIS

- The majority of pharyngitis is viral, benign, and self-limiting
- Epi: EBV and CMV are common, most common bacterial spp. is *Strep*
- Decision to swab for a rapid *Strep* test can be determined by the Centor criteria

Group A Streptococcal (GAS) Pharyngitis
- **Centor Criteria for testing of strep pharyngitis**

Age	3–14 yo: 1	>14 yo: 0
Exudate/swelling of tonsils	Yes: 1	No: 0
Tender/swollen cervical lymph nodes	Yes: 1	No: 0
Temp >38°C	Yes: 1	No: 0
Cough	Yes: 0	No: 1

- **0–2 points:** No testing indicated. **3–5:** Consider rapid *Strep* test and cx
- Tx: Focuses on prev of complications (abscess, meningitis, acute rheumatic fever, PSGN, reactive arthritis, rheumatic heart disease [RHD]), sx mgmt, and prev of spread to others
  - PCN 250 mg BID or TID × 10 d
  - IM benzathine penicillin for 1 dose
  - Amoxicillin 50 mg/kg/d daily or BID × 10 d
  - **Alternatives:** Cephalexin 20 mg/kg/dose BID or clindamycin 20 mg/kg/d TID × 10 d (Pediatr Rev 2017;38:84)
  - **PCN allergy:** Consider cephalosporins, macrolides, and clindamycin

Acute Rheumatic Fever (Circulation 2015;131:1806)
- Complication of untreated GAS pharyngitis, occurs 2–4 wk following infection
- Dx: Jones Criteria with major and minor criteria. For sufficient diagnosis, 2 major manifestations or 1 major + 2 minor are sufficient if there is evidence of preceding GAS infection

Jones Criteria

Major Criteria	Minor Criteria
Arthritis	Fever
Carditis	Arthralgia
Sydenham chorea	↑ ESR/CRP
Subcutaneous nodules	↑ PR interval
Erythema marginatum	

- Prev GAS infection: + GAS throat cx, + rapid streptococcal antigen test, ↑ anti-streptolysin O (ASO) or anti-deoxyribonuclease B (ADB)
- Once ARF is diagnosed, echocardiogram should be done to evaluate valvular changes as ARF can lead to RHD, a progression to chronic valvular disease
  - Mitral regurgitation is the most common valvular manifestation of RHD
- Tx: Prophylactic abxs, usually monthly benzathine penicillin

Peritonsillar and Retropharyngeal Abscesses
- One of the more common complications of strep pharyngitis although still rare
- With the formation abscess, becomes polymicrobial w/ anaerobic spp.
- Sx: Odynophagia, drooling, trismus, muffling of voice, uvular deviation toward the opposite side, lymphadenopathy
- Tx: Drainage and cx of the drainage w/ ENT consultation
  - Broad spectrum abxs covering strep and anaerobes: Ampicillin–sulbactam, penicillin + metronidazole or clindamycin

Lemierre Syndrome (Laryngoscope 2009; 119:1552)
- Def: Jugular vein suppurative thrombophlebitis
- Dx: Primary infection of the oropharynx, bacteremia (+ blood cx), thrombophlebitis of the internal jugular vein, metastatic infections at ≥1 distant sites (lung, bone, liver, spleen)
  - Pulmonary abscesses with preceding pharyngitis should ↑ suspicion
- Typically caused by *Fusobacterium necrophorum* (also *Prevotella* spp., *Bacteroides* spp., streptococci, and polymicrobial)
- Tx: Ampicillin–sulbactam or penicillin + metronidazole or clindamycin

PERIORBITAL AND ORBITAL CELLULITIS

	Periorbital (Preseptal) Cellulitis	Orbital Cellulitis
Definition	Infection of the anterior of the eyelid and anterior to the orbital septum	Infection of contents of the orbit (fat and muscle) excluding the globe itself
Pathology	Trauma (minor or major such as bug bite or scratch) to the skin typically precedes the infection	Sinusitis is a leading cause of orbital cellulitis, odontogenic origin also possible
Signs & Sx	Typically no pain with ocular movement or impairment of movement although it may be subjective	Pain with ocular movement, impaired ocular movement, proptosis, loss of visual acuity
Pathogens	*Staph* and *Strep* spp.	*Staph* spp., *Strep* spp., anaerobes from upper respiratory tract, *Prevotella*, *Fusobacterium*
Tx	Ampicillin–sulbactam 200 mg/kg/d Q6H If *MRSA* concern: Clindamycin 30–40 mg/kg/d TID or TMP/SMX 12 mg/kg/d BID of trimethoprim	Ampicillin–sulbactam 200 mg/kg/d Q6H. If *MRSA* suspected, vancomycin 40–60 mg/kg/d QID + piperacillin–tazobactam 240 mg/kg/d TID or ceftriaxone 50 mg/kg QD
Complications	Rare, preseptal cellulitis can also rarely lead to orbital cellulitis	Subperiosteal abscess, orbital abscess, cavernous sinus thrombosis, intracranial extension

ENDOCARDITIS

Infective Endocarditis (Am J Med 1994;96:200)
- Relatively rare in pediatrics compared with adults
- More prevalent in children with congenital heart disease
- Diagnosis of IE utilizes the modified **Duke criteria** which has major and minor points:
  - **Major criteria:**
    - Positive blood cx with typical microorganisms consistent w/ IE from 2 separate cx: *S. aureus*, viridans streptococci, *S. gallolyticus*, HACEK (*Haemophilus, Aggregatibacter, Cardiobacterium, Eikenella, Kingella*)
    - Persistently blood cx: Of organisms that are typical causes of IE (≥2 >12 hr apart) or of organisms that are commonly skin contaminants (3/4 cx or majority of >4 cx)
    - Single positive blood cx for *Coxiella burnetii* or phase 1 IgG antibody titer >1:800
    - Echocardiogram w/ vegetation, abscess, or new partial dehiscence of prosthetic valve
    - New valvular regurgitation (increase or change in preexisting murmur)
  - **Minor criteria:**
    - Predisposition: IV drug use or predisposing heart condition
    - Fever >38°C
    - Vascular phenomena: Major arterial emboli, septic pulmonary infarcts, mycotic aneurysm, intracranial hemorrhage, conjunctival hemorrhages, or Janeway lesions
    - Immunologic phenomena: Glomerulonephritis, Osler nodes, Roth spots, or rheumatoid factor
    - Microbiologic evidence: Positive blood cx that do not meet major criteria or serologic evidence of active infection if organism consistent with IE

Diagnosis
- **Definite diagnosis:**
  - Pathologic criteria: Microorganisms demonstrated by cx or histology in vegetation, embolized vegetation, or an intra-cardiac abscess specimen
  - Clinical Criteria: 2 major criteria or 1 major and 3 minor, or 5 minor
- **Possible diagnosis:** 1 major criteria and 1 minor or 3 minor criteria
- **Rejected diagnosis:** Firm alternate diagnosis is made or resolution of clinical manifestations after 4 or fewer days of abxs or no pathologic evidence of IE in surgery or autopsy after abxs therapy for 4 d or less, or criteria above not met

Tx
- Tailor to the specific pathogen and susceptibilities should be done
- Empiric tx: Cover gram-positive organisms such as *Staph* and *Strep* spp. Ceftriaxone 100 mg/kg daily is a good choice (covers atypical organisms)
- If *MRSA* is suspected, add vancomycin 20 mg/kg/dose Q8–12H
- Narrowing of abxs is recommended once able
- Duration of therapy should start the 1st day of negative blood cx and can be up to 6 wk of therapy parenterally (if virulent pathogen, prosthetic valve)
- 4 wk of tx may be appropriate in certain cases if pathogen is not virulent and/or it is an infection of a native valve

PNEUMONIA

- The majority of pneumonias in pediatric pt are caused by viruses with RSV being predominant
- Other viral causes include human metapneumovirus, parainfluenza, rhinovirus, adenovirus
- For 3-wk–3-mo old, *Chlamydia trachomatis* from maternal transmission should be considered (staccato cough, tachypnea, hyperinflation)
- Mycoplasma pneumonia affects school-aged children and occurs in cycles
- Due to widespread vaccination, *Haemophilus influenzae* pneumonia is not as common
- *Strep* is the most common pathogen, causing the majority of bacterial pneumonia
- *Staph* pneumonia can also occur and result in necrotizing pneumonia

Diagnosis
- Sx: Fever, tachypnea, hypoxemia, crackles on exam
- CXR, SpO_2, and can consider *Strep* urine antigen
- CT can be considered if there is concern for empyema and/or loculations

Management
- Hospitalization: Hypoxemia, dehydration or inability to take oral, moderate to severe respiratory distress, toxic appearance, underlying conditions that may predispose to more serious infection, complications such as empyema, effusion or abscess, outpatient tx (worsening or no response for 2–3 d) or inability of family to treat as an outpatient

Tx
- Outpatient oral tx of bacterial pneumonia w/ amoxicillin (90 mg/kg/d div BID)
- Initial parenteral tx can be ampicillin 150–200 mg/kg/d Q6H or ceftriaxone 50 mg/kg daily and then transition to oral regimen
- Mycoplasma pneumonia tx: Azithromycin 10 mg/kg day 1, 5 mg/kg days 2–5

Complications
- Untreated pneumonia → parapneumonic effusions (fluid accumulation 2/2 inflammation) → secondary bacterial infection → empyema
- Empyema may require thoracentesis and placement of chest tube
  - If loculated and severe, may require VATS to break up the loculations

GASTROENTERITIS

- Def: Stool frequency of ≥3/d or ↑ usual amount of stool frequency typically by ≥2× (J Infec Dis 2013;208:790)
- Vomiting usually initial sx
- In the developed/immunized world, the majority of cases are viral
  - Norovirus > rotavirus (especially in unimmunized)
  - Consider parasites (*Giardia*, amoebas) if + travel hx
- **Bacterial gastroenteritis**
  - Sx: Age >2, gross blood or mucus in stool, high fever (>40°C), tenesmus, severe abdominal pain, ↑ bands, and + exposures (Brit Med J 2007;334:35)
  - Pathogens: *E. coli*, *Campylobacter*, *Shigella*, *Salmonella*
- Dx: Stool studies with viral PCR, bacterial stool cx, and looking for ova and parasites
- Complications: Dehydration, electrolyte disturbances, and in severe cases hypovolemic shock

- Tx is mainly supportive with fluid resuscitation with oral rehydration therapy or parenteral fluids. Abx are not routinely used as may increase risk of HUS
- Abxs may be warranted if there is confirmed infection of nontyphoid *Salmonella* AND with severe illness such as severe diarrhea, high and/or persistent fever, and need for hospitalization (Pediatr Neonatol 2013;53:193)

MESENTERIC LYMPHADENITIS

- Def: Enlargement of LNs 2/2 usually infectious etiology – a common cause of abdominal pain in pediatric patients
- Dx: Enlarged LNs in the abdominal and retroperitoneal w/ CT, US, or MRI
- Etiology: *E. coli, Salmonella,* and *Shigella* spp., *Yersinia.* Viral causes include enterovirus, adenovirus, and lymphoproliferative viral infections (e.g., EBV). Noninfectious inflammation (e.g., IBD) can also be a cause
- Tx: Supportive care, treat underlying condition if indicated

APPENDICITIS

- Appendicitis is one of the most common reasons for acute surgical intervention in pediatrics
- Male predominance
- Common pathogens of perforated appendicitis: *E. coli, Bacteroides,* α-hemolytic strep
- Sx: Fever, migratory abdominal pain from umbilicus to the right lower quadrant, nausea, vomiting, anorexia, rebound tenderness, leukocytosis
- Physical exam maneuvers such as Rovsing, obturator, and iliopsoas can be helpful, do not r/o appendicitis if absent

Diagnosis
- Pediatric appendicitis score:
  - 1 point each for anorexia, nausea or vomiting, migration of pain, fever >38°C, leukocytosis (>10,000), and neutrophils plus bands (>7,500)
  - 2 points for pain with cough, percussion or hopping, and right lower quadrant tenderness
- If PAS is 7 or greater, surgical consultation is recommended
- Recommendations are to perform an abdominal US. If US is not diagnostic and clinical suspicion is still high, a CT scan with PO and IV contrast is warranted
- MRI can also be done in lieu of CT which can decrease radiation exposure

Tx
- Piperacillin–tazobactam 100 mg/kg/dose Q8H for preoperative abx
- Surgical removal of appendix

OSTEOMYELITIS

- In pediatric patients, osteomyelitis is almost always caused by acute hematogenous spread (*Principles and Practice of Pediatric Infectious Diseases.* 5th ed. 2018:480)
- Long bones (femur, humerus, tibia) are common sites
- Due to the anatomy, infants <18 mo can have their infection spread to the epiphysis and growth plate and if left untreated can lead to joint space infection
- By 2 yr of age, the cartilaginous growth plate prevents extension of infection from the metaphysis (*Principles and Practice of Pediatric Infectious Diseases.* 5th ed. 2018:480)
- Preexisting conditions can result in specific pathogens for osteomyelitis. Patients with hemoglobinopathy such as sickle cell disease are at risk for *Salmonella* osteomyelitis

Diagnosis
- Positive blood cx
- ↑ ESR, CRP, leukocytosis
- MRI is most accurate test. XR is the best initial test
- Aspiration of the infected bone should also be performed to isolate the pathogen
- *Staph* spp. is most common cause of acute hematogenous osteomyelitis along with GBS. *E. coli,* other gram negatives, and *Kingella kingae* are other considerations

Tx
- Tx should be pathogen and susceptibility specific
- Empiric tx: Nafcillin 100 mg/kg/d QID (MSSA) or vancomycin 30 mg/kg/d BID (MRSA)
- Clindamycin has superb bioavailability especially with bone penetration only in the pediatric population and can be used for oral therapy after initial parenteral
- *K. kingae* osteomyelitis should be covered with cephalosporins such as ceftriaxone

SEPTIC ARTHRITIS

- Due to hematogenous spread, trauma, or contiguous spread of osteomyelitis
- Most common pathogens: *Staph*, GBS, and enteric gram-negative pathogens, *K. kingae* (Pediatr Infect Dis J 2013;32:1296)
- >90% of septic arthritis is monoarticular
- Polyarticular infections can be seen w/ *N. gonorrhoeae*, *N. meningitides*, and *Salmonella* spp.
- The knee is the most common joint affected, followed by the hip and ankle

Diagnosis
- Labs: CRP, ESR, CBC w/ diff, blood cx
- Imaging:
  - First test: XR
  - US to evaluate for fluid for joint aspiration
- Therapeutic and diagnostic joint aspiration for cell counts, culture (surgical wash out still necessary to prevent joint destruction)
  - Synovial fluid leukocyte count >50,000 with neutrophil predominance is likely septic arthritis despite negative synovial cx
- Screen sexually active adolescents for sexually transmitted infections

Tx
- Initial empiric coverage should cover *MSSA* and *Strep*
- If *MRSA* is suspected, vancomycin or clindamycin should be added
- If *Neisseria* suspected, ceftriaxone should be added

SKIN AND SOFT TISSUE INFECTIONS

Cellulitis
- An infection of the skin involving the dermis and subcutaneous tissue typically caused by a break in the protective skin barrier
- GAS and *Staph* most common

Erysipelas
- Superficial skin infection affecting the upper dermis and lymphatics
- Characterized by painful, bright red, shiny edematous plaques
- Causative pathogen is mostly GAS but other *Strep* spp. also possible. Rarely, *Staph*

Impetigo
- Common infection characterized by honey-colored or gold-colored crust and is contagious
- Risk factors: Poor hygiene, crowded living conditions, humidity, skin trauma
- Causative agents: *Staph* or GAS. Anaerobes have also been isolated on cx
- Localized impetigo can be treated topically with mupirocin with severe infections requiring oral medications

Common Pathogens	Tx (7–10-d Duration)
MSSA	Cephalexin: 25–50 mg/kg/d BID Dicloxacillin: 25–50 mg/kg/d Q6H
MRSA	Clindamycin: 40–60 mg/kg/d Q6–8H Sulfamethoxazole–trimethoprim: 8–12 mg/kg/d of trimethoprim Q12H Doxycycline: 2 mg/kg/dose Q12H
GAS (erysipelas)	Cephalexin: 25–50 mg/kg/d BID Clindamycin 10–20 mg/kg/d TID
Pasteurella (dog/cat bites)	Amoxicillin–clavulanate: 25 mg/kg/d BID of amoxicillin
Vibrio spp. (brackish water injury)	Tetracycline: 25–50 mg/kg/d Q6H Fluoroquinolones is also an alternative For severe infection surgical debridement is recommended

Lymphadenitis *(Principles and Practice of Pediatric Infectious Diseases.* 5th ed. 2018:139)
- Def: Inflammation and infection of an LN, distinct from lymphadenopathy – is a common soft tissue infection in pediatric patients
- Typical locations: Cervical, periauricular, and occipital LNs although epitrochlear and axillary nodes can also become infected
- Etiology
  - Usually caused by *Staph* and *Strep*
  - Less commonly 2/2 cat-scratch disease (*Bartonella henselae*) and tularemia (*Francisella tularensis*)
  - Lymphadenitis due to dental abscesses can also occur and pathogens tend to be mixed
- Dx: History and exam, US. Blood cx, CBC w/ diff, ESR/CRP should be included if systemic signs of infection
- Tx: Aspiration of the infected LN with cx and Gram stain of aspirate
  - Abx should be tailored to cx results and sensitivities of the aspirate
  - Empiric therapy: Cephalexin 50 mg/kg/d BID (covers *Strep*, *MSSA*)
  - If there is suspicion for *MRSA*, clindamycin 30–40 mg/kg/d
  - Duration of tx is 7–10 d after source control
- Complications: Lymphangitis, red linear streaking on the skin 2/2 inflammation lymphatics

URINARY TRACT INFECTION

- Urinary tract infections (UTI) are a common cause of fever in newborns
- Should be evaluated promptly in newborns as they can rapidly progress to bacteremia
- Cystitis = infection in the bladder
- Pyelonephritis = involvement of the kidneys, has higher morbidity
  - Complications from untreated pyelonephritis: Renal abscesses, renal scarring → HTN & CKD
- Rarely, xanthogranulomatous pyelonephritis – a process that arises from inflammation & obstruction with extension into the perinephric fat – can occur, typically due to *Proteus* and *E. coli* infection (*Medicine* 1979;58:171)
- Uncircumcised boys have a greater risk for UTIs than circumcised boys during the 1st yr of life. During this time period, boys have more UTIs than girls
- Sx: Fever, flank pain, N/V, abdominal pain, frequency, incontinence, dysuria
- Most common pathogens: *E. coli*, followed by *Klebsiella, Proteus, Pseudomonas* (recurrent and history of hospitalization), and *Enterobacter* spp.
  - Consider enterococcus in infants w/ abnormal urinary tracts, recent instrumentation
  - Gram-positive organisms such as *S. saprophyticus* are rare but possible
  - *S. aureus* rarely causes UTI; thus if it is isolated in the urine, pursuing the primary source of infection is warranted (*Principles and Practice of Pediatric Infectious Diseases.* 5th ed. 2018:343)
- Viral causes of UTIs such as adenovirus should also be considered with positive symptoms but negative urine cx

Diagnosis
- UA and cx of sterile urine specimen (usually catheter)
- UA: Pyuria (5 WBC per high power field), + Gram stain, + leukocyte esterase, + nitrite (some bacteria, e.g., *Pseudomonas*, do not produce nitrites)
- Urine cx: (Gold standard) Diagnostic if ≥100,000 CFUs. Pyuria + 50,000 CFUs may be considered sufficient for diagnosis

Tx
- Tx should be tailored to cx susceptibilities
- Empiric tx should cover local pathogens and resistance patterns, e.g., ceftriaxone 50 mg/kg daily
- If enterococcus is suspected: Ampicillin (1–2 g Q4–6H) is recommended
- Patients w/ frequent UTIs: Tailor initial empiric tx to previous urine cx susceptibilities

Management (*Pediatrics* 2014;133:394)
- Renal and bladder US are recommended in patients after acute phase of illness has passed and who are:
  - ≤2 yo with first febrile UTI **or** children of any age with recurrent febrile UTIs **or** children of any age with UTI and family history of renal/urologic disease **or** poor growth **or** hypertension **or** children who do not respond to appropriate abx therapy

- A voiding cystourethrogram – which is a more invasive test than US – should be considered on patients who are:
  - Any age with two or more febrile UTIs **or** children of any age with first febrile UTI **and** with any anomalies on renal US **or** a fever >39 with a pathogen other than *E. coli* **or** poor growth **or** hypertension

SEXUALLY TRANSMITTED INFECTIONS

Chlamydia
- *Chlamydia* spp. are an obligate intracellular gram-negative and nonmobile pathogen
- Causes a wide range of diseases in perinatal, oculogenital, lymphogranuloma venereum (rare in the United States) and trachoma infections
- Chlamydia is a reportable disease and sexual partners should also be tested and treated
- Sx: Include urethral discharge and dysuria, genital ulcers and lymphadenopathy, scrotal or pelvic pain
- Dx: Cx or nucleic acid amplification test (NAAT) of tissue swabs or dirty urine sample
- Tx:
  - Doxycycline 100 mg BID for sexually transmitted chlamydia in nonpregnant adults
  - Azithromycin 1-g single dose which can also be used in pregnant adults
  - Fluoroquinolones and amoxicillin can also be used if there are allergies
- Complications from untreated chlamydia infection: Pelvic inflammatory disease (PID), Epididymitis, prostatitis, reactive arthritis, and also sterility

Gonorrhea
- *N. gonorrhoeae* is a gram-negative diplococcus pathogen
- Causes a wide range of symptoms including urogenital infection, pharyngitis, perinatal infection, and also disseminated gonococcal infection
- Gonorrhea is a reportable disease and increases the risk of infection by other sexually transmitted infections (STI's). Coinfection with other STI's are common
- Sx: Urethral and vaginal discharge, pharyngitis in pharyngeal infections, anorectal discharge and bleeding
- Disseminated gonococcal infection can results in arthritis, tenosynovitis, and dermatitis
- Diagnosis can be done with cx or NAAT with tissue swabs or dirty urine sample
- Due to the extremely high prevalence of abx resistance and cotransmission of other STI such as chlamydia, recommended tx is with ceftriaxone 250 mg IV or IM once with azithromycin 1 g PO once (rx of chlamydia)
- Complications of untreated gonorrhea: Disseminated gonococcal infection, PID, endometritis, salpingitis, tubo-ovarian abscesses, sterility

Syphilis
- Caused by *Treponema pallidum*, a tapered, thin spiral bacilli with corkscrew locomotion
- It is spread through congenital infection or sexually transmitted
- There are three distinct stages of syphilis with its own manifestations and symptoms
  - Primary syphilis is characterized by a painless indurated ulcer or chancre on the skin or mucus membranes and it usually appears 3 wk after exposure
  - Secondary syphilis occurs 1–2 mo later and is characterized by a maculopapular rash including the palms and soles, general lymphadenopathy, fever, headaches
  - Tertiary syphilis occurs 1–30 yr later and is manifested with aortitis (cardiovascular syphilis), nodular lesions throughout various tissue sites (gummatous syphilis), and CNS involvement (neurosyphilis)
- If neurosyphilis is suspected, a lumbar puncture must be performed for diagnosis
- Diagnosis is made initially with a nontreponemal test followed by A treponemal test
- Tx: Benzathine penicillin (penicillin G) should be used for primary and secondary disease. Alternatively, doxycycline 100 mg BID can be used in allergic cases. Neurosyphilis and syphilis infection during pregnancy can only be treated with penicillin G and those with allergies will need desensitization prior to tx

Pelvic Inflammatory Disease (PID) (Am J Obstet Gynecol 1992;166:519)
- Untreated STIs can lead to PID with 40% of infection due to *Chlamydia* and *N. gonorrhea*
- Chlamydia is the most common, gonorrhea is the 2nd most common
  - Bacterial vaginosis can facilitate ascension of other pathogenic organisms
  - Rarely, *Mycoplasma genitalium* can be a cause
- Risk factors: High-risk sexual behavior, unprotected sex, multiple sex partners, drug or alcohol abuse, early sexual activity
- Complications of PID: Fitz-Hugh–Curtis syndrome (perihepatitis), tubo-ovarian abscesses, and sterility

- **Minimum criteria:** Patients who are sexually active and experiencing pelvic or lower abdominal pain, if one of the minimum criteria is met, empiric tx should be initiated
  - Uterine tenderness
  - Adnexal tenderness
  - Cervical motion tenderness
- **Additional criteria:** Can help support the diagnosis of PID
  - Fever (>38.3°C)
  - Mucopurulent cervical/vaginal discharge
  - Lab diagnosis of gonorrhea or chlamydia infection
  - Increased inflammatory markers (CRP, ESR)
  - WBCs on microscopy of vaginal secretions
- **Definitive criteria**
  - Endometrial biopsy with histopathologic evidence of endometritis
  - Imaging diagnosis (MRI, US)
  - Laparoscopic abnormalities consistent with PID
- Tx
  - If there is any concern that patient is unable to complete outpatient tx, hospitalization is recommended
  - Parenteral: Cefotetan (2 g IV Q12H) or cefoxitin (2 g IV Q6H) + doxycycline (100 mg BID) OR clindamycin (900 mg IV Q8H) + gentamicin (2 mg/kg loading)
  - Outpatient: Ceftriaxone (250 mg IM) + doxycycline (100 mg BID) +/– metronidazole (500 mg BID)

HIV (Human Immunodeficiency Virus)
- Given widespread screening and antiretroviral therapy, HIV incidence in the pediatric population is decreasing
- Special consideration should be given to pediatric patients who have not had prenatal care, refugees, immigrants, or any patient whose significant risk factors are based on history
- In patients 12 yr and younger, their symptomology classification is based on the presence of exam findings and also the presence of infections
- Diagnosis of HIV should be done with confirmatory testing. Once diagnosis has been confirmed, initial workup should include investigation for coinfection with other viruses, genotyping of the virus, and viral load

HIV Classification in Pediatrics

HIV in Patients 12 yr and Younger	HIV in Patients 13 yr and Older
Category N: Not symptomatic	HIV/AIDS definition
Category A: Mildly symptomatic	HIV+ with CD4 count <200
Category B: Moderately symptomatic	HIV+ with AIDS-defining illness
Category C: Severely symptomatic	

See CDC website for the specific list of infections

- In HIV+ patients, opportunistic infections include Pneumocystis jiroveci pneumonia, mycobacterial infections, CMV infection, toxoplasmosis, progressive multifocal leukoencephalopathy, cryptosporidiosis
- Tx is tailored specifically to virus susceptibilities and require a combination of different classes (cART, combination antiretroviral therapy)
- Different tx classes include: Nucleoside/nucleotide reverse transcriptase inhibitors, nonnucleoside reverse transcriptase inhibitors, protease inhibitors, entry inhibitors, and integrase strand transfer inhibitors
- Patients with severe immunosuppression from HIV with an underlying infection who initiate antiretroviral therapy are at risk for immune reconstitution inflammatory syndrome (IRIS)

TUBERCULOSIS

- Caused by a slow growing, highly fastidious, acid-fast bacilli *Mycobacterium tuberculosis*
- **Exposure** occurs when patient has had significant contact ("shared air") with another patient with infectious tuberculosis
- **Infection** means *M. tuberculosis* has invaded the lung but not resulted in signs/symptoms. Testing with tuberculin skin test (TST) or interferon gamma release assays (IGRA)

- **Disease** occurs when intrathoracic or extrathoracic signs/symptoms caused by the bacteria are present (radiographic manifestations such as lung parenchyma or lymph-adenopathy) (*Principles and Practice of Pediatric Infectious Diseases*. 5th ed. 2018:4134)
- In developed countries, diagnosis can be done with a TST or IGRA. IGRA can be used to confirm TB infection in a BCG-vaccinated patient with a positive TST result
- Pulmonary tuberculosis is the most common manifestations of TB but may not have signs or symptoms even on chest XR aside from fever and a mild cough
- Extrapulmonary manifestations of TB include osteomyelitis, pericarditis, disseminated and miliary TB, meningitis, gastrointestinal, and also renal disease
- Specimen collection – for sensitivity testing – requires use of expectoration of sputum
- For pediatric patients who are unable to perform expectoration, gastric aspiration done in the early morning when the child has been fasting can also be performed.
- HIV testing is also recommended in patients with suspected TB or undergoing TB testing
- Tx should be tailored to the susceptibility profile of the pathogen and requires direct observed therapy (DOT). Local public health authorities should be contacted and informed as well
- 1st-line agents include isoniazid, rifampin, pyrazinamide, and ethambutol

VIRAL INFECTIONS

Human Herpesvirus

	Disease	Tx/Mgmt
HSV 1 & HSV 2	Genital, mucocutaneous, keratoconjunctivitis, encephalitis	Acyclovir, Valacyclovir
Varicella zoster virus	Varicella (Chickenpox)	Vaccination, supportive
Epstein–Barr virus (HHV 4)	Mononucleosis	Supportive, may require sports clearance due to splenomegaly
Cytomegalovirus (HHV5)	Congenital CMV, mononucleosis	Ganciclovir is approved for use in certain diseases. Mononucleosis is mainly supportive
HHV 6/7	Roseola	Supportive
Kaposi sarcoma associated (HHV 8)	Kaposi sarcoma, multicentric Castleman disease, lymphoma	None

Hepatitis B (*Principles and Practice of Pediatric Infectious Diseases*. 5th ed. 2018:1108)
- Hepatitis B virus (HBV) is a double-stranded DNA virus belonging in the family of hepadnaviridae and is responsible for causing hepatitis B in humans
- Transmission: Percutaneous, sexual, perinatal. Found in blood, vaginal secretions, semen, saliva
- Worldwide HBV infection represents a high burden of morbidity and mortality but transmission is low in the US due to hepatitis B vaccination
- There is no cure for hepatitis B but tx options exist
- Hepatitis B infection can be divided into acute infection, chronic infection, and resolved infection (recovery phase of chronic infection. Each stage has corresponding serology listed in the chart below
- HBs-Ag: HBV surface antigen. Anti-HBs: HBV surface antigen antibody. Anti-HBs IgM: HBV surface antigen IgM antibody. Anti-HBc: HBV core antibody

	HBs-Ag	Anti-HBs	Anti-HBs IgM	Anti-HBc
Acute infection	+	–	+	+
Chronic infection	+	–	–	+
Past infection, recovered	–	+	–	+
Vaccinated (immune)	–	+	–	–

- In the acute infection, symptoms can be asymptomatic or fulminant hepatitis. Signs and symptoms include nausea, vomiting, abdominal pain, jaundice, dark urine, hepato-megaly or splenomegaly. There are also elevated liver enzymes (AST, ALT) and hyper-bilirubinemia
- Fulminant hepatitis is uncommon but can lead to death in acute infection
- Chronic infection can progress to liver disease leading to cirrhosis, liver failure, and hepatocellular carcinoma (HCC)

- Extrahepatic manifestations of HBV infection cryoglobulinemia, glomerulonephritis, polyarteritis nodosa, polyradiculoneuritis, and even thyroid dysfunction
- Tx: Pediatric patients with normal LFTs can be monitored. Patients who have persistently elevated LFTs should be treated
- Tx options include: Interferonα-2b, pegylated interferonα-2a, lamivudine, adefovir, entecavir, tenofovir, and telbivudine
- Tx of HBV infection can prevent progression of liver disease, fibrosis, and HCC

Hepatitis C (*Principles and Practice of Pediatric Infectious Diseases.* 5th ed. 2018:1139)
- Hepatitis C virus (HCV) belongs in the single-stranded RNA family of Flaviviridae
- There are multiple genotypes of the virus and the prevalence is relatively location specific
- Transmission: Blood exposure and perinatal transmission are most common in pediatrics
- Infection in pediatric patients is mostly asymptomatic, signs and symptoms are very mild and similar to other hepatitis infections
- Dx: HCV infection is confirmed w/ NAAT along with genotyping
- Current approved tx options include pegylated interferon α-2a and ribavirin
- Other HCV txs are sofosbuvir, ledipasvir, simeprevir but are not yet approved for children

VECTOR-BORNE DISEASES

Lyme Disease
- Caused by a spirochete and fastidious pathogen *Borrelia burgdorferi*
- Spread via bites form the tick, commonly the *Ixodes* genus. Deer are common hosts for the adult ticks but are not the reservoir for the bacteria
- Small mammals such as the white-footed mouse serve as natural reservoir for the bacteria
- Highly endemic areas in the U.S. include the Northeast and Midwest with reported cases also in the West Coast
- Lyme disease is typically divided into three phases with distinct findings and tx: (*Principles and Practice of Pediatric Infectious Diseases.* 5th ed. 2018:984)

	Diagnosis	Findings	Tx/Mgmt
Early Lyme	Serology typically negative and diagnosis is centered on history & exam	Erythema migrans with central clearing bulls-eye appearance, possible vesicles	Doxycycline 4 mg/kg/d BID 14 d Alternative: Amoxicillin 50 mg/kg/d TID 14 d
Early disseminated Lyme	Serology (IgM and IgG) along with history & exam	Multiple erythema migrans on body, facial nerve palsy, heart block	Facial nerve palsy: Doxycycline 4 mg/kg/d BID 14 d Meningitis: Ceftriaxone 100 mg/kg/d 14 d or penicillin G Q4H 14 d *Patients with heart block, IV abx are indicated until heart block has resolved
Late Lyme	Serology (IgM and IgG) along with history & exam	Intermittent/persistent arthritis, encephalopathy/polyneuropathy	Same abx as above in early disseminated Lyme

Rocky Mountain Spotted Fever (RMSF) (*Principles and Practice of Pediatric Infectious Diseases.* 5th ed. 2018:955)
- Causative agent is *Rickettsia rickettsii*, a obligate intracellular gram-negative rod
- Infection causes small-vessel vasculitis resulting in widespread organ damage
- RMSF is spread via bite of an infected tick – American dog & Rocky Mountain wood tick are the primary vectors in the U.S.
- Symptoms typically develop 2–10 d after bite with onset of fever, headache, nausea, vomiting, and generalized myalgia and the hallmark generalized maculopapular rash
- The rash is composed of discrete blanching macules and can also be absent during illness
- If untreated, disease can rapidly progress to septic shock and multiple-organ damage such as hepatic and renal failure, heart block, coma, and death

- Diagnosis is often misdiagnosed due to its initial nonspecific symptoms and can be confirmed with serology, PCR, or immunohistochemical staining and may require special lab methods
- Labs: Hyponatremia, hypoalbuminemia, anemia, thrombocytopenia
- Tx: Doxycycline at 2.2 mg/kg Q12H or 100 mg BID for 7–10 d

FEVER OF UNKNOWN ORIGIN

- Fever of unknown origin (FUO) in the pediatric population is defined as presence of a fever 38.3°C or greater on several occasions, 3 wk in duration, and an uncertain diagnosis after 1 wk of intensive evaluation
- Approximately half of children referred for FUO do not meet the fever and exclusion criteria
- As with all diseases, FUO requires careful assessment of history and physical exam which will then guide the proper serologic, imaging or biopsy
- Potential noninfectious causes, pathogens, and general disease processes that can mimic FUO are listed in the chart below and should be ruled out prior to making the FUO diagnosis: (Principles and Practice of Pediatric Infectious Diseases. 5th ed. 2018:120)

Noninfectious Causes	Specific Pathogens	Diseases
Kawasaki disease	Salmonella spp.	Malaria
Kikuchi–Fujimoto disease	Bartonella spp.	Endocarditis
Castleman disease	Mycobacterium spp.	Intraabdominal abscess
Familial Mediterranean fever (FMF)	Leptospira spp.	Retroperitoneal abscess
Periodic fever, aphthous stomatitis, pharyngitis, & cervical adenitis (PFAPA)	Rickettsia, Ehrlichia, Anaplasma	Osteomyelitis
Inflammatory bowel disease	C. burnetii	Odontogenic infections
Sarcoidosis	Yersinia enterocolitica	Histoplasmosis
Malignancy	EBV, CMV, HIV	Blastomycosis
Autoimmune disorders	Enterovirus	Toxoplasmosis
Hyperthyroid	Arbovirus	Leishmaniasis
Pulmonary embolism		
Medication reaction		
Munchausen by proxy		

ANTIMICROBIAL CHART

ANTIMICROBIAL 11-13

Class	Abx	Pathogen Treated	Notes
Penicillin	Penicillin G (IV) Penicillin V (PO)	Most Strep, Treponema (syphilis)	
Amino-penicillin	Ampicillin (IV) Amoxicillin (PO)	Strep, Enterococcus, Listeria	
Antistaphylococcal penicillin	Methicillin, oxacillin, nafcillin (IV) Dicloxacillin (PO)	Strep, MSSA	No coagulase Staph
β-lactam + β-lactamase inhibitors	Ampicillin/sulbactam Amoxicillin/clavulanate	MSSA, gram negatives, anaerobes (Serratia, Proteus, Enterobacter, Citrobacter)	
	Piperacillin–tazobactam	MSSA, gram negatives, anaerobes (Serratia, Proteus, Enterobacter, Citrobacter), Pseudomonas	
Cephalosporins	Cefazolin (IV) Cephalexin (PO)	MSSA, Strep, E. coli, Proteus, Klebsiella	
	Cefuroxime (PO/IV)	MSSA, Strep, E. coli, Proteus, Klebsiella, Haemophilus, Enterobacter, Neisseria	
	Ceftriaxone, cefotaxime (IV) Cefpodoxime (PO)	MSSA, Strep, E. coli, Proteus, Klebsiella, Neisseria, Haemophilus, Acinetobacter, Citrobacter, Enterobacter	Gram-positive coverage less effective vs. 1st generation cephalosporins

	Cefepime (IV)	MSSA, Strep, gram negative + Pseudomonas	Poor anaerobe coverage, preferred for neutropenic fever
	Ceftaroline (IV)	MRSA, VRSA, Strep, gram negatives	No Pseudomonas and ESBL coverage
Carbapenems	Imipenem–cilastatin, meropenem, ertapenem (IV)	Gram positive & negative including Pseudomonas, anaerobes, ESBL	No MRSA, VRE; Ertapenem does not cover Pseudomonas
Monobactam	Aztreonam (IV)	Aerobic gram negatives, Pseudomonas	Poor gram positive and anaerobe coverage
Macrolides	Erythromycin, clarithromycin, azithromycin (PO, IV)	Chlamydia, Mycoplasma, Legionella, Helicobacter, Bordetella	
Tetracyclines	Doxycycline (PO, IV)	MSSA, MRSA, Rickettsia (RMSF), Borrelia (Lyme), Vibrio (vibriosis), Francisella (tularemia), Brucella (brucellosis), Bacillus (anthrax), Coxiella (Q fever)	
Lincosamides	Clindamycin (PO, IV)	MSSA, MRSA, Strep, anaerobics	No Enterococcus, covers anaerobes above diaphragm
Aminoglycosides	Gentamicin, tobramycin, Amikacin (IV)	Aerobic gram negatives + Pseudomonas	No activity vs. gram positives, but can be used for synergy
Fluoroquinolones	Ciprofloxacin (PO, IV)	Gram negatives + Pseudomonas, Bacillus	No gram positives (lacks Strep)
	Levofloxacin (PO, IV)	MSSA, Strep, gram negatives + Pseudomonas, Bacillus, Chlamydia, atypicals	
	Moxifloxacin (PO, IV)	Gram positive, atypicals, anaerobe coverage	No Pseudomonas or Strep coverage
Sulfonamides	Sulfamethoxazole–trimethoprim (PO, IV)	MSSA, MRSA, Strep, Pneumocystis, Nocardia, Toxoplasmosis, gram negatives	No Pseudomonas coverage
Lipoglycopeptides	Vancomycin (IV), DAPTOMYCIN (IV)	MSSA, MRSA, Enterococcus, Clostridium (PO)	Not as effective for MSSA (use cephalosporins or penicillins)
Oxazolidinones	Linezolid (PO, IV)	MSSA, MRSA, Enterococcus, VRE	Bacteriostatic
Nitroimidazoles	Metronidazole (PO, IV)	C. difficile, Helicobacter, anaerobes, protozoans (Trichomonas, Entamoeba)	Covers anaerobes below diaphragm
Antifungals			
Azoles	Fluconazole (PO, IV)	Preferred for nonsevere Candida infections	
	Itraconazole (PO, IV)	Preferred for histoplasmosis	
	Voriconazole (PO, IV)	Preferred for aspergillosis	
Echinocandins	Caspofungin (IV)	Preferred for severe Candida infections	
Polyenes	Amphotericin B (IV)	Cryptococcus, histoplasmosis, blastomycosis, coccidioidomycoses	

EPILEPSY

(Pediatr Rev 2013;34:333–342)

Definition
- An individual is considered to have epilepsy when any of the following exists (ILAE, 2014)
  - ≥2 unprovoked seizures more than 24 hr apart
  - Diagnosis of an epilepsy syndrome
- Types of seizures: Generalized, focal (partial), epileptic spasms

DDx
- Epileptic seizure, psychogenic (nonepileptic) seizure, GER (Sandifer syndrome), breath-holding spell, tic, complex migraine, shuddering attack, syncope

Workup
- **History:** The key to diagnosis – details of behavior before, during, and following an episode; video of event is useful
- **Physical exam:** Pay special attention to eyes (congenital ocular defects, retinal changes), skin (signs of neurocutaneous disorder), abdomen (hepatosplenomegaly suggestive of glycogen storage disease), cardiac (possible cardiogenic cause of episodes)
- **EEG:** Most useful if done within 24 hr of seizures, should be both awake + sleeping EEG
- **Neuroimaging:** Useful if structural abnormality is suspected as the basis of seizures (congenital malformation, neoplasm, infectious/inflammatory, hypoxic-ischemic insult); MRI is more sensitive than CT
- **Laboratory testing:** If above negative, consider specialist consult for evaluation for underlying metabolic, genetic, immune-mediated, or neurodegenerative disorders

Treatment
- AED initiation – broad spectrum (both focal and generalized): Keppra, Depakote, Topamax; narrow spectrum (focal): Carbamazepine, oxcarbazepine
  - Specific seizure types: Ethosuximide for absence epilepsy; valproate for juvenile myoclonic epilepsy; ACTH for infantile spasms
- Status epilepticus
  - Start with lorazepam 0.1 mg/kg; repeat in 10 min if seizures persist
  - If status persists, load with fosphenytoin 20 mg/kg
  - If status persists, load with phenobarbital 20 mg/kg
  - Consider midazolam drip

FIRST UNPROVOKED SEIZURE

How likely are seizures to recur?	• Majority of recurrences happen within 1st 1–2 yr • Only ~10% of children go on to experience >10 seizures
What factors increase recurrence risk?	• Underlying etiology • Idiopathic: Recurrence risk 30–50% by 2 yr • Remote symptomatic (CP, MR, hx trauma): Recurrence risk >50% by 2 yr • Abnormal EEG
What if the 1st seizure is prolonged?	• 10–12% of 1st unprovoked seizures present in status • Recurrence risk after status is no different than brief seizure, but is more likely to have status vs. brief seizure in the future
Does treatment after a 1st unprovoked seizure prevent recurrence?	• Treatment with AED after a 1st seizure ↓ risk of seizure recurrence (though no pediatric evidence), but likely does not change long-term prognosis • Need to balance likelihood of recurrence with potential side effects of medications

WEAKNESS

(Fenichel's Clinical Pediatric Neurology. 7th ed. 2013;170–194)

Definition
- Weakness = decreased ability to voluntarily and actively move muscles against resistance

DDx
- **Acute weakness:** Infection (GBS, myositis), neuromuscular blockade (botulism, tick paralysis), stroke (ischemic, hemorrhagic), periodic paralysis, metabolic disease, Todd's paralysis (post seizure)
- **Progressive proximal weakness:** SMA, muscular dystrophy, myasthenia, inflammatory myopathy (dermatomyositis, polymyositis), GM2 gangliosidosis (hexosaminidase A deficiency), metabolic myopathy, endocrine myopathy
- **Progressive distal weakness:** Motor neuron disease, neuropathy, myopathy

Workup
- **History:** Timing, trauma, headache, seizure, fever, diet, medications/toxins
  - Neuromuscular disease → slow motor development, easy fatigability, frequent falls, abnormal gait (steppage, toe-walking, waddling), specific disability (arm elevation, climbing stairs, hand grip, rising from floor)
- **Physical exam:** Thorough neurologic exam (CN, sensation, coordination, DTRs, rising from seated position – look for Gower sign, gait); MSK exam (muscle bulk, tone, strength)
- **Neuroimaging:** Any focal weakness suggestive of CNS lesion warrants prompt CT/MRI
- **EMG/nerve conduction studies**

Treatment
- Management depends on etiology, regardless should watch respiratory function (some etiologies can be associated with diaphragmatic weakness)

	Upper motor neuron	Lower motor neuron			
	CNS	**Anterior Horn Cell**	**Peripheral Nerve**	**NMJ**	**Muscle**
Strength	Normal/↓	↓	↓	↓	↓
Tone	↑/↓	↓	↓	Normal/↓	↓
DTRs	↑/Clonus	↓	↓	Normal/↓	Absent/↓
Muscle Mass	Normal (may have disuse atrophy)	Proximal atrophy	Distal atrophy	Normal or atrophied	Proximal atrophy, distal pseudo-hypertrophy
Muscle Fasciculations	Absent	Present	Absent	Absent	Absent
Sensation	Normal	Normal	↑/↓	Normal	Normal

THE HYPOTONIC INFANT

(Fenichel's Clinical Pediatric Neurology. 7th ed. 2013;147–169; Pediatr Rev 2009;30:e66–e76)

Definition
- Hypotonia = diminished resistance of muscles to passive stretching
  - Weakness = decreased ability to move muscles against resistance
  - While weak infants are always hypotonic, hypotonia may exist with normal strength

DDx
- **Central causes:** HIE, intracranial hemorrhage, intracranial infection, genetic/chromosomal disorders (T21, Prader–Willi), congenital hypothyroidism, inborn errors of metabolism, metabolic disease

- **Peripheral causes**
  - anterior horn cell – infantile SMA, traumatic myelopathy
  - peripheral nerve – CMT
  - NMJ – congenital myasthenia, infantile botulism, Mg toxicity, aminoglycoside toxicity
  - Muscle – congenital myopathy

Workup
- **Hx:** Prenatal/perinatal, developmental, and family history
- **Px:** Assess tone (head lag, horizontal/vertical suspension, appendicular tone); comprehensive neuro exam and assessment for dysmorphic features
- **Labs:** Sepsis evaluation, electrolytes (including LFTs, ammonia, glucose, CK), TORCH titers, screening for inborn errors of metabolism (plasma amino acids, urine organic acids, lactate, pyruvate, acylcarnitine profile), karyotype/molecular genetic testing
- **Neuroimaging:** MRI is a valuable tool if CNS abnormality is suspected

Treatment
- Treatment should be tailored to underlying cause; in general, therapy is supportive

---

SCHEMATIC APPROACH TO HYPOTONIA

(Paediatrics & Child Health 2005;10:397–400)

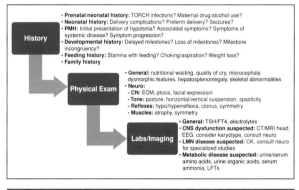

DEMYELINATING DISEASES

GUILLAIN–BARRÉ SYNDROME (GBS)

(Pediatr Rev 2012;133:164–171)

- **Epidemiology:** AIDP is the most common sub-type of GBS (90% of cases) and most common cause of acute flaccid paralysis in healthy infants and children
- **Pathogenesis:** Antecedent infection → immune response → cross-reacts with myelin sheath due to molecular mimicry
  - Campylobacter infection is the most commonly identified precipitant (30% of cases in US)
- **Sxs:** Paresthesias in the toes followed by LE weakness (gait difficulty or refusal to walk) that ascends over hr to d to include the arms, face, and diaphragm
- **Px:** Diminished or absent DTRs
- **Eval:**
  - LP: Elevated CSF protein level (>45 mg/dL) without an elevated WBC count (albuminocytologic dissociation)
  - Neuroimaging: Gadolinium enhancement of the spinal nerve roots on MRI
  - EMG: Conduction block (evidence of demyelination)
- **Management:** IVIG as soon as possible; steroids are not indicated
- **Prognosis:** Most patients reach nadir of function in 2–4 wk, followed by gradual return of function over subsequent wks to mos; mortality 3–4%, usually due to respiratory failure

ACUTE DISSEMINATED ENCEPHALOMYELITIS (ADEM)

(Pediatrics 2002;110:e21)

- **Epidemiology:** Uncommon; 80% of cases occur in children under 10 yo
- **Pathogenesis:** Viral infection → generates auto-immune response due to molecular mimicry
  - Most common precipitant = viral URI, some cases are post-immunization
- **Sxs:** Abrupt onset encephalopathy (confusion, excessive irritability, AMS) +/– fever, neck stiffness, hemiparesis, ataxia, cranial neuropathies, and/or spinal cord dysfunction
- **Evaluation:**
  - Labs: Usually show leukocytosis and ↑ ESR/CRP
  - LP: CSF studies may show pleocytosis and/or elevated protein
  - Neuroimaging: MRI T2 and FLAIR sequences may show diffuse hyperintense lesions mostly in cerebral white matter; T1 hypointense lesions are rare (more suggestive of MS)
- **Management:** High-dose IV glucocorticoids; data from small case series suggest that IVIG may be beneficial for patients who fail to respond to IV glucocorticoids
  Prognosis: Most children fully recover, usually slowly over 4–6 wk

MULTIPLE SCLEROSIS (MS)

(J Child Neurol 2012;27:1378 1383)

- **Epidemiology:** Rare in peds, ~5% of cases present at 18 yo, <1% present before 10 yo; more common in females (F:M = 2:1)
- **Pathogenesis:** Dysregulation of the immune system leads to CNS injury in genetically susceptible individuals; inflammation, demyelination, and axonal degeneration are the major pathologic mechanisms that cause clinical manifestations
- **Sxs:** Nonspecific, but common symptoms include sensory disturbance, weakness, vision loss, gait disturbance, vertigo, bowel/bladder dysfunction
  Children may be more likely to present with isolated optic neuritis, an isolated brainstem syndrome, or encephalitic symptoms (evidence limited)
- **Evaluation:**
  - McDonald Diagnostic Criteria – need to see lesion dissemination in time and space on MRIs – need both of the below
    - One or more T2 lesions in at least 2 of 4 MS-typical regions (periventricular, juxtacortical, infratentorial, or spinal cord)
    - Simultaneous presence of asymptomatic gadolinium-enhancing and nonenhancing lesions at any time, or a new T2 and/or gadolinium-enhancing lesion on follow-up MRI
  - LP: Presence of oligoclonal IgG bands different from any such bands in serum; increased IgG index (CSF IgG to CSF albumin ratio compared to serum IgG to serum albumin ratio)
- **Management:**
  - Acute Tx = methylprednisolone daily x 5 d. Consider IVIG or plasma exchange if inadequate response to steroids
  - Disease-modifying therapy (DMT) = interferon β and glatiramer acetate – reduce relapse rates and may reduce progression of disability. Limited data in Peds
- **Prognosis:** Relapsing-remitting course in >90% of pediatric cases (intermittent attacks of disability followed by partial or complete recovery to baseline functioning)

HEADACHES

(Pediatr Review 2012;33(12):562)

- Initial Evaluation of Headaches in Children
  - Thorough history – timing, pattern, triggers, frequency, location, assoc sxs, duration, alleviating/exacerbating factors
    - Look for signs of secondary headache syndromes (recent trauma, sinus issues, medication effects, recent procedures such as LP), neurocutaneous disorders, systemic disease (lupus, hypothyroidism)
    - FH (migraines have genetic component), SH (stressors, drugs, EtOH, mood)
    - Lifestyle (diet, exercise, sleep, hydration) – consider a headache diary
    - Try to ID triggers – medications (i.e., tetracyclines), dietary triggers (EtOH, drugs, caffeine, chocolate)

- Physical exam – basics + the following:
  - Palpation of face, neck, and shoulders – assess for nuchal rigidity, muscular or bony tenderness, trigger points, allodynia
  - Skin exam for systemic disease, cutting behavior or neurocutaneous disease; oral exam for signs of dental disease
  - Neuro exam (including fundoscopy to evaluate for papilledema)
- Red flag symptoms (concerning for ↑ ICP) – sleep-related headache, lack of FH, headache <6 mo, confusion, abnormal neuro exam, lack of visual aura or vomiting, associated with cough/urinary/defecation, recurrent focal headache, exclusive occipital headache, progressive headache, or change in type of headache
  - If any of the above, consider brain MRI; CT if concerned for hemorrhage or fracture; specialist consult
- Basic Management – primarily lifestyle changes – improve sleep hygiene, ↑ sleep, ↓ caffeine (<3/wk), adequate hydration, regular exercise; manage mood as needed
  - Medication – in children, OTC ibuprofen, naproxen, or acetaminophen is typically effective
  - Complimentary medicine – biofeedback, relaxation, hypnosis, acupuncture may also be effective
  - Physical therapy can be effective with muscle pain and tension causing headaches

MIGRAINES

- Epidemiology: 1–3% in children <7 yo; 8–23% in adolescents; F > M
  - Most common type of headache that leads to medical evaluation
- Pathophys: Unclear – due to complex interactions between neural and vascular symptoms, no longer thought to be due to isolated vasoconstriction
- RFs: FH, stress, anxiety, poor sleep, frequent medication use
- Sxs: Severe headache (usually lasting 30–60 min) +/– photophobia or phonophobia
  - Often assoc with anorexia, nausea, vomiting. Other sxs include dizziness, blurry vision, abd pain, flushing, sweating, pallor
- Aura: Pre-migraine scotomata, transient blurry vision, zig-zag lines, or scintillations
  - Usually occur <30 min prior to headache and last 5–20 min
  - Other types of auras can include sensory changes, confusion, weakness, amnesia, or aphasia
- Treatment
  - Abortive – NSAIDs 1st line, triptans can be used if child can identify headache right away
  - Prophylactic – TCAs, AEDs, and β-blockers can be used
    - Should be chosen on an individual patient basis with consideration of possible comorbidities

TENSION HEADACHE

- Epi: Most common type of headache, less intense than other types
  - May be episodic (<15 d per month) or chronic (>15 d per month)
- Sxs: Described as a "band-like," pressure or tightening in the head
- Pathophys: Similar to migraine, but also include muscle pain and tension in neck and shoulders
- Mgmt: Thorough history – identify stressors, depression, or other possible triggers
  - Management of muscle pain and tension
  - NSAIDs may also provide relief

TRIGEMINAL AUTONOMIC CEPHALAGIAS (TACs)

- Includes cluster headaches, paroxysmal hemicranias, and short-lasting unilateral neuralgiform headache attacks with conjunctival injection and tearing (SUNCT)
- Epi: Rare in children
- Sxs: Brief (few seconds), one-sided, stabbing headache in 1st division of trigeminal nerve
  - Can be associated with ipsilateral eye redness, tearing, nasal congestion, eyelid swelling, rhinorrhea, eyelid swelling, forehead or facial sweating, miosis or ptosis
- Mgmt
  - Can have secondary causes, children should undergo neuroimaging (however most will be normal)
  - Rare and limited data, oxygen may be effective as an abortive agent in chronic attacks

NEUROCUTANEOUS SYNDROMES

TUBEROUS SCLEROSIS

(Pediatr Rev 2017;38(3):119)

- Epi: 1/6,000 worldwide
- Cause: Mutation in TSC1 or the TSC2 gene (results in same phenotype); complete penetrance but variable expression. 50% of cases are new mutations
- Clinical findings
  - Hypopigmented macules: "ash leaf" spots, >3 in different regions of body (BMJ Case Rep 2013; 2013)
    - Other skin lesions include angiofibroma, collagenous plaques, and the shagreen patch
  - Other features: Approximately 50% of children with rhabdomyoma have TSC, seizures can occur at any age, but often present in the 1st 2 yr (seizures in the 1st 12 mo, can present as infantile spasms or partial seizures)
- Diagnosis: Requires 2 major criteria or 1 major + 2 minor criteria
  - Major criteria: Hypomelanotic macules (≥3 at least 5 mm in diameter), angiofibroma (≥3), ungual fibroma, Shagreen patch, retinal hamartomas, cortical dysplasias, subependymal nodules, subependymal giant cell astrocytoma, cardiac rhabdomyoma, lymphangioleiomyomatosis
  - Minor criteria: "Confetti" skin lesions, dental enamel pits (≥3), intraoral fibromas (≥2), retinal achromic patch, multiple renal cysts, nonrenal hamartomas
- Management
  - Surveillance for early diagnosis of complications (seizures, renal lesions, cognitive impairment)
    - Annually – ophthalmology exam, check GFR, BP, developmental screening, skin exam, dental exam (ideally every 6 mo)
    - Every 1–3 yr – MRI, EEG, MRI abdomen
    - Every 3–5 yr – Echo, EKG

NEUROFIBROMATOSIS TYPE 1

- Epi: 1/3,000 people worldwide; no known ethnic, racial or geographic predilection
- Cause: AD mutation of NF1 gene; 50% of cases are new mutations; complete penetrance with variable expression
- Diagnostic criteria (at least 2 of the following): 6 or more cafe-au-lait macules >5 mm before puberty or 15 mm after puberty, axillary/inguinal freckling, two or more neurofibromas, characteristic skeletal dysplasia (long bone or sphenoid wing), optic glioma, iris Lisch nodules, affected 1st-degree relative, Noonan syndrome
- Workup: NF1 genetic testing is 95% sensitive for syndrome
- Long-term risks: Risk of pheochromocytoma, moya-moya syndrome, scoliosis, long bone dysplasia
- Management: Long-term surveillance to monitor for complications
  - Regular MRIs to assess for plexiform neurofibromas
  - Annual ophthalmology exams to screen for optic gliomas until at 6–7 yo
  - BP monitoring (due to risk of renal artery stenosis)
  - Cognitive development should be watched closely

NEUROFIBROMATOSIS TYPE 2

- Epi: 1/30,000
- Cause: AD mutation of NF2
- Features: Bilateral vestibular schwannomas (90–95%), meningiomas or spinal tumors (up to 90%), eye lesions (i.e., cataracts) up to 81%, skin lesions (i.e., cutaneous tumors)
- Sxs: Tinnitus, hearing loss, poor balance, sometimes facial nerve issues
- Mgmt: Surgery prn for tumors
  - Children of affected parents should be followed by audiology and have a brain MRI by adolescence

STURGE–WEBER

- Epi: Estimated 1/30,000
- Sxs: Port-wine stain on the face, in association with leptomeningeal angiomatosis
  - Risk of seizures, strokes, and glaucoma (highest risk when upper division of trigeminal nerve is involved)
- Mgmt: MRI preferably after 1 yr of age in those with port-wine stain
  - If leptomeningeal involvement → ASA to ↓ risk of stroke

ATAXIA TELANGIECTASIA

- Definition: Multisystem, degenerative disorder characterized by ataxia, oculocutaneous telangiectasia, immunodeficiency and a high incidence for neoplasia
- Cause: Mutation in ATM gene which aids in DNA repair
- Sxs
  - Infants – tremors of head, unsteadiness of gait
  - Early school years → progressive global ataxia + slurred, scanning, dysarthric speech in early school years
  - <10 yo – loss of DTRs, impairment of position and vibratory sensation; cutaneous manifestations (telangiectasia)
  - Adolescence → choreoathetosis, dystonic posturing, gaze apraxia, progressive dementia
- Complications: Major defects in cellular and humoral immunity, highly sensitive to ionizing radiation

VON HIPPEL–LINDAU

(Nelson Textbook of Pediatrics 2016;596;2874)

- Epi: 1/36,000
- Cause: AD mutation in VHL (tumor suppressor gene), 80% of patients have affected parent
- Definition: multisystem disease affecting cerebellum, spinal cord, retina, kidney, pancreas, and epididymis
- Sxs
  - Neuro – cerebellar hemangioblastomas and retinal angiomas → sxs of intracranial pressure in early adulthood
    - Some patients can be present with proprioception, gait disturbances, or bladder dysfunction from spinal cord hemangioblastomas

CONCUSSION

(Pediatr Rev 2012;33(9):398; Bradley's Neurology in Clinical Practice 2016;61:860)

- Definition: Minor head injury resulting in altered mental status, +/– LOC. GCSF typically 14–15, no focal neurologic deficits or evidence of fractures
- Epi: Common, 600,000 ED visits per year. Mostly from falls, MCVs, pedestrian incidents, sports
- Second-impact syndrome: Rare – diffuse cerebral edema from 2nd head injury soon (few wks) within 1st head injury – usually fatal
- Management: Graduated return to play, brain rest
  - Remove child from all sports while signs and symptoms ongoing
  - Once symptoms improve can start gradual return to sports starting with low-level physical activity
    - If >15 min of sxs initially, should have at least 1 wk w/o sxs prior to return
  - Brain rest: Minimization of visual and auditory stimuli and rest from physical activity
- Post-concussion syndrome: Prolonged sxs after initial concussion
  - Symptoms vary – headaches, dizziness, nausea, memory disturbance, fatigue, depression, sleep problems, difficulty concentrating, and mental "fogginess"
  - Mgmt: Sertraline and anti-migraine medications have been shown to be effective
    - Patient may benefit from biofeedback, CBT, or psychotherapy for changes in cognition and memory

MOVEMENT DISORDERS

(Pediatr Rev 2015;36(3):104)

- Definitions
  - Tic: Nonrhythmic, repetitive, and intermittent muscle contractions resulting in "stereotyped" movements
  - Tremor: Sinusoidal oscillation about a central point
  - Dystonia: Concurrent agonist and antagonist muscle contractions → abnormal twisting and posturing
  - Chorea: Near-continuous irregular movements with a writing or dance-like quality
  - Athetosis: Similar to chorea but with larger amplitude
  - Stereotypy: Consistent, rhythmic, repetitive movements without clear purpose (i.e., finger rubbing, hand flapping, head shaking, mouth posturing, vocalizing, and rocking behavior)
  - Myoclonus: Rapid jerks, which can occur singly or in clusters

ATAXIA

(Pediatr Rev 2015;36(3):105)

- Definition: Lack of muscle control during voluntary movements
- Cause: Usually cerebellar dysfunction, but can also be due to proprioceptive sensory loss (typically related to peripheral nerve of posterior spinal column disease of the spinal cord)
- Sxs: Dysmetria, difficulty controlling tempo and amplitude of movements and impaired ability to generate rapid, alternating movements

TICS/TOURETTE SYNDROME

(Pediatr Rev 2010;31(6):223)

- Types
  - Transient tics: <1 yr – motor or vocal – usually milder, not always associated with other conditions – can occur in up to 25% of children
  - Chronic tic disorder: >1 yr – motor or vocal (but not both) – often assoc with other comorbid conditions such as OCD and ADHD
  - Tourette syndrome: >1 yr – phonic + motor tics – tics can be mild and easily overlooked
    - Epi: 1%, M:F 4:1
- Pathophysiology: Strong genetic influence, although unclear inheritance pattern
  - Environmental factors: Sleep insufficiency and stress
- Diagnosis: Clinical – no need for labs or imaging
- Management: Primarily education (reversing misconceptions and myths), treatment of comorbid conditions
  - Comprehensive behavioral intervention for tics (CBIT) – a behavior-based strategy to reduce tics
  - Pharmacologic – primarily if tics significant and bothersome to child
    - α_2-agonists – can reduce tics and treat comorbid ADHD or insomnia
    - Atypical neuroleptics – can reduce tics and treat comorbid aggression

CEREBRAL PALSY

(Nelson Textbook of Pediatrics 598:2896)

- Definition: group of permanent disorders of movement and posture causing activity limitation, due to nonprogressive disturbances in the developing fetal or infant brain
  - Often accompanied by disturbances of sensation, perception, cognition, communication and behavior as well as epilepsy and secondary musculoskeletal problems
- Initial evaluation of children with cerebral palsy
  - Thorough history, including risk factors (i.e., prematurity, trauma at birth, history of anoxic brain injury, in utero exposures)
  - Imaging – MRI of brain, can also MRI spinal cord if concern for spinal cord pathology
  - Hearing and visual function testing
  - Consider genetic evaluation in patients with congenital malformations or evidence of metabolic disorders

- Epidemiology: 3.6/1,000 children, M:F 1.4:1
  - NOTE: most common and costly form of chronic disability that begins in childhood
- Classifications
  - Spastic hemiplegia – ↓ spontaneous movements on the affected side
    - Can show hand preference at a very early age, arm more involved than leg
    - 1/3 of patients have a seizure disorder (usually presents within 2 yr); 25% of cognitive abnormalities
  - Spastic diplegia – hypertonia and spasticity of the lower extremities – 35% of CP
    - RF – damage to immature white matter between 20–34 wk GA
    - Approx 15% of cases result from in utero lesions in infants who deliver at term
    - Most common neuropathologic finding is PVL (visualized >70% of cases)
  - Spastic quadriplegia – most severe form – marked motor impairment of all extremities, intellectual disability and seizures are very common
    - May have swallowing difficulties leading to aspiration pneumonia
    - PVL and multicystic cortical encephalomalacia are most common lesions
- Treatment/Management: Interdisciplinary approach (neurodevelopmental, neurology, PT, OT, speech, developmental psychologist, etc.) to optimize function and quality of life
  - Education for parents and families for managing daily activities
  - Assistance with communication using adaptive technologies
  - Spasticity → benzodiazepines and baclofen
  - Surgical interventions may be necessary as children get older to help with contractures

RESPIRATORY COMPLAINTS BY SYMPTOM

(Nelson Textbook of Pediatrics. 20th ed. Ch 384–385, 391)

Symptom	Differential Diagnosis	Evaluation
Tachypnea **Infant:** >60 **Toddler:** >40 **Pre-schooler:** >34 **School-aged:** >30 **Adolescent:** >20	• Compensation for ↓ **tidal volume:** Airway obstruction, pain/splinting, restrictive lung dz, pneumothorax • Compensation for ↓ **O_2:** VQ mismatch, ↓ FiO_2, ↓ diffusion capacity, shunt, anemia • Compensation for **metabolic acidosis:** Sepsis, RTA, DKA • CNS mediated: Fever, anxiety, toxicity	Assess airway, oxygenation, metabolic status, pain, fever, toxicity/ingestions, CXR, full lung exam, equal lung sounds, PE risk factors, infectious w/u, BMP, ± ABG, ± tox panel (see "PICU")

Stridor	• Inspiratory = extrathoracic
	  • Croup, laryngo- or tracheomalacia, tracheitis, epiglottitis, RPA, laryngeal web/cyst, vocal cord paralysis, subglottic stenosis, foreign body (FB), intraluminal tumor, cystic hygroma, angioedema, traumatic intubation, laryngospasm (hypocalcemic tetany), psychogenic
	• Expiratory = intrathoracic
	  • Mimics asthma but tracheal/bronchial origin: Tracheomalacia, vascular rings, bronchomalacia, extrinsic compression, FB, psychogenic
		Determine degree of airway compromise first. CXR ± AP/lateral neck films, w/u for infectious etiology (CBC, viral PCR), bronchoscopy for persistent sx or FB, CT if suspect extrinsic compression, barium swallow for vascular compression/tumor/GERD, EGD or pH probe for GERD, PFTs

Wheezing	• Acute: Asthma/RAD, bronchiolitis, anaphylaxis, toxic inhalation, meds (BB, ASA, indomethacin), aspiration • Extrinsic airway compression: Vascular ring, lymphadenopathy • Intrinsic compression: FB, tumor • Metabolic abnormalities: Hypocalcemia, hypokalemia	Assess respiratory status and airway. Consider trial of bronchodilator (albuterol ± SAMA). If no change or severe symptoms consider CXR. If more chronic: PFTs, pH probe, fluoroscopy, bronchoscopy
Cough	• Acute: Infection, FB, PE, inhaled irritant • Chronic: Asthma, allergic rhinitis, & postnasal drip, reflux, TB, CF, bronchiectasis, toxic exposure (cigarette smoke), CHF, meds (ACE-I), ILD, habit • Recurrent w/ infection: CF, TE fistula, immunodeficiency, ciliary dyskinesia, anatomic disorders, sickle cell anemia	Assess for allergic rhinitis on exam, always ask about poss aspiration/FB, consider CXR, sputum culture if suspect infection, CT scan if suspect bronchiectasis or ILD, trial of antacid if c/w GERD

WHEEZING

(Nelson Textbook of Pediatrics. 20th ed. Ch 391.1; Pediatr Rev 2014;35(7))

• Def: High-pitched, "whistling" sound auscultated – can be inspiratory or expiratory
• Two common natural courses
  • Viral trigger, nonatopic, low risk for asthma in later years
  • Multiple trigger, atopy-associated, persists into later childhood and often adulthood

- Differential for wheezing is broad and should be considered prior to diagnosis of asthma
  - FB aspiration (sudden onset), vocal cord dysfxn (teenager, inspiratory > expiratory difficulty), bronchiolitis, dysphagia/aspiration (sxs associated with feeding), immotile cilia syndrome, chronic bronchiectasis, CF, immunodef (>2 pneumonias in a year), vascular rings/slings, TE fistula, tracheobronchomalacia, tumors/lymphadenopathy, inhalation injuries, many others

ASTHMA

(Pediatr Rev 2014;35(7); EPR3: Guidelines for Diagnosis and
Management of Asthma, NIH 2007)

- Pathophys: Airway hyperresponsiveness → mucus production + chronic inflammation with intermittent bronchospasm → reversible airway obstruction and air trapping → sxs of asthma (wheezing, chest tightness, cough, shortness of breath)
- Most kids symptomatic by 6 yo

Diagnosis
- Key history to obtain: Episodes of wheezing, cough (worse at night), chest tightness, allergies, identifiable trigger(s) leading to symptoms, symptom pattern, family hx
  - Triggers: Viral URI, exercise, weather Δ, tobacco/smoke exposure, environmental allergens (dust mites, pet dander, cockroaches, pollution), cold or hot air, perfumes, drugs (i.e., ASA, β-blockers), med nonadherence/misunderstanding
- Exam: Wheezing, prolonged expiratory phase (assess w/ normal breathing & forced exp), ↑ WOB, hyperexpansion, ↑ RR
- PFTs should be obtained starting at age 6 (discussed at end of chapter). Normal spirometry does not rule out asthma
- Peak expiratory flow not recommended for dx (due to variability), but may have a role in monitoring
- CXR: normal but may show hyperinflation or peribronchial thickening
- Allergy testing (skin or in vitro) indicated for persistent asthma or asthma associated with obvious triggers
- Asthma predictive index (of those who are (+), ~2/3 develop asthma) for children 0–4, if:
  - 3 or more wheezing episodes per year
  AND
  - 1 major criteria: Eczema or parental asthma
  OR
  - 2+ minor criteria (allergic rhinitis, wheezing unrelated to colds, eosinophil count >4%) (Curr Opin Allergy Clin Immunol 2011;11(3):157–161)
- Consider alt dx if no response to standard therapy or symptoms are difficult to control
- Cough variant asthma: Cough may be only manifestation, particularly in young children

Asthma Classification				
	Intermittent	**Mild Persistent**	**Moderate Persistent**	**Severe Persistent**
Sxs or albuterol use	<2/wk	>2 d/wk, not daily	Daily	Throughout day
Nighttime sxs	None	1–2/mo	3–4/mo	>1/wk
Lung function	FEV1 nl between exacerbations, (>80% predicted)	FEV1 >80% predicted	FEV1 = 60–80% predicted	FEV1 <60% predicted
Mgmt	Albuterol prn	Low-dose ICS, cromolyn, or montelukast	Medium-dose ICS, + LABA/ montelukast	High-dose ICS + LABA/ montelukast

Treatment
- Based on severity: Determine current impairment (frequency and severity of symptoms) and risk (frequency of exacerbations, speed of deterioration, access to care, need for steroids). See criteria and stepwise approach above
- Recommend trigger avoidance
- Medications:
  - Rescue medications: Short-acting β2-agonist (SABA) usually albuterol (Proair, Proventil); levalbuterol (Xopenex) theoretically may have less tachycardia but this is not supported by the evidence; can combine with inhaled anticholinergic (ipratropium)

- Controller medications:
  - Inhaled corticosteroids (ICS): Budesonide (Pulmicort), fluticasone (Flovent), beclomethasone (QVAR). Use w/ spacer & rinse mouth to prevent thrush
    - Regular use of nebulized budesonide more effective than budesonide only as needed (Arch Dis Child 2008;93:654–659)
    - Note: DPIs (dry powder inhalers) usually not usable in kids <5 yo
    - Daily use of budesonide not superior to intermittent use in preschool children with wheezing (N Engl J Med 2011;365:1990)
    - Beclomethasone (w/ albuterol) as recue may be used as stepdown for children with mild asthma (Lancet 2011;377:650)
    - Doubling dose of ICS w/ URI not effective in preventing exacerbation (J Allergy Clin Immunol 2011;128:278)
    - 2 trials in NEJM in 2018, in adults quadrupling dose of ICS w/ onset of sxs ↓ severe exacerbations. Quintupling in study of 5–11 yo had no benefit and showed possible harm (↓ linear growth) (N Engl J Med 2018;378:891–910)
  - Long-acting β2-agonist (LABA): Salmeterol, formoterol. Do not use as mono-therapy (may ↑ asthma-related mortality), only with ICS. In adolescents & adults (not children), LABAs combined w/ low/med dose ICS may be beneficial for poorly controlled asthma (Cochrane 2010;CD005533; Chest 2006;129:15)
  - Leukotriene receptor antagonists (LTRAs): Montelukast (Singulair), zafirlukast (Accolate), zileuton (Zyflo)
    - LTRAs provide modest improvement in lung fxn when used as monoRx in children as young as 5 & in asthma control outcomes (other than lung fxn) in pts as young as 2 (EPR3: Guidelines for Diagnosis and Management of Asthma, NIH 2007)
    - Fluticasone vs. montelukast: Fluticasone more effective in improving lung fxn, asthma sxs, and rescue albuterol use (J Pediatr 2005;147:213–220)
    - Montelukast can offer protection from exercise induced bronchospasm (Treat Respir Med 2004;3:9; Ann Allergy Asthma Immunol 2001;86:655)
  - Long-acting antimuscarinic (LAMA): Tiotropium (Spiriva). Equivalent to flutica-sone/salmeterol for step-up therapy in asthma (N Engl J Med 2010;363:1715)
  - Anti-IgE: Omalizumab (Xolair) for allergic asthma and has shown good efficacy when used as add-on to standard tx (J Allergy Clin Immunol 2009;124:1210; N Engl J Med 2011;364:1005–1015)
  - Mast cell stabilizer: Cromolyn (Intal), nedocromil (Tilade). Not used regularly but have shown efficacy for allergic asthma (Chest 1996;109(4):945–952)
  - Theophylline (methylxanthine) is rarely used due to narrow therapeutic window, side effects (arrhythmias, szs, n/v, hypokalemia), and lack of efficacy in studies
- Asthma action plan: Written care instructions for what to do at baseline & w/ ↑ sxs
  - Providing asthma action plan ↓ risk of exacerbations and ↓ oral steroid course (J Am Board Fam Med 2015;28(3):382–393)
- Indications for outpatient pulmonology referral:
  - Hx of life-threatening exacerbation, complicating conditions (i.e., aspergillosis, nasal polyps, VCD), additional diagnostic testing (i.e., complete PFTs, provocative chal-lenge, bronchoscopy), consideration of immunotherapy, frequent exacerbations requiring systemic steroids, hx suggests occ/environmental exposure provoking or contributing

Asthma Exacerbations/Status Asthmaticus
- Refer "Emergency Medicine" on respiratory emergencies for management including discussion of therapy escalation, HeliOx, NIPPV, intubation, and auto-PEEP

BRONCHIOLITIS
(N Engl J Med 2016;374:62–72; Pediatrics 2014;134(5):e1474–e1502)

- Episodes of wheezing in infants <12–24 mo of age due to viral illness
- Mucous and edema in smaller airways causes obstruction and air trapping → localized atelectasis leads to ↑WOB due 2/2 to VQ mismatch (lower resp tract infxn)
- Viral culprits: RSV 50–80%, rhinovirus 5–25%, paraflu (usually type 3) 5–25%, coronavirus 5–10%, metapneumovirus 5–10%, adenovirus 5–10%, influenza 1–5%, enterovirus 1–5%
  - Can be caused by mycoplasma bacterial infection
- Hospitalization for bronchiolitis linked w/ asthma (Am J Respir Crit Care Med 2000;161(5):1501–1507)

WHEEZING 13-3

Evaluation

- History: Assess for risk factors for severe dz: Young age (most hospitalization in <5 mo of age), BPD, prematurity, CHD (pHTN or CHF – unable to ↑ CO in response to infection)
  - Typical symptoms: Low-grade fever, nasal congestion, and rhinorrhea for 2–4 d → lower resp sxs (~peak day 3–5)
- Exam: Δs over time; URI sxs, wheezing, rhonchi, cough, ↑ RR, ↑ WOB, crackles, ↓ O₂ sat
- Diagnosis: Clinical; no need for routine labs or imaging unless toxic or high-grade fever
  - Viral testing may be helpful (i.e., oseltamivir if flu +)

Treatment (Pediatrics 2014;133(3):e730–e737)

- When to hospitalize: Poor feeding, dehydration, mod–severe resp distress, apnea, O₂ sat <95%, RR >70, unable to receive supportive care at home (Am J Dis Child 1991; 145(2):151–155)
- Supportive care; supplemental O₂ for SpO₂ </= 90%, IV fluids if dehydrated (↑ needs 2/2 ↑ insensible losses), npo for ↑ RR to ↓ aspiration risk
- Nasal suctioning (not deep suctioning), hand washing, contact precautions
- Saline nebs (0.9% & 3%) are safe & effective, not recommended in ED settings, ↓ LOS w/ saline nebs reported (Cochrane 2008;CD006458; Pediatr Pulmonol 2010;45(1): 36–40)
- Not recommended: Albuterol (Cochrane 2014; CD001266), epinephrine nebs (N Engl J Med 2003;349:27), systemic glucocorticoids (Cochrane 2008:CD004878)
  - Albuterol may improve symptom scores but no effect on resolution, hospitalization, LOS

Prevention

- Palivizumab (anti-RSV IgG) indicated during RSV season for infants <12 mo who are:
  - Born <29 wk
  - Born <32 wk w/ chronic lung dz or required O₂ for 1st 28 d of life
  - Cyanotic congenital heart disease (Pediatrics 2014;134(2):e620–e638)

RESPIRATORY INFECTIONS

PNEUMONIA

(IDSA guidelines: Clin Infect Dis 2011;53(7):e25–e76; JAMA 2017;318(5):462–471)

- **Def:** Lung infection at the level of alveoli caused by virus, bacteria, or other pathogens
- Most common pathogens by age:
  - Newborns: GBS, *Chlamydia* (afebrile), gram-negative enteric
  - 1–3 mo: Viruses, *Chlamydia trachomatis*, *Ureaplasma urealyticum*, *Bordetella pertussis*
  - 1–12 mo: Viruses, *S. pneumo*, *H. influenzae*, *Staph*, *Moraxella catarrhalis*
  - 1–5 yo: Viruses, *S. pneumo*, *M. pneumo*, *C. pneumo*
  - >5 yo: *S. pneumo*, *M. pneumo*, *C. pneumo*

Evaluation

- **Hx:** Nonspecific; cough, fever, dyspnea, pleuritic pain, abdominal pain. Infants may p/w fussiness and ↓ po intake; fever alone may be presenting sx in young children
- **Exam:** Tachypnea (>60 if <2 mo, >50 if 2–12 mo, >40 if 1–5 yo), respiratory distress, cough, fever, crackles, ↓ breath sounds, egophony, dull to percussion, + wheezing
- **CXR:** (Pediatr Rev 2008;29:e5)
  - Unilateral: Bacterial, aspiration (RML/RLL, pneumonitis vs. infectious), mycobacterial
  - Bilateral ("multifocal"): Atypical bacteria (*Mycoplasma*), viral, neonatal (if afebrile more likely *Chlamydia*; if febrile more likely GBS)
  - Recurrent (same location): Suggests anatomic abnormality (FB, obstructive mass, CCAM, sequestration, focal bronchiectasis); oropharyngeal incoordination w/ aspiration and TE fistula also possible in this setting
- **Diagnosis:**
  - Lung ultrasound (Pediatrics 2015;135(4):714–722)
  - Other testing: Viral swabs, CBC w/ diff, inflammatory markers (CRP, ESR, procalcitonin), blood cultures; urine antigens have high false-positive rate in children

Treatment

- When to hospitalize: Sepsis physiology, respiratory distress, SpO₂ <90%, infants <6 mo w/ suspected bacterial infxn, suspected or documented *MRSA*, inability to comply with outpatient therapy, history of chronic illness or immune compromise, effusion/empyema

- Amoxicillin for mild illness that does not require hospitalization
  - Respiratory fluoroquinolones (levofloxacin, moxifloxacin) in adolescents can be used
- Ceftriaxone or cefotaxime initially in hospitalized children, tailor therapy based on microbiology data as available
  - Vancomycin or clindamycin added if staphylococcal infection suspected

Complications
- Pulmonary: Effusion or empyema, pneumothorax, lung abscess, bronchopleural fistula, necrotizing pneumonia, respiratory failure
  - Empyema
  - Parapneumonic effusion
- Metastatic: Meningitis, CNS abscess, pericarditis, endocarditis, osteomyelitis, septic arthritis
- Systemic: Sepsis, HUS

PERTUSSIS

(Epidemiology and Prevention of Vaccine-Preventable Diseases. 13th ed. Ch 16)
- Highly contagious, toxin-mediated infection 2/2 to *Bordetella pertussis*
- 50% <1 yr hospitalized; complications: Convulsions, apnea, encephalopathy, death

Evaluation
- **Hx/Exam:** Uncontrollable, violent cough >2 wk; after coughing fits sufferers often take deep breaths with a "whooping" sound, apnea seen in infants
  - Incubation period: Commonly 7–10 d, with a range of 4–42 d
  - Catarrhal stage (1–2 wk): Coryza, sneezing, low-grade fever, mild cough
  - Paroxysmal stage (1–10 wk): Bursts of numerous, rapid coughs and difficulty expelling thick mucus; more common at night; posttussive emesis
  - Convalescent stage (weeks to months): Gradual recovery
- **Diagnosis:** Nasopharyngeal swab or aspirate for culture, PCR, and/or direct fluorescent assay

Treatment
- Supportive + antibiotics (azithromycin, erythromycin, or TMP-SMX)
  - Abx eradicate organism in secretions → ↓ communicability; may modify course (if early)

Immunization *(Pediatrics 2009;123:1446; JAMA 2000;284:3145; JAMA 2006;296:1757)*
- Included in childhood vaccination as DTaP, Tdap given at age ≥7
- Children of parents who refuse immunization are at ↑ risk relative to vaccinated children
- Geographic pockets of exemptors pose a risk to the whole community

HEMOPTYSIS

(Pediatr Pulmonol 2004;37(6):476–484; Pediatr Rev 1996;17(10):344–348)
- Bleeding from either pulmonary or bronchial circulation; more severe if bronchial

Common	• Respiratory infection esp tracheobronchitis. Also associated with TB, aspergilloma, endemic mycoses • Aspirated FBs (especially chronic) • Bronchiectasis (especially in CF) • Tracheostomy-related
Uncommon	• Trauma (accidental and nonaccidental) • Congenital heart disease • Pulmonary HTN • PE • AVMs • Lane–Hamilton syndrome (in setting of celiac disease) • intrathoracic endometriosis (catamenial hemoptysis)

Rare	• Tumor (often metastatic)
	• Primary bleeding diathesis
	• Immunocompromised esp following transplant (BM or solid organ)
	• Pulmonary-renal syndromes (vasculitis vs. cavitary lesions)
	• Idiopathic pulmonary hemosiderosis (IPH)
	• Heiner syndrome (associated with cow's milk allergy)
	• Acute idiopathic pulmonary hemorrhage of infancy
Mimics	• Epistaxis/oral/upper-airway bleeding
	• Hematemesis → consider getting pH of sample to differentiate

Evaluation

Adapted from Pediatr Pulmonol 2004;37:476.
CF, cystic fibrosis; BAL, bronchoalveolar lavage; HLM, hemosiderin-laden macrophages.

- **History:** Sxs highly variable. Focal hemorrhage may feel like warmth or "bubbling"
- **Labs/imaging:** CBC, reticulocytes, coags, UA, pulmonary renal syndrome w/u (ANA/anti-GBM/ANCA), sputum sample, PPD
- **Imaging:** CXR, CT with contrast, ECG
- **Bronchoscopy** (+ BAL): May reveal hemosiderin-laden macrophages 3 d to 1 wk after bleed

Management
- Treat underlying cause once identified
- Mild hemoptysis: No immediate treatment required
- Massive hemoptysis: Provide O_2, decubitus position (w/ bleeding side down to promote oxygenation), selective intubation or mainstem bronchus on nonbleeding side, bronchial artery embolization, rigid bronchoscopy, surgical resection

DISEASES OF THE PLEURAL SPACE

PNEUMOTHORAX

(Pediatr Rev 2008;29(2):69–70; N Engl J Med 2000;342:868;
Pediatr Emerg Care 2012;28(7):715–720)

- Air leak in pleural space → pleural pressure > lung pressure → partial/complete lung collapse
- Risk factors for primary spontaneous ptx: Male, tall/thin body habitus, smoking, age 16–24. Also very common in newborns (estimated 1 in 2 births) but <1% are symptomatic
- **Types**
  - Traumatic (penetrating or blunt chest trauma), thoracentesis, barotrauma, CVC placement
  - Spontaneous (nontraumatic): Primary (no underlying predisposing lung disease) vs. secondary due to complication of asthma, CF, necrotizing pneumonia, connective tissue dz
  - Tension (life threatening): Tissue at air-entry point acts as one-way valve, allows air to enter but not exit → complete lung collapse & mediastinal shift to contralateral side → decreased venous return → decreased cardiac output

Evaluation

- **History:** Sudden onset dyspnea and pleuritic chest pain or pain in ipsilateral shoulder, typically at rest or with minimal exertion. May be preceded by popping sensation. Pain often resolves within 24 hr even when pneumothorax persists
- **Exam:** Hyperresonant chest to percussion, decreased fremitus, diminished breath sounds. Exam may be normal or tachycardia only with small PTX (<15% hemithorax)
  - Tension: Absent BS with tracheal shift away from affected side, JVD, hypotension, tachycardia, pulsus paradoxus
- **Diagnosis:** CXR taken in the upright position, lateral decubitus w/ affected side up
  - Other diagnostic modalities: Transillumination in infants, ultrasound ("barcode sign"), CT
- **Treatment**
  - Most reabsorb spontaneously in days to weeks
  - Asymptomatic or small: Observation ± "nitrogen washout" to speed absorption (100% O_2 via NRB at ≥15 L/min); no further tx needed if CXR at 24 hr shows stable/smaller size
  - Large (>30% hemithorax) or symptomatic or secondary to other process: Chest tube placed in midaxillary line, 4th–5th intercostal space (tube courses over the rib)
  - Tension: Immediate needle aspiration followed by chest tube
  - Surgical intervention (VATS w/ or w/o bullous resection and pleurodesis) for recurrent or bilateral PTX, not responsive to therapy (air leak >4 d), or high risk (divers and pilots)
  - Anticipatory guidance: Smoking cessation, avoid air travel for 1 wk following resolution, avoid exertion and physical contact until fully resolved, complete avoidance of deep sea diving and flying in small unpressurized aircrafts
  - Recurrence of primary spontaneous PTX usually occurs within 6 mo–2 yr

PLEURAL EFFUSION

(Pediatr Rev 2017;38(4):170–181)

- **Types:**
  - Transudate: Altered Starling forces
    - Increased pulm venous pressure: CHF, PE
    - Decreased colloid osmotic pressure: Nephrotic syndrome, liver disease
  - Exudate: Leaky vasculature, dense fluid
    - Caused by pleural inflammation & ↑ capillary permeability ± impaired lymphatic drainage 2/2 to infectious processes, malignancy, inflammatory disorders
      - Parapneumonic is the most common type of effusion & occurs usually in children hospitalized with CAP; most common organisms isolated = S. pneumo, S. aureus, GAS but may also occur in viral or atypical pneumonia
      - Most common pleural-based metastasis in childhood: Nephroblastoma, Wilms tumor, hepatoblastoma, malignant germ cell tumors, rhabdomyosarcoma
  - Chylothorax: Postoperative, birth trauma (extension of spine), or congenital (Noonan, Turner, Down); L-sided effusion if thoracic duct abnormality above T5 (R-sided if below)

Evaluation
- **Hx:** Pleuritic chest pain, dyspnea, cough, signs/sxs/history of pneumonia
- **Exam:** ↓ breath sounds, dullness to percussion, decreased tactile fremitus
- **Imaging:**
  - CXR: Perform supine and upright to demonstrate whether fluid changes position
    - AP will detect ≥400 mL, lateral decubitus may detect ≥50 mL w/ proper placement
  - US
  - CT if loculation, abscess, or malignancy suspected
- **Workup – Thoracentesis:**
  - Always obtain following studies on fluid: Total protein, LDH, glucose, cell count + diff, cultures (aerobic ± anaerobic ± fungal)
  - Light criteria: If any of the following present effusion is exudative; protein e:s (effusion to serum ratio) >0.5, LDH e:s >0.6, LDH >2/3 upper limit of normal of serum
    - Exudate w/ WBC >10,000, low glucose (<50% blood glucose), pH <7.30 likely infectious
    - If hct >50% serum hct effusion is a hemothorax; suspicious for malignancy but can occur w/ infection, PE, trauma, others
    - Other studies: Cholesterol/TG for chylothorax, amylase for esophageal rupture, adenosine deaminase (>40 U/L is 90% sensitive for TB), galactomannan (aspergillus)

Treatment
- Treat underlying cause ± fluid evacuation
- Transudate may be treated w/o drainage, repeat thoracentesis for sx relief, diuretics
- Hemothorax: Smaller bleeds require evacuation to prevent pleural adhesions; larger bleeds (blood transfusion >20 mL/kg or blood loss of >3 mL/kg/hr) require urgent thoracotomy
- Chylothorax: Medium-chain triglyceride diet to decrease lymph flow, TPN if needed; other tx options include thoracic duct ligation/embolization and chemical pleurodesis
- Indications for chest tube: Frank pus, + culture data, pH <7.20, large effusion in setting of sepsis; when output <30 mL/d & sxs improve, chest tube can be removed

CYSTIC FIBROSIS

(Pediatr Rev 2014;35(5); Pediatr Rev 2009;30(8); J Cyst Fib 2016;15(2)147–157)

- ↓ or absent chloride channel function due to CFTR gene mutation (7q31.2) → dehydrated secretions → mucus plugging → end-organ damage (progressive lung disease, pancreatic insufficiency, liver disease)
- >1,900 mutations categorized into 6 classes; 70% of people with CF have at least 1 copy of ΔF508 and 50% have 2 copies
- Most common recessive genetic dz in Caucasians; 1/25 carriers, 1/2,500 affected
- ~1,000 new cases per year; 70% diagnosed before age 2
- Current median survival time is 41 yr

Evaluation
- **History:**
  - Recurrent sinopulmonary infections, steatorrhea, FTT, salty skin, clubbing, nasal polyps, FTT, chronic cough
    - ~15–20% neonates w/ delayed passage of meconium, meconium plug syndrome, or meconium ileus; rectal prolapse possible in untreated children b/w 6 mo–3 yr
- **Diagnosis:** Presence of 1+ of the following: Chronic recurrent sinopulmonary disease, nutritional/GI abnormalities, male urogenital abnormalities, salt depletion syndrome
  - Newborn screening (all states in the U.S. now screening): Measures immunoreactive trypsinogen (IRT), if ↑ then repeat or genetic testing; some areas perform IRT + DNA screen initially
  - Sweat test (pilocarpine iontophoresis): Need 2 separate tests for dx, measures chloride concentration of sweat with ≥60 mEq/L positive (J Pediatr 2008;13:S4)
  - Genetic testing currently screens for 23 most common known mutations
  - Stool fecal elastase <500 indicates pancreatic exocrine insufficiency

Treatment
- DMARDs now available: Ivacaftor for the class III mutation G551D (~5% of cases), lumacaftor/ivacaftor for ΔF508; most recent is tezacaftor/ivacaftor also for ΔF508
- **Lung disease**
  - Appropriate isolation to prevent spread of resistant organisms
    - B. cepacia, P. aeruginosa, MRSA

- Airway clearance: Chest PT, positive expiratory pressure, vesting, routinely done in combination w/ nebulized therapies (dornase, hypertonic saline, β2-agonists) (Coch Rev 2003;3:CD001127; N Engl J Med 2006;354:229; Cochrane Rev 2005;4: CD003428)
- Eradication of *P. aeruginosa*: Inhaled tobramycin, colistin, aztreonam (Cochrane Rev 2006:CD004197)
- Chronic inflammation: High-dose ibuprofen, azithromycin. ICS w/o benefit unless treating asthma component (J Pediatr 2007;151:249; Cochrane Review 2007;4: CD001505; Cochrane Rev 2004;2:CD002203)
- Severe hemoptysis: Bronchial artery embolization, lobectomy
- Respiratory failure, heart failure 2/2 pulmonary HTN: Lung (± heart) transplantation
- **Pulmonary exacerbations** of CF diagnosed based on interval ↑ in sxs (fatigue, cough, ↑ sputum production) + interval worsening of PFT parameters (FEV_1 commonly used & monitored routinely during tx)
  - Tx involves aggressive airway clearance + abx (often IV)
- **ENT:** Nasal polyps (15%), recurrent sinusitis → nasal saline rinses, nasal polypectomy
- **GI:** Meconium ileus (10%), distal ileal obstructive syndrome (DIOS, 10–15%), rectal prolapse
  - Osmotic laxatives, stool softeners, gastrografin enema for DIOS w/ near-complete obstruction; prokinetic agents generally not helpful
  - Pancreatic exocrine insuff (85%), chronic pancreatitis, vit ADEK def, malnutrition/FTT → pancreatic replacement enzymes, ADEK vit, high-fat/high-protein diet
  - Biliary cirrhosis (2%) → ursodiol
  - Hyponatremia → hydration, sodium chloride supplements
- **Endocrine:** CF-related diabetes → insulin; osteopenia/osteoporosis → vit D
- **Reproductive:** Male sperm transport defects (95% M infertility), amenorrhea/thick cervical mucus (20% F infertility) → in vitro fertilization

DISEASES OF THE UPPER AIRWAY

OBSTRUCTIVE SLEEP APNEA
(Pediatrics 2012;130(3):576–584)
- **Def:** Intermittent partial or complete upper airway obstruction while sleeping → frequent sleep arousals and/or gas-exchanged abnormalities
- Prevalence peaks around 2–8 yo; corresponds with peak adenotonsillar size
- Risk factors: Adenotonsillar hypertrophy, obesity, AA race, craniofacial anomalies, neuromuscular d/o
- 27% of children have habitual snoring, but OSA only affects 2–3% of children (i.e., 16–25% of children who snore will also have OSA)

Evaluation
- **History:**
  - Nighttime: Snoring, witnessed apnea or snorting episodes, cyanosis, sweating, disturbed sleep, enuresis, sleep walking, periodic limb movement
  - Daytime: Difficulty waking up, moodiness, FTT, developmental delay, ADHD (Pediatrics 2003;111:554–563), daytime sleepiness (less prominent in children bc they are better able to preserve sleep architecture despite apneic events)
- **Exam:** Mouth breathing, adenoidal facies, hyponasal speech
- **Diagnosis:** Polysomnography (PSG) – apnea hypopnea index (AHI): 5–15/hr = mild; 15–30/hr = moderate; & >30/h = severe. Hypopnea is a 50% reduction in airflow × 2 breaths with associated arousal or 3% desat
  - Obstructive apnea is airflow obstruction × 2 breaths with arousal or 3% desat
  - Central hypoventilation syndrome 2/2 PHOX2B gene mutation (the Ondine curse)

Treatment
- Weight loss if obese
- Rx: Intranasal steroids, leukotriene receptor modifiers (Pediatrics 2006;117:e61–e66)
- Tonsillectomy and adenoidectomy – can be curative but less effective in children with severe OSA, those who are obese, and in those with + family hx of OSA or asthma
  - Inpatient postop monitoring (≥24 hr) if: Severe OSA, craniofacial syndromes, or age <3
- CPAP
- Hypoglossal nerve stimulation

LARYNGOMALACIA

(Pediatr Rev 2006;27:e33)

- "Floppy" tissue above vocal cords that falls into airway w/ inspiration
- Most common cause of stridor in infants (~65–75% of all cases)

Evaluation
- **Hx:** Symptoms (typically stridor) appearing during 1st 2 mo of life
  - May be mistaken for congestion, sxs worsen w/ crying, agitation, URI; improve w/ prone
- **Exam:** Stridor w/ features above; ~10% w/ severe obstruction causing biphasic stridor
  - May coexist with other airway malformations
- **Diagnosis:** Flexible laryngoscopy and/or bronchoscopy

Treatment
- Self-limited condition, usually resolves w/o rx by 12–18 mo of age
  - When to refer: FTT, feeding difficulty, respiratory distress/apnea/hoarseness, cyanosis, atypical clinical course/persistent stridor, sleep disturbances
- Surgical: Supraglottoplasty, tracheostomy

TRACHEOMALACIA

(Pediatr Rev 2006;27:e33)

- Weakness of the airway cartilage that results in "floppiness" of airway
  - Positive intrathoracic pressure causing intrathoracic trachea to collapse and obstruct on expiration; extrathoracic trachea may collapse on inspiration
- May be secondary to compression by mediastinal mass or vascular rings/slings

Evaluation
- **Hx:** Wheeze often is expiratory, central, low-pitched, and homophonous + possible stridor; as opposed to wheezing heard in asthma (diffuse, high pitched)
  - Symptoms improve in prone position
  - History of wheezing that does not change or worsens w/ β2 agonists
- **Diagnosis:** Imaging (CXR, CT w/ contrast), airway fluoroscopy, bronchoscopy

Treatment
- Treat coexisting conditions such as GERD
- Nasal CPAP can help maintain airway patency temporarily
- Aortopexy or tracheostomy for long-term relief of obstruction
- Most improve spontaneously by 6–12 mo of age if primary tracheomalacia

---

UPPER AIRWAY OBSTRUCTION

(Nelson Textbook of Pediatrics. 20th ed. Ch 384–387)

Causes
- **Infectious**
  - Croup (laryngotracheobronchitis): Viral infxn; presents w/ stridor, barky cough, fevers
  - Epiglottitis: Rare but potentially lethal; fevers, sore throat, dyspnea, rapid obstruction
  - Others: Laryngitis (hoarseness), bacterial tracheitis, retropharyngeal/peritonsillar abscess
- **Noninfectious**
  - FB aspiration: Typical symptom is violent paroxysms of coughing; classic CXR findings include air trapping on involved side w/ mediastinal shift to opposite side
  - Allergic croup
  - Laryngospasm (severe episodic laryngospasm in neonates 2/2 SCN4A mutation)
- **Chronic/persistent obstruction**
  - Papillomas (seen in neurofibromatosis) & endobronchial/endotracheal neoplasms
  - Laryngeal/tracheal webs
  - Vocal cord dysfunction
  - Cyst formation (bronchogenic cysts, laryngoceles)
  - Extrinsic compression: Mediastinal mass, vascular ring, thyroid hypertrophy
  - Others: TE fistula, Pierre–Robin syndrome, Cri-du-chat syndrome, tracheomalacia, laryngomalacia, subglottic stenosis, congenital hemangiomas

LOWER AIRWAY DISEASE

CHILDHOOD INTERSTITIAL LUNG DISEASE (CILD)

(Pediatrics 2016;137(6):1)

- **Def:** Conditions associated with abnormalities of interstitium, alveoli, or airway compartments
- Diffuse developmental disorders: Primary disorders – without lung transplantation, these tend to be fatal
  - Acinar dysplasia
  - Congenital alveolar dysplasia
  - Alveolar capillary dysplasia assoc. with misalignment of pulmonary veins (ACDMPV)
    - Associated with markedly dilated bronchial veins due to prominent R → L intrapulmonary vascular shunt; often associated with CV, GI, or GU anomalies as well
- Alveolar growth abnormalities: Most common cause of cILD in infants – secondary
  - Pulmonary hypoplasia in setting of oligohydramnios, abdom wall defects, or neuromuscular dx
  - Prematurity (chronic neonatal lung disease)
  - Chromosomal abnormalities
  - Congenital heart disease
- Neuroendocrine cell hyperplasia of infancy (NEHI): Unknown etiology, presents <1 yo with ↑ WOB and imaging showing scattered hyperinflation
  - DDx confirmatory via lung biopsy
- Pulmonary interstitial glycogenosis (PIG): Presents in 1st few weeks of life with respiratory distress and diffuse interstitial infiltrates with scattered hyperinflation
  - **Bx:** Interstitial thickening by immature vimentin positive mesenchymal cells
  - Can be diffuse PIG (isolated, PIG alone) vs. patchy PIG (assoc. with underlying lung growth disorder)
  - **Prognosis:** Good for diffuse PIG; bad for patchy PIG
- Surfactant dysfunction disorders – due to mutations within genes encoding proteins involved in surfactant function

BRONCHOPULMONARY DYSPLASIA (BPD)

(Nelson Textbook of Pediatrics. 20th ed. Ch 384–387)

- **Def:** Chronic lung disease arising during neonatal period characterized by persistent O_2 requirement ≥28 d postnatally
  - Severity graded mild, mod, severe based on GA and degree of O_2 requirement
  - Prematurity results in incomplete development of lung vasculature and airways

Evaluation

- **Hx:** As above with persistent O_2 requirement, possible hx of prolonged mechanical ventilation, prematurity, low birth weight
- **Exam:** Varies by severity; tachypnea, ↑ AP diameter 2/2 air trapping, retractions, wheezes + coarse crackles (commonly heard even at baseline state, fixed wheezes suggest subglottic stenosis or large airway malacia), fine crackles 2/2 fluid, possible evidence of cor pulmonale
- **Diagnosis:** Persistent O_2 requirement as defined above as well as:
  - Born <32 wk: Mild if on RA by 36 wk, mod if <30% FiO_2 at 36 wk, severe if >30%
  - Born >32 wk: Mild if on RA by 56 d, mod if <30% FiO_2 at 56 d, severe if >30%
    - Correlation b/w severe BPD & albuterol responsiveness, ↑ hospitalizations
  - **Exacerbations of BPD:** 2/2 viral illnesses, extrapulmonary infxns, weather Δ, smoke exposure, reflux; characterized by ↑ WOB, worsening baseline findings, resp distress

Treatment

- β-agonists if wheezing and + effect with use
- Optimal O_2 sat goal unclear, should keep above 90% with supplemental O_2 prn
- Diuretics (loop, thiazides, spironolactone)
- ↑ calories due to ↑ consumption from chronic resp insufficiency
- Infxn prevention (see "RSV immunoprophylaxis" in "NICU")

PULMONARY FUNCTION TESTS

(Nelson Textbook of Pediatrics. 20th ed. Ch 373–374)

- Spirometry = Assessment of voluntary air flow and volumes
  - Usually includes total lung volumes, maximal expiratory volumes, expiratory pressures, and diffusing capacity
- Indications: To establish, follow, quantify, or define the nature of pulmonary dysfunction
- Ages: Most useful data begins at age 4/5 – child must be able to follow instructions to take a deep breath and then blow out completely for at least 3 s in children <10 yo and at least 6 s in those >10 yo

Review Basics of Breathing

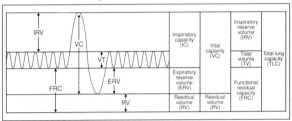

Spirometry Interpretation (Am Fam Physician 2014;69(5):1107–1115)
- Shape of curve – the shape of the curve can help identify restrictive vs. obstructive processes (as shown below)
  - Restrictive processes → relatively normal flows, but ↓ volume
  - Obstructive processes → ↓ flows and ↓ volume with scooped out appearance

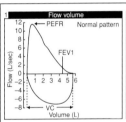

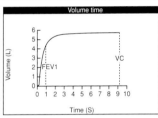

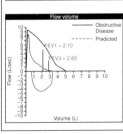

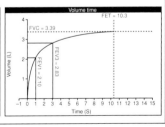

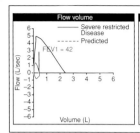

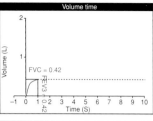

(Adapted from Gold WM. Pulmonary function testing. In: Murray JF, Nadel JA, eds. *Textbook of respiratory medicine.* 3rd ed. Philadelphia: Saunders, 2000:805)

- Value interpretation
  - Report will include "actual", "predicted" and "% predicted" values
    - Predicted values are based on age, gender, race, and height
  - Assess FVC, FEV1, and FEV1/FVC
    - If FEV1/FVC >0.7 and FVC ↓ (<80% predicted) → restrictive impairment
    - If FEV1/FVC <0.7 and FEV1 ↓ (<80% predicted) → obstructive impairment
      - If obstructive impairment, consider bronchodilator challenge. Positive if FEV1 ↑ by at least 12%. Can aid in diagnosis of asthma, but if negative does not rule out asthma.

URINALYSIS

OVERVIEW

(Pediatr Clin North Am 2006;53:325; Pediatric Ann 2013;42:45–51)

- Indications for UA
  - Gross hematuria
  - Periorbital and pedal edema (r/o proteinuria or renal etiology)
  - Urinary frequency, dysuria, and secondary nocturnal enuresis (r/o UTI, nephrolithiasis)
  - Polyuria and polydipsia
  - Suspected renal diseases (HTN, FH of CKD)

Urine Dipstick Test Finding	Nonpathologic Causes	Pathologic Causes
Specific gravity (low)	Polydipsia	DI, renal tubular dysfunction
Specific gravity (high)	Dehydration	Volume depletion
pH (low)	High-protein diet	Acidosis
pH (high)	Low-protein diet; recent meal	RTA (inappropriate renal response); UTI (i.e., *Proteus*)
(+) Blood (can represent RBCs, Hgb, myoglobin)	Menses, traumatic catheterization, exercise	Glomerular d/o, tubular d/o, UTI, calculi, hypercalcemia, urinary tract trauma, tumor, rhabdo, hemolysis
(+) Protein	Orthostatic proteinuria, fever, exercise	Glomerular disorders, tubular disorders, UTI
(+) Glucose	Renal glycosuria (SGLT2 transporter defect)	Diabetes mellitus, Fanconi anemia
(+) Ketones	Restricted carbohydrate intake	Diabetic ketoacidosis, starvation, EtOH
(+) Bilirubin	None	Hepatitis, biliary obstruction
(+) Urobilinogen	Low amounts: systemic abx rx	Hepatitis, intravascular hemolysis
(+) Nitrite	None	UTI (enterobacteriaceae only)
(+) LE (from PMNs)	Fever, poor specimen quality	UTI, glomerulonephritis, pelvic inflammation, sterile pyuria

(Pediatr Clin North Am 2006;53:325)

HEMATURIA

(Pediatr Ann 2013;42:45–51, Curr Opin Pediatr 2008;20:140–144; Arch Pediatr Adol Med 2005;159:353; Urol Clin J North Am 2004;31:559)

- Macroscopic (visible to naked eye): Incidence in ED 1.3 per 1,000 patients
  - Etiologies: 38% idiopathic, 22% hypercalciuria, 15% IgA nephropathy, 4% structural abnormalities (in a study of 228 patients) (Arch Pediatr Adol Med 2005;159:353)
  - Workup
    - History: UTI symptoms, recent rash/sore throat, pain, trauma (including self-manipulation), FH, color, duration, where in stream is the blood
    - Microscopic exam of spun sediment to confirm presence of RBCs (coloration of urine can occur with bile, myoglobin, beets, blackberries, rifampin, porphyrins, chloroquine, and others)
    - No RBC casts or dysmorphic cells: Concern for urinary infection/urologic issue; consider renal/bladder US, CT and/or cystoscopy
    - Presence of proteinuria, RBC casts, and deformed RBCs raise concern for glomerular disease – see **"GN/Nephritic and Nephrotic Syndromes"**
- Microscopic: 1–2% incidence in children 6–15 yo
  - Definition: >5 RBCs per HPF (always confirm with microscopic eval)
  - Etiology:
    - Asymptomatic microscopic hematuria – 342 patients – 81% idiopathic, 15% hypercalciuria, 1% PSGN (Arch Pediatr Adol Med 2005;159:353)
    - Additional etiologies summarized in table below

- **Workup:**
  - Repeated UA with microscopy 2–3 times over several months without preceding exercise, 1st morning sample preferred with microscopy w/i 2 hr
  - Significant if 3 urine analyses are positive for >5 RBCs/HPF over with rechecks
  - False positives: Oxidizing agents (like bleach) in sample
  - False negatives – High SG or high ascorbic acid
  - Red flags: Recent skin infection/sore throat; edema; HTN; decreased urine output; rashes; arthralgias; constitutional symptoms; weight loss; current medications; FH of hematuria, renal calculi or kidney disease
  - Parent UA for hematuria
  - If significant hematuria and/or concerning history: Test CMP, complement (C3 and C4) levels, CBC and consider ASO titer, ANA/DNA binding antibody, ANCA and tests for hepatitis and referral to nephrology – **see "Nephritic/nephrotic syndromes"**

	Glomerular	Nonglomerular
History		
Dysuria	None	Urethritis, cystitis
Systemic complaints	Edema, fever, pharyngitis, rash, arthralgia	Fever with UTI
Pain	Flank pain (IgA nephropathy)	Calculi (CVA pain, radiating to groin)
Trauma	None	Bright-red urine
Family history	Deafness (Alport syndrome), FH of renal failure	Renal calculi history
Physical Exam		
HTN	Often (+)	Unlikely
Edema	(+)/(−)	(−)
Abdominal mass	(−)	Wilms tumor, polycystic kidney
Urinalysis		
Color	Brown, tea, cola	Bright red
Proteinuria	Often (+)	(−) (RBCs can cause some – should resolve with clearance of RBCs)
Dysmorphic RBCs	(+)	(−)
RBC casts	(+)	(−)
Crystals	(−)	May be present in calculi

(Pediatr Ann 2013;42:45–51)

PROTEINURIA

(Pediatr Ann 2013;42:45–51)

- All proteinuria should be rechecked to confirm resolution or determine etiology
- Etiology:
  - Transient proteinuria: Fever, seizures, cold exposure, epinephrine administration, congestive heart failure, serum sickness
  - Orthostatic proteinuria: Benign, but can persist for years
  - Glomerular disease: Minimal change, postinfectious glomerulonephritis (PIGN), HSP nephritis, IgA nephropathy, MPGN, membranous nephropathy, lupus nephritis (LN), Alport syndrome, vasculitis, HIV-associated nephropathy, sickle cell disease
  - Tubulointerstitial disease: Interstitial nephritis, Fanconi syndrome, reflux nephropathy, medications (aminoglycosides, penicillin, lithium), ischemic tubular injury, renal hypoplasia, dysplasia
- Workup:
  - History: Systemic illnesses, fever preceding detection of proteinuria, UTI, FH of renal diseases, deafness
  - Exam: Height & weight, blood pressure, edema, rash, arthritis, absent nail lunulae & absent patellae (nail patella syndrome), eye exam (SLE/HTN), genital exam (Denys–Drash)
  - Initial eval
    - Start with spot urine protein to creatinine ratio (~equivalent to 24 hr protein)
    - If urine protein:Cr elevated → 1st morning UA w/ repeat urine protein:Cr ratio × 3 or 24-hr urine protein, BMP (lytes, Cr, BUN, albumin), cholesterol
    - Be aware that urine dipstick tests only tests albumin and it is concentration dependent – if only look at UA in morning, will be concentrated urine, and can "over-read" protein level. Dilute urine can miss proteinuria

	Protein mg/24 hr	Mg/m²/hr	U P:C (mg/mg)
Adults			
Normal	<150		<0.2
Nephrotic range	2,000–3,000		>2.0
Children			
Normal <2 yo		<4	<0.5
Normal >2 yo		<4	<0.2
Nephrotic range		>40	>2.0

(Pediatr Ann 2013;42:45–51)

- If concerning – second pass labs/imaging – see "Nephritic/nephrotic syndromes"
  - Serum C3, C4, antistreptolysin antibodies, consider ANA, dsDNA, ANCA, hepatitis tests
  - Consider renal US and likely referral to nephrology
- Indications for renal biopsy
  - Nephrotic range proteinuria
  - FH of chronic glomerulonephritis or unexplained renal failure
  - Associated hematuria and red blood cell casts – except with acute poststrepto-coccal glomerulonephritis (APSGN)
  - Low C3 concentration (except with APSGN)
  - HTN and/or elevated serum creatinine concentration (except with ASPGN)
  - Persistent nonorthostatic proteinuria for more than 1 yr

ACUTE KIDNEY INJURY

(Pediatr Rev 2014;35:1; Kidney Int 2007;71(10):1028–1035; Kidney Int 2012;2(8):1–128)

- Definition
  - Acute decrease in GFR → ↑ serum creatinine. Cr increase can be delayed by as much as 48 hr after kidney damage

pRIFLE		
Stage	**Change in Estimated Cr Clearance**	**Urine Output**
Risk of kidney injury	Decrease by 25%	<0.5 mL/kg/hr for 8 hr
Injury to kidney	Decrease by 50%	<0.5 mL/kg/hr for 8 hr
Failure	Decrease by 75% or <35 mL/min/1.73 m²	<0.5 mL/kg/hr for 24 hr/anuria for 12 hr
Loss of kidney function	Failure for >4 wk	
End-stage kidney disease	Failure for >3 mo	

(Kidney Int 2007;71(10):1028–1035)

KDIGO Modification		
Stage	**Change in Estimated Cr**	**Urine Output**
I	Increase by 0.3 mg/dL during 48 hr/increased 150–200%	<0.5 mL/kg/h for 8 hr
II	Increase > = 200–300%	<0.5 mL/kg/h for 16 hr
III	Increase > = 300%, serum cr >4 mg/dL or dialysis or estimated GFR <35 mL/min/1.73 m²	<0.5 mL/kg/h for 24 hr or anuria for 12 hr

(Kidney Int 2012;2(8):1–128)

- Epidemiology (Pediatr Rev 2014;35:1; Am J Kidney Dis 2005;45(1):96–101)
  - Developed countries: Volume depletion and primary renal disease (HUS, glomerulonephritis)
  - Developing countries: Volume depletion, infection, and primary renal disease
  - Hospitalized patients in developed countries: Secondary causes that are multifactorial (heart disease, sepsis, and nephrotoxic drug exposure)
  - NOTE: Term neonates only have 25% of their adult GFR and reach mature GFR at ~2 yo

- Etiology (Pediatr Rev 2014;35:1)
  - Prerenal:
    - Reduced blood volume: GI loss, renal loss (DI, diuretics), hemorrhage, insensible loss (burn patients)
    - Redistributed blood volume: Cirrhosis, nephrotic syndrome, malnutrition, protein-losing enteropathy, increased leaking from blood vessels (SIRS/sepsis)
    - Loss of vascular tone (systemic vasodilation): Sepsis/anaphylaxis
    - Decreased blood delivery to kidneys: Decreased cardiac output, heart disease
    - Increased resistance to flow: Renal artery stenosis, abdominal compartment syndrome
  - Postrenal: Bilateral ureteral obstruction, bilateral obstructive renal calculi, or clots w/i bladder
  - Intrinsic renal:
    - Tubular injury: Acute tubular necrosis (often after prerenal or medication), glomerulonephritides
    - Interstitial nephritis: Allergic (antibiotics, PPIs – only 15% with classic triad with eosinophilia, fever, and rash), HUS (schistocytes, thrombocytopenia, elevated LDH)
- Diagnostic evaluation (Pediatr Rev 2014;35:1; Am J Kidney Dis 2005;45(1):96–101)
  - Complete H&P
  - Labs: U/A with microscopy, UNa or Uurea (if on diuretics), UCr, CMP, CBC with diff
    - Fractional excretion of sodium (FENa) = (Urine Na/plasma Na)/(Urine Cr/plasma Cr) – inaccurate if on diuretics (though if <1 on diuretics, patient is very volume deplete)
    - Fractional excretion of urea (FEUrea) = (Urine urea/BUN)/(Urine Cr/plasma Cr)
    - Consider albumin, cholesterol, serum complement, ANA, streptococcal serologies, toxicology screen, US, CT
  - **See algorithm on next page**

Lab Value	Prerenal	Intrinsic
Urine SG	>1.02	≤1.01
Urine Na	<20 mEq/L	>40 mEq/L
FENa	<1% (neonates <2%)	>2% (neonates >2.5%)
FEUrea	<35%	>50%
Urine osmolality	>500 mOsm/kg	<350 mOsm/kg
BUN:Cr ratio	>20	10–15

- Therapy (Pediatr Rev 2014;35:1; Am J Kidney Dis 2005;45(1):96–101)
  - Etiology dependent
    - Oliguria, hypotension, or instability: 20 mL/kg bolus of isotonic fluids unless underlying cardiac etiology
    - Could consider diuretics (mixed literature) after sufficient volume resuscitation, but no evidence that they alter course of AKI, need for renal replacement or mortality. No data to support use of dopamine. Consider fenoldopam. No role for mannitol
    - Once volume resuscitated, but remain oliguric: Give fluids to match insensible losses – consider avoidance of K and Phos in fluids if they remain oliguric
  - Avoid nephrotoxic agents and dose all medications per CrCl
  - Renal replacement (dialysis, CVVH) for AEIOU – **A**cid–base disturbance, **E**lectrolyte abnormality, toxin **I**ngestion, volume **O**verload, & complications of **U**remia (pericarditis, encephalopathy)
- Prognosis (Pediatr Rev 2014;35:1; Am J Kidney Dis. 2005;45:96–101)
  - Depends on etiology: Worse if multiorgan involvement; >50% mortality if ≥3 organs are involved; ~10% pediatric pts w/ AKI develop CKD in 1–3 yr
  - Should have long-term follow-up with either PCP or specialist if severe AKI

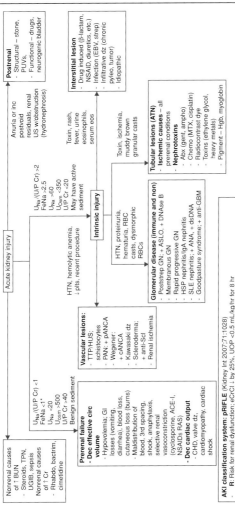

Nonrenal causes of ↑ BUN
- Steroids, TPN, UGIB, sepsis
Nonrenal causes of ↑ Cr
- Rhabdo, bactrim, cimetidine

Acute kidney injury

Anuria or inc postvoid residuals, renal US w/obstruction (hydronephrosis)

Postrenal
- Structural – stone, PUVs,
- Functional – drugs, neurogenic bladder

$U_{Na}/(U/P\ Cr) <1$
$FeNa <1^*$
$U_{Na} <20$
$U_{osm} >500$
$U/P\ Cr >40$
Benign sediment

$U_{Na}/(U/P\ Cr) >2$
$FeNa >2.5$
$U_{Na} >60$
$U_{osm} <350$
$U/P\ Cr <20$
May have active sediment

Toxin, rash, fever, urine eosinophils, serum eos

Intrinsic injury

Interstitial lesion
- Drug induced (β-lactam, NSAID, diuretics, etc.)
- Infection (EBV, strep)
- Infiltrative dz (chronic pyelo, tumor)
- Idiopathic

Prerenal failure
- **Dec effective circ volume**
  - Hypovolemia, GI losses (vomiting, diarrhea), blood loss, cutaneous loss (burns)
  - Maldistribution of blood, 3rd spacing, shock, anaphylaxis, selective renal vasoconstriction (cyclosporine, ACE-I, NSAIDs, RAS)
- **Dec cardiac output**
  - CHD, valve dz, cardiomyopathy, cardiac shock

HTN, hemolytic anemia, ↓ plts, recent procedure

HTN, proteinuria, hematuria, RBC casts, dysmorphic RBCs

Toxin, muddy brown granular casts

Vascular lesions:
- TTP/HUS; schistocytes
- PAN: + pANCA
- Wegener; + cANCA
- Kawasaki dz
- Scleroderma; + anti-Scl
- Renal ischemia

Glomerular disease (immune and non)
- Poststrep GN; + ASLO, + DNAse B
- Membranous GN
- Rapid progressive GN
- HSP nephritis/IgA nephritis
- SLE nephritis; + ANA; + dsDNA
- Goodpasture syndrome; + anti-GBM

Tubular lesions (ATN)
- **Ischemic causes** – all prerenal conditions
- **Nephrotoxins**
  - Abx (gent, ampho)
  - Chemo (MTX, cisplatin)
  - Radiocontrast dye
  - Toxins (ethylene glycol, heavy metals)
  - Pigment — Hgb, myoglobin

* Other causes of FeNa <1%: Vascular occlusion, glomerulonephritis, vasculitis, early postrenal failure, pigment nephropathy, radiocontrast nephropathy, hepatorenal syndrome

AKI classification system: pRIFLE (Kidney Int 2007;71:1028)
- **R**: Risk for renal dysfunction; eCrCl ↓ by 25%, UOP <0.5 mL/kg/hr for 8 hr
- **I**: Injury to kidney; eCrCl ↓ by 50%, UOP <0.5 mL/kg/hr for 16 hr
- **F**: Failure of kidney; eCrCl ↓ by 50% or <35 mL/min/1.73 m², UOP <0.3 mL/kg/kr for 24 hr or anuric × 12 hr
- **L**: Loss of kidney function; persistent failure >4 wk
- **E**: End-stage renal disease; persistent failure >3 mo

AKI 14-5

CHRONIC KIDNEY DISEASE

- Definition (Pediatr Rev 2014;35:1)
  - Two independent criteria:
    - Kidney damage for 3 mo or longer as defined by structural or functional abnormalities of the kidney, with or without decreased GFR, manifested by either pathologic abnormalities or markers of kidney damage, including abnormalities in the composition of the blood or urine or abnormalities in imaging studies
    - GFR <60 mL/min/1.73 m^2 for 3 mo or longer, with or without kidney damage
  - 5 stages (for >2 yo): **GFR (mL/min/1.73 m^2)**
    - Stage 1 – >**90**; stage 2 – >**60**; stage 3 – >**30**; stage 4 – >**15**; stage 5 (kidney failure)
- Epidemiology (Pediatr Rev 2014;35:1)
  - CKD: 82 cases/1 million/yr; ESRD – 15 cases/million/yr
- Etiologies: Glomerulopathies (33%), urologic anomalies or infections (25%), hereditary nephropathies (16%), hypoplasia or dysplasia (11%), and vascular disorders (5%)
- Complications/comorbidities (Pediatr Rev 2014;35:1)
  - HTN, HLD, altered glucose metabolism, obesity, anemia, abnormal electrolytes, malnutrition, bone disease, acidosis, neurocognitive impairment, social stressors, vit D deficiency, and secondary hyperPTH
  - Cardiovascular events
    - Arrhythmias (19.6%), valvular heart disease (11.7%), cardiomyopathy (9.6%), and cardiac death (2.8%)
  - Infections prompt up to 45% of hospital admissions in 1 series
  - Growth retardation is a major complication, degree matches age of onset of CKD, likely due to effect on GH & IGF-1 axis; treatment with nutritional support +/– GH therapy
- Prognosis (Pediatr Rev 2014;35:1; Pediatr Nephrol 2008;23:705; J Am Soc Nephrol 2005;16:2796)
  - 10-yr survival for adolescent-onset ESRD is 80%
  - Lifespan of pediatric patient dependent on dialysis and unable to receive a transplant is reduced by 50 yr
  - Proteinuria, low hematocrit, hypoalbuminemia, hypocalcemia, hyperphosphatemia, hyperparathyroidism are all associated with rate of progress to ESRD, as is age at diagnosis and the diagnosis itself
  - Glomerular disorders (including FSGS) increase risk of progression to ESRD
- Management (Pediatr Rev 2014;35:1; Advances in CKD 2017;24:6; N Engl J Med 2009;361:1639; Cur Op Peds 2010;22:170)
  - ESCAPE trial: Fixed-dose ACE-inhibitor + additional antihypertensives – tight MAP (<50th percentile) slowed loss of GFR compared to MAP target of 50th–90th percentile
  - R-A blockade may also benefit by ↓ proteinuria, correction of acidosis, hyperuricemia
  - Treat complications: Goal Hgb 11–13 – treat with Epo, iron repletion with goal of ferritin >100 ng/mL or trans sat >20%, vit D, growth hormone, phosphate binding, modified diets with increased calories
  - Immunizations
    - Special attention should be paid to immunizations against hepatitis B and Streptococcus pneumoniae (normal 13-valent and additional 23-valent after age 2 and minimum 8 wk after receiving 13-valent)
    - Avoid live-attenuated vaccines if immunosuppressed
  - Renal replacement with dialysis; ultimate goal is renal transplantation

RENAL TUBULAR ACIDOSIS

- Definition (Int J Biochem Cell Biol 2005;37:1151)
  - Metabolic acidosis 2/2 impaired renal acid excretion
- Clinical manifestations (Int J Biochem Cell Biol 2005;37:1151)
  - Often p/w hyperchloremic metab acidosis w/ nml/near-nml AG & w/o diarrhea
  - Can also present with hypokalemia, medullary nephrocalcinosis, recurrent calcium phosphate stone disease, growth retardation/rickets
- Etiologies
  - Isolated tubular defects can be due to drugs, autoimmune disease, obstructive nephropathy, or any cause of medullary nephrocalcinosis
  - Can be genetic, associated with deafness, osteoporosis, or ocular abnormalities

- Workup: BMP (all present with albumin-corrected nonanion gap metabolic acidosis [NAGMA]), urine pH, urine anion gap (UAG + UNa + UK − UCl), FE HCO_3
  - NOTE: UAG only valid if UNa >25 and no evidence of ↑ unmeasured urinary anions (DKA, glue sniffing, D-lactic acidosis, chronic Tylenol use, neonates)
- Classification/diagnosis/etiology/treatment (Pediatr Rev 2017;38:11; Pediatr Rev 2001;22:8; Int J Biochem Cell Biol 2005;37:1151)
  - **Distal (Type 1 RTA)**: Failure of distal tubule to secrete H+ into lumen – results in decreased ammonium excretion (can't acidify urine)
    - Patient presentation: Can present with nephrocalcinosis due to low urine citrate and high urine Ca, vomiting, dehydration, poor growth, rickets, and/or hypokalemia
    - Diagnosis: urine pH (>5.5) ↑ UAG with normal UA
    - Etiology: Acquired (lithium, amphotericin, and sickle cell disease) or due to auto-immune dz (Sjögren syndrome/SLE)
    - Treatment: Bicarbonate replacement, typically 1–3 mEq/kg/d
  - **Proximal (Type 2 RTA)**: Impairment in HCO_3 reabsorption
    - Patient presentation: Can have full Fanconi syndrome (hypophosphatemia, renal glucosuria, aminoaciduria, tubular proteinuria, and proximal RTA) with growth failure and episodes of hypovolemia and bone abnormalities, can have hypokalemia, hypophosphatemia
    - Diagnosis: Urine pH can vary and can have negative or positive urine anion gap. Likely proximal with positive UAG, urine pH <5.5, and fractional excretion of bicarbonate 5–15%. Likely proximal with negative UAG and fractional excretion of bicarbonate >5% (if fractional excretion of bicarbonate is <5%, likely loss from nonrenal source like diarrhea)
    - Etiology: Fanconi syndrome (most commonly caused by cystinosis), medication induced (acetazolamide, ifosfamide, platinum-based chemotherapy, topiramate, aminoglycosides), hereditary fructose intolerance, Wilson disease
    - Treatment: Bicarbonate supplementation: 10–30 mEq/kg/d of HCO_3
  - **Type 4 RTA**: Hyperkalemia due to defect in aldosterone production or aldosterone receptor sensitivity
    - Patient presentation: NAGMA and hyperkalemia
    - Etiology: ACEI/ARBs, potassium sparing diuretics, TMP-SMX, heparin, pentamidine, and NSAIDs. Other causes include sickle cell nephropathy, adrenal insufficiency, and obstructive nephropathy. More rare causes include genetic causes (pseudohy-poaldosteronism type I and Gordon syndrome), amyloidosis, and transplant
    - Diagnosis: Albumin-corrected NAGMA, hyperkalemia, UAG positive, urine pH <5.5, fractional excretion of bicarbonate <5%
    - Treatment: Cessation of causative agent (d/c offending drug, relieve obstruction, hydrate). Low K diet. Can treat primary hypoaldosteronism with mineralocorti-coid replacement (fludrocortisone 0.1–0.3 mg/d), loop diuretics, or cation exchange resins

HYPERTENSION

- Definitions (Pediatrics 2017;140(3):1–72)

Upper Limit of Category	1–13 yo	>13 yo
Normal BP	90th percentile	120/80 mmHg
Elevated BP	95th percentile	<129/80 mmHg
Stage 1 HTN	95th percentile + 12 mmHg	<139/89 mmHg
Stage 2 HTN	>95th percentile + 12 mmHg	>140/90 mmHg
White coat HTN	Normotensive outside medical setting, but HTN in office	
Masked HTN	Normotensive in office, but HTN outside medical setting	

- Risk factors: Obesity, male, Hispanic or African American, FH aortic coarctation, some medications
- Screening/diagnosis (Pediatrics 2017;140(3)1–72)
  - ≥3 yo: Screen annually or at every visit if RFs as above
  - Screen <3 yo if: Hx of prematurity (<32 wk), SGA or VLBW, NICU stay, congenital heart disease, concern for renal disease, FH of congenital renal disease, hx of transplant (solid organ, BMT), medications, concern for ↑ ICP
  - Any high BP (>90th percentile) should be rechecked via manual BP. Average of two manual measurements should be used to assign a BP category per definitions above

- Diagnosis of HTN (Pediatrics 2017;140(3):1–72)

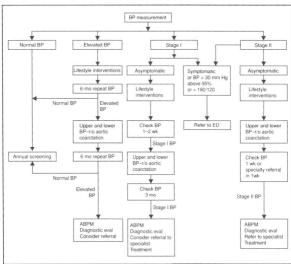

- Primary HTN: Most common – no obvious etiology/idiopathic
- Secondary HTN
  - Causes: MANY (see table below) – renal and renovascular disease most common
  - NOTE: Kids >6 yo do not need extensive workup if FH, obesity, and no concerning hx or px

Systemic	Diagnoses	Workup
Cardiac	Aortic coarctation	Echocardiogram
Endocrine	Pheochromocytoma, congenital adrenal hyperplasia, 11β-hydroxylase deficiency, 17α-hydroxylase deficiency, familial hyperaldosteronism, Cushing syndrome, iatrogenic excess glucocorticoid, hyperthyroidism, hyperparathyroidism	TSH, Free T4 Serum renin/aldosterone Cortisol level, Corticotropin Adrenal imaging Plasma & urine steroids
Renovascular	Renal artery stenosis, fibromuscular dysplasia, neurofibromatosis, renal vein thrombosis, Wilms tumor	Doppler renal US Serum renin/aldosterone CTA, MRA, angiography UPT
Drugs Environmental	OCPs, CNS stimulants, corticosteroids, pseudoephedrine, cocaine, methamphetamine, anabolic steroids, lead	Urine drug screen Lead level
Renal Parenchymal Dx	Renal scarring (recurrent UTI, VUR), glomerulonephritis, PCKD, obstructive uropathy	CBC, BMP UA, urine protein:Cr ratio Renal US

- Diagnostic evaluation (Pediatr Rev 2017;38(8):369–382)
  - Hx: Perinatal, nutrition, physical activity, psychosocial, and family history
  - Px: Height, weight, BMI – look for findings consistent with the underlying secondary cause for HTN. Examples:
    - Tachycardia, proptosis, thyromegaly → hyperthyroidism
    - Acne, hirsutism, moon facies → Cushing syndrome
    - Abdominal mass → Wilms tumor, neuroblastoma
    - Palpable kidneys → PCKD
    - Ambiguous or virilized genitalia → CAH
    - Epigastric or flank bruit → RAS

- Labs (Pediatrics 2017;140(3):1–72)
  - Get a UA, BMP, and lipid panel in every patient with HTN
  - In obese patients (BMI >95%), also get Hgb A1c and ALT/AST
  - Additional labs based on findings suspicious for secondary HTN (table)
- Imaging (Pediatrics 2017;140(3):1–72)
  - Echocardiography recommended at the time of medication initiation
  - Renal US recommended for age <6 yo or abnormal UA or renal function
  - Doppler renal US recommended for evaluation of RAS in children ≥8 yo who are not obese and have other suspicion for renovascular HTN (bruit, significant diastolic HTN, kidney size discrepancy)
  - NOTE: CTA/MRA are more sensitive and specific for RAS and may also be considered
- Management of HTN (Pediatrics 2017;140(3):1–72)
  - Goal of therapy is to prevent or ↓ end-organ damage and CV dx in adulthood
  - Target SBP and DBP is <90th percentile or <130/80 in adolescents
  1. Lifestyle modification: DASH diet, exercise 3–5×/wk
  2. Pharmacologic Tx: If lifestyle mods fail, stage II HTN, symptomatic HTN, or HTN with DM/CKD
     - Start with a single agent: ACEI, ARB, long-acting CCB, or thiazide are first choices
     - If CKD, proteinuria, or DM → start with ACEI or ARB as first line
- Hypertensive emergency (Pediatrics 2017;140(3):1–72)
  - Should be concerned if BP ↑ >30 mmHg above the 95th percentile (although can have sxs at lower BP)
  - Sxs: Encephalopathy, seizure, visual Δ, shortness of breath, peripheral edema, hematuria, ↓ UOP, tremor, nausea, vomiting
  - Acute, severe hypertension is secondary HTN until proved otherwise (need full evaluation)
  - Tx: Use short-acting anti-HTN agents
    - Severe and life-threatening HTN → can use esmolol (β-blocker), hydralazine (vasodilator), labetalol (α- and β-blocker), nicardipine (CCB), sodium nitroprusside (vasodilator)
    - Severe and not life threatening → clonidine (central α-agonist), fenoldopam (dopamine receptor agonist), isradipine (CCB), minoxidil (vasodilator)
    - Goal: Reduce by no more than 25% of planned reduction in first 8 hr, remainder over next 12–24 hr. Short-term goal is ~95th percentile

NEPHROTIC SYNDROME

- Definition (Pediatr Rev 2015;36;117–126)
  - Characterized by proteinuria, hypoalbuminemia, edema, and HLD due to ↑ permeability of glomerular filtration barrier (GFB)
- Epidemiology (Pediatr Rev 2015;36;117–126): Incidence = 2–7/1,00,000 children
- Pathogenesis (Nelson Textbook of Pediatrics. Ch 527, 2521–2528)
  - Can be idiopathic (primary), secondary to systemic disease, or genetic/hereditary
  - All forms → effacement of podocyte foot processes in the GFB as a result of different immune and non-immune insults → protein spillage into urine
- Etiology (Nelson Textbook of Pediatrics. Ch 527, 2521–2528)

Primary	Age (yr)	Progression to Renal Failure?	Renal Pathology	Remission After Steroids
Minimal change (MCNS) (~85% of pediatric NS)	2–6	No	Foot process fusion	90%
Focal segmental glomerulosclerosis (FSGS)	2–10	Yes (most w/i 10 yr)	• Foot process fusion • Focal sclerotic lesions • IgM, C3 deposition	15–20%
Membranous nephropathy (MN)	40–50	Yes (50% in 10–20 yr)	• Thickened GBM, spikes • Fine granular IgG • Subepithelial deposits	Resistant

| Membranoproliferative glomerulonephritis (MPGN) | 5–15 | Yes (most w/i 5–20 yr) | Type 1
• Mesangial and subendothelial deposits of IgG and C3 along GBM
Type 2
• Lobulation
• Dense deposits of C3 only in the mesangium | Resistant |

Secondary	Hereditary
• Infection: Endocarditis, hepatitis B&C, HIV, syphilis, toxoplasmosis, EBV, malaria • Drugs: Captopril, NSAIDs, pamidronate, interferon, lithium, heroin • Immunologic: Vasculitis, food allergy, serum sickness • Malignancy: Lymphoma, leukemia, solid tumors	• Congenital nephrotic syndrome • Diffuse mesangial sclerosis • Denys–Drash syndrome • Diseases which may include nephrotic syndrome: Charcot–Marie–Tooth, Jeune syndrome, Cockayne syndrome, alpha1-antitrypsin deficiency, Fabry disease, glycogen storage disease, Hurler syndrome, sickle cell disease

- Clinical manifestations (*Nelson Textbook of Pediatrics.* Ch 527, 2521–2528): 4 major clinical criteria
  - Proteinuria (>3.5 g/24 hr or urine protein:Cr ratio >2)
  - Hypoalbuminemia (<2.5 g/dL)
  - Edema (periorbital and gravity dependent)
  - Hyperlipidemia (cholesterol >200 mg/dL)
- Diagnosis (Pediatr Rev 2015;36:117–126)
  - Urine studies: UA (proteinuria, +/– hematuria), urine protein:Cr ratio
  - Labs: BMP, lipid profile, albumin
    - Depending on clinical presentation → C3, ANA, CBC, infectious serologies (Hep B, Hep C, HIV, etc.)
- Complications/comorbidities (Pediatr Rev 2015;36:117–126)
  - Thrombosis: Intravascular depletion, urinary loss of antithrombotic factors, ↑ in hepatic production of procoagulant factors
  - Infection: Urinary loss of immunoglobulins (Ig) ↑ risk for bacterial infection with encapsulated organisms (S. pneumoniae, H. influenzae, GBS)
  - Dyslipidemia: Change in oncotic pressure from loss of albumin → ↓ in catabolism and ↑ in production of cholesterol and LDL in the liver
  - Renal dysfunction: Renal hypoperfusion secondary to intravascular depletion, sepsis, or diuretic use
- Management
  - Corticosteroids
    - In most cases can tx empirically w/o renal bx as 80% of children respond to steroids (Kidney Int 2012;2:163–171)
    - Consider nephrology consultation and biopsy prior to initiation of corticosteroids if age <1 or >10–12, gross hematuria, elevated Cr, or signs of autoimmune disease (rash, arthralgias, fevers) (Pediatr Rev 2015;36:117–126)
    - Biopsy should be obtained in children with NS unresponsive to steroids after 8 wk (Kidney Int 2012;2:163–171)
  - Immunosuppressant therapy (mycophenolate mofetil, calcineurin inhibitors, cyclophosphamide, rituximab) indicated for (Pediatr Rev 2015;36:117–126):
    - Steroid-resistant nephrotic syndrome (SRNS): NS unresponsive to steroids after initial course (8–12 wk)
    - Steroid-sensitive nephrotic syndrome (SSNS) with frequent relapse: ≥2 relapses w/i 6 mo after therapy or ≥4 relapses in a 12-mo period (Kidney Int 2012;2:163–171)
      - Risk factors for frequent relapse: Shorter time to 1st relapse, number of relapses in 1st 6 mo, younger age, males, prolonged time to first remission, infection at time of 1st relapse, hematuria at presentation
    - Steroid-dependent SSNS: Relapse during steroid taper or w/i 2 wk of discontinuation
  - Consider genetic testing in patients <1 yr or SRNS (30% have genetic cause)
  - Treatment of complications of NS:
    - Diuretics (for edema)
    - ACE-I/ARBs to help reduce proteinuria and slow progression of CKD
    - Pneumococcal vaccination (prevent pneumococcal PNA)

- Prognosis
  - SSNS (Pediatr Nephrol 2013;28:415–426)
    - Majority of cases are MCNS with good prognosis and low rates of progression to ESRD
    - Natural course is relapse and remission
  - SRNS (Kidney Int 2012;2:172–176)
    - Generally poor long-term prognosis
    - 43% have 10-yr renal survival in multidrug-resistant SRNS (J Am Soc Nephrol 2017;28:3055–3065)

GLOMERULONEPHRITIS/NEPHRITIC SYNDROMES

Definition (Lancet 2005;365:1797–1806)
- Syndrome classically defined by hematuria, proteinuria, hypertension, and renal failure caused by inflammation w/i the glomerulus due to a wide range of disorders

Etiologies
- Membranous nephropathy (Pediatr Nephrol 2018;33:463–472)
  - Epi: Rare in children, 1–5% prevalence
  - Immune complex disease usually presenting as nephrotic syndrome
  - Histology: Thickening of the GBM, immune deposits in the subepithelial space
  - Primary: Autoimmune disease caused by antibodies against endogenous podocytic antigens
    - PLA_2R1, NEP (neonatal), and BSA (early childhood)
  - Secondary: Hepatitis B/C, EBC, SLE, syphilis, malaria, medications
- C3 glomerulopathy (C3G) (Pediatr Nephrol 2017;32:43–57)
  - Pathophys: Complement deposition due to defect in alternative complement pathway
  - Labs: Usually low C3, but normal C3 does not rule out
  - Dx: Made by kidney biopsy showing C3-dominant IF staining
  - Prognosis: 50% of patients with C3G progress to ESRD in 10–15 yr
- Immune complex–mediated MPGN (Am J Kidney Dis 2015;66:359–375)
  - Dx: Made by kidney biopsy showing Ig + C3 deposits on IF staining
  - Causes: Infection (Hep B/C, TB, protozoal diseases), autoimmune (SLE, mixed cryoglobulinemia, Sjögren syndrome), monoclonal gammopathies (MGUS, MM, CLL), genetic forms
  - Labs: Low/normal C3, low C4
- IgA nephropathy (N Engl J Med 2013;368:2402–2414)
  - Epi: More common in males
  - Pathogenesis: Due to abnormal glycosylation of IgA resulting in formation of immune complexes
  - Sxs: 75% of children and adolescents present with gross hematuria in the setting of URI/GI infection
  - Dx: Renal bx shows IgA-dominant deposits in the glomerular mesangium on IF staining
  - Prognosis: If kidney function normal at diagnosis → 90% 10-yr renal survival
- Henoch–Schönlein purpura (HSP) nephritis (Pediatr Nephrol 2015;30:245–252)
  - Epi: 30–50% of patients with HSP
  - Pathogenesis: Glomerular deposition of immune complexes containing IgA1
  - Sxs: Palpable purpura, joint pain, abdominal pain, hematuria
  - Dx: Renal bx similar to IgA nephropathy, serial UAs (nephritis may develop up to 6 mo from initial HSP presentation)
- Anti-GBM disease (Goodpasture) (J Autoimmun 2014;48–49:108–112)
  - Epi: 1:1,000,000, rare before puberty
  - Pathophys: Autoantibodies formed against $\alpha 3$ chain of type-IV collagen → immune complex small vasculitis affecting glomerular and/or pulmonary capillaries
  - Rx: Renal bx – linear deposits of IgG +/− C3 along the GBM on IF staining
  - Labs: Anti-GBM antibodies (+) in serum or on bx
  - Prognosis: Poor – rapidly progressive – <33% of patients have 6 mo preserved renal function
- PIGN (Paediatr Int Child Health 2017;4:240–247)
  - Common cause of acute GN in children, classically poststrep but can be due to other infxns
  - Pathophys: Immune complex formation → deposition in glomeruli → glomerular injury

- Labs: (+) ASO titers or anti-DNase B titers; low C3 – recovers by 6 wk
- Prognosis: Good, progression to ESRD is rare
- ANCA-associated vasculitis (Pediatr Nephrol 2018;33:25–39): Small to medium vessel vasculitides characterized by necrotizing inflammation associated with ANCA autoantibodies
  - Granulomatosis with polyangiitis (GPA)
    - Labs: cANCA (PR3-ANCA) (+)
    - Clinical: Multiple-organ involvement – primarily ENT + pulmonary + renal. Can also involve MSK, GI, eyes, skin, and nervous system
    - Path: Necrotizing vasculitis with granulomas
  - Microscopic polyangiitis (MPA)
    - Labs: pANCA(MPO-ANCA)
    - Path: Necrotizing vasculitis without granulomas
    - Clinical: Multiple-organ system involvement usually
    - Renal limited vasculitis
      - Absence of vasculitis in other organs
      - 80% have ANCA (usually MPO)
  - LN (Rheum Dis Clin North Am 2013;39:833–853)
    - Epi: 0.72 cases per 100,000 children (prevalence of LN varies with race and exposures)
    - Dx: Requires renal bx classification (I–VI) based on pathology
    - Prognosis: 77–93% 5-yr renal survival; worse in males and non-Caucasians

Clinical Presentation
- Acute nephritic syndrome arch → hematuria (RBC casts), proteinuria, renal impairment, HTN (Arch Intern Med 2001;161:25–34)
- Rapidly progressive glomerulonephritis (Lancet 2005;365:1797–1806)
  - Symptoms of nephritic syndrome with rapid progression to renal failure in days to weeks
  - Pathology typically shows extensive glomerular crescent formation

Diagnosis (Arch Intern Med 2001;161:25–34)
- History/physical: Look for signs of system illness (fever, rash, arthritis, infection, abd pain, nausea, vomiting), recent illness, or FH
- Labs
  - Labs: BMP, C3, C4, anti-DNA antibodies, ANA, ANCA, cryoglobulins, hep B/C, antiglomerular basement membrane antibody, streptozyme, blood cultures
  - Urine: UA, urine protein:Cr ratio
  - Imaging: Renal US (evaluate kidney size, signs of scarring or fibrosis)
  - For definitive diagnosis, obtain kidney biopsy

Management (Lancet 2005;365:1797–1806)
- BP control
- Proteinuria → ACEI
- Corticosteroids/immune suppression
- Dialysis if needed

Prognosis (Lancet 2005;365:1797–1806)
- Glomerulonephritis is the 3rd most common cause of end-stage renal disease in the U.S.
- Disease course and progression to ESRD varies by etiology
- Rapidly progressive GN, IgA nephropathy, membranous GN, and LN have been found to have high rates of progression to renal failure
- Early diagnosis and intervention is important to slow disease progression

URINARY CALCULI

Definition (Pediatr Rev 2010;31:179)
- Urolithiasis = stones at any location w/i the urinary tract
- Nephrolithiasis = stones formed in the kidney
- Nephrocalcinosis = deposition of Ca salts in the renal parenchyma (usually associated with underlying metabolic disorder)

Epidemiology (Pediatr Rev 2010;31:179)
- Incidence increased in pediatric population, though still much lower than adults
- RFs: Male, Caucasian

Etiology/Pathogenesis (Pediatr Rev 2010;31:179; Nelson Textbook of Pediatrics. Ch 547; 2600–2604)

Type of Stone	Frequency	Etiology	Urine pH	Imaging
Calcium oxalate	45–65%	• Hyperoxaluria (calcium oxalate): 1° and 2° hyperoxaluria, enteric hyperoxaluria (↑ gut absorption) • Hypercalciuria (calcium oxalate and phosphate): ↑ gut absorption, distal RTA, hyperparathyroidism, loop diuretics, vit D excess, sarcoidosis, ketogenic diet, immobilization	>7	Radiopaque
Calcium phosphate	14–30%	• Hypocitraturia (calcium oxalate and phosphate): ketogenic diet, hypokalemia, metabolic acidosis, chronic diarrhea • Hyperuricosuria (calcium oxalate)	>7	Radiopaque
Struvite (magnesium ammonium phosphate)	13%	• UTI (Proteus, Klebsiella, E. coli, Pseudomonas, S. marcescens, Citrobacter, Morganella) • Foreign body • Urinary stasis (e.g., neurogenic bladder)	>8	Radiopaque
Cystine	5%	• Cystinuria: Rare autosomal recessive disorder of the renal tubule that prevents absorption of cystine, which precipitates and forms calculi	<6	Radiolucent
Uric acid	4%	• Hyperuricosuria: Lesch–Nyhan syndrome, G6PD, myeloproliferative disorders, chemotherapy, high-protein diet, metabolic syndrome, ketogenic diet	<6	Radiolucent

Clinical Manifestations (Pediatr Rev 2010;31:179)
• Severe, colicky flank pain with radiation to the groin
• Gross hematuria, dysuria, urgency, frequency
• Passage of stones or gravel-like sediment in urine

Diagnosis (Pediatr Rev 2010;31:179; JAMA Pediatrics 2015;169:964–970)
• History: Sxs, prior history of renal or GI disease, HF, recent immobilization
  • Medications (vit D, Ca, vit C, topiramate, diuretics)
  • Dietary history: Na intake, Ca intake, ketogenic diet
• Px: Growth, evidence of spina bifida, or metabolic disease
• Labs
  • Acutely: UA, urine cx, BMP
  • Outpatient: Above + serum uric acid, ALP, urine Ca:Cr ratio, urine spot cystine
    • 24-hr urine collection
      • Volume, Cr clearance, Ca, Phos, oxalate, uric acid, citrate, cystine, pH
  • All recovered stones should be sent for lab analysis
• Imaging
  • Noncontrast CT: Gold standard, highest Se. Radiation exposure is high
  • US: 1st choice +/– plain film (can assess for stone, obstruction, and hydronephrosis with minimal radiation)

Acute Management (Pediatr Rev 2010;31:179)
• IV fluids (flush the kidneys)
• Medications: α-blockers (i.e., tamsulosin) to facilitate stone passage; NSAIDs +/– opiates for pain mgmt

- Have patient strain all urine to catch the stone for later analysis
- Surgical tx (Nelson Textbook of Pediatrics 547;2600–2604)
  - Indications: Complete obstruction, sepsis, inability or unlikely to pass (stone typically >5 mm in size), severe pain, failure of conservative mgmt
  - Procedural options: Lithotripsy, ureteral stent, percutaneous nephrolithotomy, laparoscopic removal

Prevention/Long-Term Therapy (Pediatr Rev 2010;31:179; JAMA Pediatr 2015;169: 964–970)
- Increase fluid intake
  - Goal urine output >750 mL/d in infants, >1 L/d in ages 1–5 yr, >1.5 L/d in ages 5–10 yr, >2 L/d in children >10
- Diet: Low sodium or "no added salt" diet, avoid excess animal protein, normal Ca intake
  - If hyperoxaluria, also avoid high-oxalate foods, avoid high-fat foods, avoid excessive vit C
- Medications (guided by results of 24-hr urine collection)
  - If hypocitraturia, hyperoxaluria, hyperuricosuria, or cystinuria → potassium citrate
  - If hypercalciuria → HCTZ and amiloride
  - If hyperuricosuria → allopurinol

CONGENITAL RENAL MALFORMATIONS

(NeoReviews 2016;17;e18–e27)
- Incidence: 0.3–1.6 in 1,000 births and make up 30–50% of all pediatric ESRD
- Classification of malformations

Renal Parenchyma	Embryonic Migration	Urinary Collecting System
Renal agenesis	Renal ectopy	Duplicated collecting systems
Renal dysgenesis	Fusion anomalies	Renal pelvis
• Dysplasia	• Horseshoe kidney	• UPJ obstruction
• Hypoplasia		Ureter
• Cystic disease		• Megaureter
Supernumerary kidney		• Ectopic ureter
Renal tubular dysgenesis		• VUR
Genetic cystic kidney disease		Bladder
		• Bladder exstrophy
		• Prune belly syndrome
		Urethra
		• Posterior urethral valves
		• Urethral atresia

Renal Parenchyma
- Renal agenesis: Mesonephric duct fails to develop → absent kidney, ureter, trigone, and vas deferens (in males)
  - Incidence of unilateral renal agenesis is 0.05%; bilateral is incompatible with life
  - Can be associated with VACTERL syndrome
  - Workup: Consider VCUG because VUR incidence is higher in patients with renal agenesis
  - Renal US, BP, kidney function monitored closely
- Renal dysgenesis
  - Dysplasia: Kidney is made up of undifferentiated tissue with loss of normal renal corticomedullary differentiation
    - If cysts are present with dysplasia, it is called cystic dysplasia (see below)
  - Hypoplasia: Small, nondysplastic kidney with fewer calyces and nephrons
    - Bilateral renal hypoplasia → ESRD during the 1st decade of life
    - Tx: Supportive, monitor renal function closely, tx HTN if present, ACEIs can slow progression of disease
  - Cystic disease
    - Multicystic dysplastic kidney (MCDK): Entire kidney affected by nonfunctional cysts which displace renal tissue
      - Incidence: 1 in 2,000 births; bilateral is usually incompatible with life
      - Most common cause of abdominal mass in newborns

- The cystic kidney involutes over time (50% completely gone by age 5)
- ↑ risk of VUR in the unaffected kidney
- Mgmt: Serial renal US, serial monitoring of renal function, proteinuria, and BP
- Genetic cystic kidney disease – polycystic kidney disease (PKD)

Embryonic Migration

- Renal ectopy: Kidney is not in normal position
  - Can be in the pelvis, thorax, or cross the midline and lie above or below the opposite kidney
  - Associated with increased incidence of urologic anomalies including cryptorchidism, hypospadias, agenesis of the uterus and vagina
  - Workup: VCUG, consider CT or MRI to find ectopic kidney, monitor renal function regularly
- Fusion anomalies: Horseshoe kidney – kidneys are fused at lower poles and rotated anteriorly
  - Incidence: 0.4–1.6 in 10,000 births
  - Pathophys: Kidney becomes trapped by the inferior or superior mesenteric arteries at the level of the lumbar spine
  - Associations: Turner syndrome, trisomy 13, trisomy 18, and trisomy 21
  - Workup: VCUG (evaluate for VUR), consider nuc med scan to r/o obstruction if hydronephrosis without VUR

Urinary Collecting System

- Duplicated collecting system: Common congenital anomaly – more common in females
  - Prognosis: ↑ risk of UTI
- Anomalies of the renal pelvis
  - Ureteropelvic junction (UPJ) obstruction: Between renal pelvis & ureter
    - Incidence: 1 in 500–1,500 births; M:F 2:1
    - Sxs: Presents anytime from birth to adulthood w/ abdominal mass, abd pain or flank pain, gross hematuria, recurrent UTI, or incidentally noted hydronephrosis on imaging
    - Dx: Diuretic renography
    - Indications for surgical repair are loss of kidney function, frequent infections, nephrolithiasis, or severe pain
- Anomalies of the ureter
  - Ectopic ureter: Ureter opens in a different location than the bladder
    - Common sites are urethra, vagina in girls, or seminal vesicles in boys
    - 80% are associated with a duplicated collecting system
    - F:M 6:1
    - Dx: Made via US, CT, or MRI if necessary
  - Ureterocele: Cystic ballooning of ureter which may cause obstruction and hydro-nephrosis
    - When obstruction is present, surgical mgmt is indicated
  - VUR (see "VESICOURETERAL REFLUX")
- Anomalies of the bladder
  - Prune belly syndrome (Eagle–Barrett syndrome): Renal + urethral + urethral anomalies
    - Pathophys: Poor development of the abdominal muscles → "wrinkling" of the abdomen aka "prune belly"
    - Incidence: 3.8/100,000 live births; more common in males
      - Associated with tetralogy of Fallot, VSD, trisomy 18, and trisomy 21
    - Urinary tract abnormalities include large ureters, distended bladder, VUR
- Anomalies of urethra
  - Posterior urethral valve (PUV): Thin flaps of tissue in the posterior urethra → dilation of the bladder and bilateral hydroureteronephrosis
    - Most common type of lower urinary tract obstruction
    - Incidence: 1 in 5,000–8,000 male births
    - Complications: Oligohydramnios, pulmonary hypoplasia, ESRD, bladder dysfunction
    - Mgmt: Starts in neonatal period with renal US, bladder catherization (to relieve obstruction), and urology consult
      - Fetal surgical intervention is possible, although there is high associated maternal and fetal morbidity

VESICOURETERAL REFLUX

- Definition (Lancet 2015;385:9965)
  - "Retrograde passage of urine from the bladder into one or both ureters of the kidneys"

Grade I	VUR does not reach renal pelvis
Grade II	VUR extends up to the renal pelvis without dilation
Grade III	Mild/moderate dilation of ureter and renal pelvis. No/slight blunting of fornices
Grade IV	Moderate dilation of ureter, renal pelvis, and calyces. Complete obliteration of sharp angle of fornices but maintenance of papillary impression in most calyces
Grade V	Gross dilation/tortuosity of ureter, renal pelvis, and calyces. Papillary impressions not visible in calyces

- Epidemiology (Lancet 2015;385:9965)
  - Affects 25–40% of children, but no need for investigation unless febrile UTI
- Diagnosis (Pediatrics 2011;138:595)
  - Febrile infants to 24 mo w/ UTI should undergo renal US to assess for anatomic abnormalities
  - Voiding cystourethrogram (VCUG) should not be performed for infant with 1st febrile UTI unless renal US shows hydronephrosis, scarring, or other signs of high-grade VUR
  - VCUG allows grading and anatomic evaluation; direct radionuclide cystography can be used for follow-up evaluation (decreased radiation exposure, but poorer anatomic detail)
  - Antenatal hydronephrosis: Follow-up with US at 1 mo (relative decrease in urinary flow in 1st mo may result in false negative if sooner) unless severe hydronephrosis noted prenatally
- Clinical manifestations (Pediatrics 2011;138:595; Ped Clin North Am 2001;48:1505)
  - Clinical consequences: UTI, reflux nephropathy, or scarring
  - Congenital ureteropelvic junction obstruction (UPJO) can present with hydronephrosis & normal renal function in asymptomatic infant
- Natural history and complications (Lancet 2015;385:9965; Ped Clin North Am 2001;48:1505; J Urol 2002;168:2594)
  - Grade I: 73% of children with dilating reflux had no or only grade I vesicoureteric reflux at the 10-yr follow-up
  - Grade I–II: Median time to spontaneous resolution was ~38 mo, grade III was 98 mo, and for grade IV–V was 156 mo
  - I & II reflux resolves in >80% of pts (10–25% resolution/yr); grade III reflux resolves in 50% (grade IV resolved in ~30%, & grade V rarely spontaneously resolves)
  - Reflux nephropathy can produce renal failure, proteinuria, and hypertension
- Management (Pediatrics 2013;132:e34–e45; Pediatrics 2017;139:5; Pediatrics 2011;138:595; N Engl J Med 2014;370:2367–2376)
  - AAP guidelines: Antibiotic prophylaxis no longer indicated for recurrent UTIs as studies have shown that prophylaxis not effective in reducing renal scars
    - RIVUR trial argues that prophylaxis is beneficial in reducing recurrent UTIs, but does not decrease renal scarring. May be beneficial to prevent recurrent infections while awaiting identification/treatment of underlying etiology
  - Grade V reflux almost always requires surgical correction; grade III/IV reflux can be managed medically unless recurrent UTIs and progressive scarring

(*Textbook of Pediatric Rheumatology.* 6th ed. 2011;Ch 13; *Nelson Textbook of Pediatrics.*
20th ed. 2015;Ch 153; *N Engl J Med* 1999;340:448–454; *Mod Rheumatology*
2009;19:219–228)

Inflammatory Markers

- Generally nonspecific, do not necessarily indicate dz, trend over time can be helpful
  - Can be elevated due to trauma, infectious, malignant, rheumatologic etiologies
- Common ones include ESR, CRP, complements, ferritin, haptoglobin, platelets, fibrinogen
  - **Erythrocyte sedimentation rate (ESR)**
    - Measures rate at which RBCs fall in a vertical tube, measured in mm/hr
    - ↑ inflammation → ↑ fibrinogen & other acute-phase reactants → ↑ rouleaux formation → ↑ faster sedimentation → ↑ ESR
    - Falsely ↓ in low-fibrinogen states, anemia, sickle cell dz, & liver/kidney dz
  - **C-reactive protein (CRP)**
    - Synthesized by liver in response to IL-6, alters cytokine release & mediates inflammation by modulating phagocyte behavior
    - Generally indicates acute inflammation, rises in 4 hr, peaks at 24–72 hr, $t_{1/2}$ ~18 hr
    - Most rheum causes w/ mild ↑. Large ↑ suggests infection, vasculitis, malignancy

Complement (C3, C4, CH$_{50}$)

- Mediate host defense & inflammation; inflammation → ↑ production or ↑ consumption
  - ↑ complement: Active phase of an illness of infection
  - ↓ complement: Immune complex formation (SLE, vasculitis, sepsis) or ↓ synthesis (liver dz, congenital def)

Antinuclear Antibody (ANA)

- Usually indirect immunofluorescence. Cells fixed to a slide incubated w/ serum to bind to nuclei → fluorescent antibody (Ab) to patient Abs added → microscopic visualization
- Titers determined by diluting patient's serum. ↑ titer = ↑ ANA presence
  - ≥1:160 considered clinically significant; no correlation w/ dz activity
- Pattern indicates target in the nucleus
  - Homogenous (nucleosome, Mi-2): SLE, drug-induced lupus
  - Speckled (Ro, La, RNP, Smith): SLE, Sjögren syndrome, mixed connective tissue disease (MCTD)
  - Nucleolar (Scl-70, U3-RNP): Systemic sclerosis
  - Centromere: CREST
- Sensitive for many autoimmune illnesses, but nonspecific:
  - In otherwise healthy people, ANA+ at 1:40 present in ~20–30%, while 1:320 in only ~3%
  - ANA may be present in patients w/ Hashimoto thyroiditis

Anti-dsDNA

- Abs that recognize native double-stranded DNA; ↑ titers correlate w/ dz activity
- Strongly associated w/ SLE, sensitivity is ~75%, while specificity ranges from 75–99%

Anti-Smith

- Small nuclear ribonucleoprotein particles (snRNPs) play a role in splicing precursor mRNA to mature RNA. The Smith proteins are critical for importation of snRNPs into the nucleus
- Presence of anti-Smith Abs highly specific for SLE (up to 100%), sensitivity only ~50%
- Correlated w/ nephritis, remain positive even after dz remission

Antiribonucleoprotein (RNP)

- Recognize specific snRNP termed U1RNP involved in splicing premessenger RNA
- Present in MCTD (presence mandatory for MCTD), SLE (~50%), RA, & Sjögren syndrome

Anti-Ro and Anti-La

- Both present in many autoimmune dzs (SLE, Sjögren syndrome, scleroderma)
- Anti-Ro (SS-A): Recognize 2 different "Ro" antigens
  - One adds ubiquitin to proteins involved in inflammation, other acts as RNA chaperone
- Anti-La (SS-B): More specific for SLE & Sjögren syndrome

Antineutrophil Cytoplasmic Antibodies (ANCA)
- c-ANCA: Diffuse staining of cytoplasm, usually against proteinase-3 (PR3), majority of GPA
- p-ANCA: Stains region around nucleus, artifact of EtOH fixation of the neutrophils, usually against myeloperoxidase (MPO, but can be others), majority of microscopic polyangiitis
- Assn w/ vasculitis: Granulomatosis with polyangiitis (GPA), microscopic polyangiitis, eosinophilic granulomatosis with polyangiitis (EGPA), & drug-induced vasculitis
  - If + for both c- & p-ANCA, consider levamisole-induced vasculitis

Rheumatoid Factor (RF)
- IgM against the Fc portion of IgG, can be + in wide variety of conditions:
  - RA, JIA, SLE, cryoglobulinemia, MCTD, infxn (hep B, endocarditis), chronic liver/lung dz
- Nonspecific but presence may indicate more aggressive course of polyarthritis

Joint Fluid Analysis

Synovial Fluid Analysis					
Condition	Color	Viscosity	WBC/mm³	PMN (%)	Culture
Normal	Yellow, clear	High	<200	<25	Negative
Traumatic	Xanthochromic, bloody	High	<2,000	<25	Negative
Chronic arthritis	Yellow, cloudy	Low	20,000	>50	Negative
Reactive arthritis	Yellow, opaque	Low	20,000	>50	Negative
SLE	Yellow, clear	Normal	5,000	10	Negative
Tuberculous	Yellow-white, cloudy	Low	25,000	50–60	Acid fast bacilli
Septic arthritis	Turbid	Low	>50,000	>75	Bacteria

ARTHRITIS

- Limitation in ROM w/ inflammation + warmth, swelling, effusion, pain, tenderness. Can be associated w/ muscle weakness & systemic signs such as fever, rash, lymphadenopathy
- Rheumatologic etiologies associated w/ AM stiffness, swelling, asymmetry, fatigue, limp, refusal to walk, leg-length discrepancy, & poor linear growth
  - Other etiologies: Infectious (acute onset, fever, recent trauma), oncologic (visible/ palpable mass, night-time awakening, abnormal CBC), or other MSK etiologies
- Initial evaluation: X-rays and/or US of affected joint(s), joint aspiration, CBC w/ diff, ESR, CRP; ANA if considering JIA

CHILD WITH A LIMP OR REFUSAL TO WALK

(Textbook of Pediatric Rheumatology. 6th ed. 2011;Ch 13&47; Nelson Textbook of Pediatrics. 20th ed. 2015;Ch 153; Rheumatology Secrets. 3rd ed. 2015)

Evaluation
- **History:** Specific points include presence & timing of pain (if present), presence of limp, recent illnesses, fever history, joint involvement
- **Exam:**
  - Joint swelling, redness, warmth, limitation in range of motion
  - Leg-length discrepancies
  - Muscle atrophy, Trendelenburg sign for hip and/or pelvis weakness
  - Scoliosis
  - Inability to walk on heels or toes localizes to foot
  - If hip pathology involved, internal rotation usually affected more than others
  - FABER test: SI joint involvement
- **Imaging:** Bilateral x-rays (+ frog-leg views w/ hips), MRI for continued pain, US if effusion
- **Lab:** ESR, CRP, CBC, blood cultures, Lyme Ab, HLA-B27, GAS antigen/cultures based on suspicion, ± joint aspiration

Diagnosis

- Pain at rest: "growing pain," infection, malignancy
- After rest and/or morning stiffness: Joint inflammation, juvenile idiopathic arthritis (JIA)
- During/after exercise: Orthopedic etiology, SCFE, osteochondritis dissecans, osteochondrosis (i.e., Köhler dz w/ tarsal navicular involvement & Freiberg dz w/ 2nd, 3rd, or 4th metatarsal involvement), apophysitis (i.e., Sever, Osgood–Schlatter, Iselin – traction apophysitis of 5th metatarsal base; Sinding–Larsen–Johansson – patellar apophysitis)
- Painless limp: Limb-length discrepancy, JIA, Legg–Calvé–Perthes
- Nocturnal pain: Bone tumors, leukemia
- Fever: Septic arthritis, osteomyelitis, discitis, myositis, leukemia, JIA
- Prior URI: Transient synovitis, aseptic synovitis, myositis, HSP, serum sickness–like rxn

Management

- Urgent referral or hospitalization for septic arthritis, osteomyelitis, tumor, unwell child

---

JUVENILE IDIOPATHIC ARTHRITIS (JIA)

(Textbook of Pediatric Rheumatology. 6th ed. 2011;Ch 13–18; Nelson Textbook of Pediatrics. 20th ed. 2015;Ch 155; Nat Reviews Rheumatol 2010;6:477–4856; Lancet 2011;377: 2138–2149; J Rheumatology 2009;36:642–650; BMC Pediatrics 2012;12:29; Arthritis Care Research 2011;63(4):465–482; Arthritis Rheum 2010;62:1824–1828)

- Required criteria: Symptom onset before 16 yr & present for at least 6 wk; distinction between subgroups based on dz expression during the 1st 6 mo
- Population prevalence is 1:1,000, risk for siblings are 1:100
- Diagnosis by physical exam, x-rays, & US; MRI sometimes beneficial
  - Indicators of dz activity: # joints involved, degree of elevation of inflammatory markers, physician assessment of dz activity, patient/parent assessment of dz activity
  - Features indicating worse prognosis: Erosions or joint space narrowing on imaging, hip or C-spine involvement, prolonged duration of illness or elevation of inflammatory markers
  - ~2–4× ↑ risk of malignancy
- Untreated → joint deformity, limb-length discrepancy, chronic pain/arthritis/uveitis
- **Uveitis:** Typically insidious & asymptomatic
  - Most likely in 1st 4 yr of dz. Risk ↓ each yr after arthritis onset. Can precede arthritis
  - Initial ophthalmologic exam should be performed w/in 1 mo of dx
  - Slit lamp exams annually in systemic JIA, more often in ANA (+) oligo/poly JIA or ANA (–) oligo/poly JIA if age of onset <7 yr

Classification of Juvenile Idiopathic Arthritis			
JIA Classification	**Clinical Criteria**	**Notable Characteristics**	**Findings**
Systemic arthritis (Still dz)	Arthritis in 1+ joints w/ fever ≥2 wk (daily for ≥3+ d) & also ≥1: Serositis, erythematous rash, lymphadenopathy, hepatomegaly, splenomegaly	Least common, 1:1 sex ratio, peak age: 2–5 yr, can involve any joints, can be destructive, can lead to MAS	Associated w/ MAS
Oligoarthritis (persistent/ extended)	Arthritis in 1–4 joints in 1st 6 mo. Types: • Persistent: ≤4 joints over course • Extended: ≥4 joints after 1st 6 mo	60% of total cases, 3× ↑ in females, bimodal (2–5 & 9–11 yr), knees & ankles commonly involved (↑ risk of ≠ limb length), assn w/ uveitis	ANA + in 75–85%, ↑ risk of uveitis if +
Polyarthritis, RF (–)	Arthritis in 5+ joints in 1st 6 mo	3× ↑ in females, peak age 2–5 yr • ANA (+): Resembles oligo JIA, asymmetric & ↑ risk of uveitis • ANA (–): Symmetric w/ shoulder, hip, DIP, & C-spine involvement	ANA + in ~40%, may have carpal/ C-spine fusion, micrognathia
Polyarthritis, RF (+)	Arthritis affecting 5+ joints in 1st 6 mo. 2+ tests for RF are + at least 3 mo apart during 1st 6 mo	6× ↑ in females, peak age 10–18, symmetric small joint involvement, systemic findings possible	RF (+) w/ slightly ↑ morbidity

Psoriatic arthritis	Arthritis + psoriasis OR Arthritis + ≥2: Dactylitis, psoriasis in a 1st-degree relative, nail-pitting/onycholysis • Can occur w/o history of psoriasis	1:1 sex ratio, bimodal (1–4 & 7–10 yr), mostly oligoarthritis but can be enthesitis, or poly/axial arthritis involving SI joint (sacroiliitis), can lead to erosive arthritis, swelling beyond joint margin → dactylitis	None
Enthesitis-related arthritis (ERA)	Arthritis + enthesitis OR Arthritis or enthesitis + ≥2: History or presence of SI or inflammatory lumbosacral pain, HLA-B27 +, arthritis onset in a male >6 yr of age, acute anterior uveitis, 1st-degree relative w/: AS, ERA, sacroiliitis w/ IBD, reactive arthritis, or acute anterior uveitis	7× ↑ in males, peak age >6 yr. Hallmark is enthesitis (inflammation of tendon/ligament insertion into bone; typically patella, Achilles, plantar fascia into calcaneus, greater trochanter, tibial tuberosity). Can develop sacroiliitis (abnormal Schober test)	HLA-B27 (+) in 80–90%, ANA & RF are negative
Undifferentiated	Fulfills criteria in none/2+ of categories		

Management
- Generally stepwise based on dz activity & response to prior tx, can jump steps if dz activity remains high despite optimal doses of DMARDs and/or NSAIDs
  - Systemic corticosteroids for control of symptoms
    - Glucocorticoid joint injections for large joints
  - NSAIDs: Naproxen, ibuprofen, indomethacin, meloxicam
  - DMARDs (typically w/ persistently active dz): Methotrexate (MTX, most commonly used), leflunomide, sulfasalazine, hydroxychloroquine
  - Other immunosuppressive drugs: Mycophenolate, azathioprine, cyclosporine
  - Biologics: TNF-α inhibitors (etanercept, adalimumab, infliximab), abatacept, rituximab, tocilizumab
  - Anakinra generally for systemic JIA
- Medication monitoring:
  - CBC, creatinine, liver enzymes, TB screening yearly if on biologics
    - NSAIDs: Check prior to starting & every 6–12 mo
    - MTX: Prior to start, 1 mo after start/dose change, & every 3–4 mo on stable dose
    - Biologics: Prior to start & every 3–6 mo
  - Steroids: Monitor for osteoporosis & growth delay
- Always consider PT, OT, & psychosocial support
- Ensure appropriate Ca/vit D in diet & aerobic exercise for preventing osteopenia
- Can consider surgery if contractures or significant pain from synovitis
- Avoid live virus vaccines while on biologic or immunosuppressive regimens

MACROPHAGE ACTIVATION SYNDROME (MAS)

(Textbook of Pediatric Rheumatology. 6th ed. 2011;Ch 14; Nelson Textbook of Pediatrics. 20th ed. 2015;Ch 155)

- Sudden onset; pancytopenia, abruptly ↓ ESR (fibrinogen consumption), lymphadenopathy, hepatosplenomegaly, coagulopathy, purpura, ↑ triglycerides, liver dysfunction, fevers
- Unknown trigger, possibly infectious; assn w/ ↓ NK cell function & low perforin expression
- Need 5 of the following 8 criteria:
  - Fever ≥38.5°C
  - Splenomegaly
  - Ferritin >500 ng/mL
  - Peripheral blood cytopenia, w/ 2+ of: Hb <9 (for infants <4 wk, Hb <10), platelets <100,000, absolute neutrophil count <1,000
  - Low or absent NK cell activity
  - Triglycerides >256 mg/dL and/or fibrinogen <150 mg/dL

- Hemophagocytosis in bone marrow, spleen, lymph node, or liver
- ↑ soluble CD25 (soluble IL-2 receptor α) 2 std dev above age-adjusted (lab-specific) norm
  - Soluble IL-2 receptor α (sCD25) levels correlate w/ dz activity
- **Treatment:** High-dose steroids, anakinra, tocilizumab; if prolonged tx required, generally use cyclosporine or etoposide

REACTIVE ARTHRITIS

(Textbook of Pediatric Rheumatology. 6th ed. 2011;Ch 39; Nelson Textbook of Pediatrics. 20th ed. 2015;Ch 157)

- Usually lower-extremity inflammatory arthritis classically w/ conjunctivitis & urethritis
- Typically follows an infection, generally a GI illness (*Campylobacter, Salmonella, Shigella, Yersinia*), but can be after respiratory or GU infections as well
  - GU (9:1 M:F), GI (1:1 sex ratio); overall 3:1 M:F
- Age distribution typically adolescents – 30s

Evaluation
- **History:** Presents ~1–4 wk after infection w/ oligoarthritis + constitutional sxs
  - Most episodes are monophasic, but can be recurrent
- **Lab:** ↑ inflammatory markers, negative serologies, ~50–60% w/ + HLA-B27

Diagnosis
- No specific diagnostic criteria, needs exclusion of other etiologies
  - Perform joint aspiration, X-rays, US, UA, gonococcal & chlamydia PCR, stool studies, Lyme serology

Management
- NSAIDs, intraarticular steroids, PT, DMARDs 2nd line for refractory dz
- Tx of urethritis ↓ risk of reactive arthritis, but tx of enteritis does not

SYSTEMIC CONNECTIVE TISSUE DISEASE

(Textbook of Pediatric Rheumatology. 6th ed. 2011;Ch 21–29; Nelson Textbook of Pediatrics. 20th ed. 2015;Ch 158–162; Rheumatology Secrets. 3rd ed. 2015)

Antibodies Associated with Connective Tissue Diseases
- SLE: ANA, anti-dsDNA, anti-Smith, anti-RNP, lupus anticoagulant, anticardiolipin, anti-β2-glycoprotein
- Drug-induced SLE: ANA, antihistone
- MCTD: ANA, anti-RNP
- Scleroderma: ANA, anticentromere, anti-RNP, anti-scl70 (topoisomerase)
- Sjögren syndrome: ANA, anti-Ro, anti-La
- Vasculitis: ANCA
- Dermatomyositis: ANA, anti-Jo-1
- JIA: ANA, RF, anti-CCP

Lab Abnormalities in Childhood CTDs	sJIA	SLE	jDM	Scleroderma	Vasculitis
Anemia	++	+++	+	+	++
Leukopenia	−	+++	−	−	−
Thrombocytopenia	−	++	−	−	−
Leukocytosis	+++	−	+	−	+++
Thrombocytosis	++	−	+	−	+
ANA	−	+++	+	++	−
RF	−	++	−	+	+
Low complements	−	+++	−	−	++
Elevated LFTs	++	+	+	+	+
Elevated muscle enzymes	−	+	+++	++	+
UA abnormalities	+	+++	+	+	++

sJIA, systemic JIA; SLE, systemic lupus erythematosus; jDM, juvenile dermatomyositis

Auto-Antibody Frequency in CTDs						
	SLE (%)	MCTD (%)	Scleroderma (%)	CREST (%)	Sjögren (%)	JIA (%)
ANA	99	100	80	80	>70	50
Anti-dsDNA	80	0	0	0	0	0
Anti-Smith	30	0	0	0	0	0
Anti-RNP	30	100	20–50	Rare	Rare	Rare
Anticentromere	Rare	Rare	10	80	Rare	0
Anti-Ro (SS-A)	30	Rare	Rare	0	70	Rare
Anti-La (SS-B)	15	Rare	Rare	0	60	Rare

MCTD, mixed connective tissue dz; CREST, calcinosis, Raynaud phenomenon, esophageal dysmotility, sclerodactyly, telangiectasias

SYSTEMIC LUPUS ERYTHEMATOSUS (SLE)

(Lupus 2004;13:829–837; J Pediatrics 2005;146:648–653; Pediatr Rev 2012;33:62–73; Acta Paediatrica 2010;99:967; *Dubois' Lupus Erythematosus and Related Syndromes.* 8th ed. 2013; Rheum Clin N Am 2007;33:267–285)

- Generally occurs after age 10, 20% of all SLE cases occur in the pediatric population
  - Female predilection in all ages, 2:1 at <10 yr of age, 5–10:1 at >10 yr of age
- Usually more severe than adult onset SLE w/ ↑ incidence of nephritis, fever, chorea, & hepatosplenomegaly. Mortality risk also higher w/ childhood-onset SLE
- Autoreactive B- & T-cells → immune complex deposition → complement system activation
- ANA ↑ sensitivity for SLE w/ poor specificity. Anti-Smith & dsDNA specific but not sensitive
- dsDNA titers correlate w/ dz activity & may herald development of renal dz
- Decreasing complements can indicate renal dz
- If associated w/ antiphospholipid Abs, up to 6× risk of venous thromboembolism
- Diagnostic criteria, need 4/11 criteria (96% sensitivity & specificity):

Revised American College of Rheumatology Criteria for Classification of SLE	
Malar rash	Fixed erythema, flat/raised, over malar eminences, spares the nasolabial folds
Discoid rash	Erythematous raised patches w/ keratotic scaling & follicular plugging; atrophic scarring may occur in older lesions
Photosensitivity	Skin rash as a result of unusual reaction to sun, can be on history or clinician observation
Oral ulcers	Oral or nasopharyngeal ulceration, usually painless, observed by a clinician
Nonerosive arthritis	Nonerosive arthritis involving ≥2 peripheral joints w/ tenderness, swelling, or effusion
Serositis	Pleuritis (convincing history of pleuritic pain or rub heard by clinician or evidence of pleural effusion) **OR** pericarditis
Renal disorder	Persistent proteinuria >0.5 g/d or greater than 3+ if quantitation not performed **OR** cellular casts (red cell, hemoglobin, granular, tubular, or mixed)
Neurologic disorder	Seizures **OR** psychosis in the absence of offending drugs or known metabolic derangement (uremia, ketoacidosis, or electrolyte imbalance)
Hematologic disorder	Hemolytic anemia (w/ ↑ retics) **OR** leukopenia (<4,000 on 2+ occasions) **OR** lymphopenia (<1,500 on 2+ occasions) **OR** thrombocytopenia (<1,00,000 in absence of offending drugs)
Immunologic disorders	Anti-dsDNA: Ab to native DNA in abnormal titer **OR** Anti-Smith: Presence of Ab to Smith nuclear antigen **OR** Positive antiphospholipid Ab on: 1. An abnormal serum level of IgG or IgM anticardiolipin Abs, or 2. A positive test result for lupus anticoagulant using a standard method, or 3. A false-positive syphilis test for ≥6 mo confirmed by additional treponemal testing
Antinuclear antibody	An abnormal titer of ANA by immunofluorescence or an equivalent assay at any point in time in the absence of drugs known to be associated w/ drug-induced lupus

Management

- Adequate rest, use of sunscreen
- NSAIDs for musculoskeletal symptoms, but monitor for renal toxicity
- Hydroxychloroquine mainly used for skin and joint symptoms
- Steroids for acute symptoms
- Immunosuppression w/ cyclophosphamide, mycophenolate, azathioprine
  - Cyclophosphamide used frequently for nephritis, CNS involvement, pulm hemorrhage
- Anti-B-cell therapies w/ rituximab & belimumab

Neonatal Lupus

- Transplacental passage of maternal SS-A/SS-B Abs; if present, risk of neonatal lupus ~2%
- Clinical manifestations
  - SS-A Abs: Rash, hepatic dysfunction, hemolytic anemia, thrombocytopenia
    - Resolves over 2–6 mo as maternal Abs are cleared
  - Congenital heart block associated with presence of anti-Ro (SS-A) and/or anti-La (SS-B)
    - Risk 1–3% w/ + SS-A/SS-B (~85% w/ CHB have + ab's); 15–18% w/ prev affected child
    - Serial prenatal USs beginning 2nd trimester, if 1st-degree block or pericardial effusion develops tx is dexamethasone or betamethasone maternal administration
    - Fetal mortality can be up to 20% due to heart block & hydrops
    - Fetal heart block is often permanent, requires pacemaker implantation

Drug-Induced SLE

- Typical drugs: Hydralazine, minocycline, doxycycline, procainamide, isoniazid, phenytoin, carbamazepine, ethosuximide, TNF-α antagonists
- Usually present w/ constitutional symptoms, arthritis/arthralgias, rash, & serositis
  - Cytopenias, nephritis, & CNS involvement are rare
- Associated w/ ANA & antihistone Abs; NOT w/ dsDNA or ↓ complements
  - Antihistone Abs are sensitive but not specific for drug-induced lupus
    - ~95% of patients w/ drug-induced SLE have antihistone but ~50% of patients w/ active SLE also have antihistone
- Typically resolves w/ offending drug discontinuation, a short course of steroids may be helpful for patients w/ serositis, NSAIDs for arthritis/arthralgias

---

DERMATOMYOSITIS

(Autoimmunity 2006;39:197–203; Lancet 2008;371:2201–2212; Curr Rheumatol Rep 2011;13:216–224)

- Inflammation of skin, GI tract, & striated muscle; no assn w/ malignancy in children
- Polymyositis extremely rare in childhood
- 2× more common in females w/ peak age of 5–14 yr

Evaluation

- Multiple clinical manifestations
  - Constitutional: Fever, fatigue, weight loss
  - Dermatologic: Photosensitivity, heliotrope rash of eyelids (75%), Gottron papules (up to 95%), rash of extensor surfaces, nailfold capillary changes, eyelid telangiectasias
  - Musculoskeletal (80–100%): Symmetric proximal muscle pain/weakness, lower-extremity weakness > upper-extremity weakness. Difficulty climbing stairs or riding a bicycle
  - Respiratory: Weakness → restrictive lung dz (up to 50%), usually manifests as ↓ DLCO
  - Can also have dysphagia (up to 40%) due to bulbar weakness
  - Can have only skin involvement without muscle involvement
  - Subcutaneous calcinosis (up to 40%) which can lead to impaired mobility & lipodystrophy (up to 40%) which is associated w/ metabolic syndrome
- **Labs:** Elevated AST, ALT, CK, LDH, aldolase; ESR, CRP, ANA may be normal
- **Imaging:** MRI may show fibrosis, atrophy, & active myositis

Diagnosis

- Gold standard is muscle biopsy showing inflammation and/or fiber necrosis, perifas-cicular atrophy, & small-vessel vasculitis

Treatment

- Generally consists of steroids w/ MTX as a steroid-sparing agent. IVIG used in refractory dz

SCLERODERMA

(Textbook of Pediatric Rheumatology. 6th ed. 2011;Ch 25; Nelson Textbook of Pediatrics.
20th ed. 2015;Ch 160; Arthritis Rheum 2006;54:3971–3978;
Best Pract Res Clin Rheumatol 2008;22:1093–1108;
Arthritis Rheum 2013;65:2737–2747)

- Abnormal collagen deposition and vasculopathy in skin & organs, characterized by skin thickening, Raynaud phenomenon, & esophageal dysmotility; associated w/ lung & renal involvement
- 3× more common in females, median age 8 yr, ~3–10% of all cases present in children
- Most patients have skin tightening, Raynaud phenomenon, arthralgias, myalgias, calcifications, dysphagia, & dyspnea
  - The skin is initially edematous, then becomes sclerotic

Noncutaneous Organ Involvement
- GI (most common): Gastroesophageal reflux, dysphagia, constipation, diarrhea, bloating
- Pulmonary: Dry cough, dyspnea; pulmonary fibrosis, & pHTN are rare; PFTs show ↑ DLCO + restriction, CXR & CT helpful to identify restrictive dz, echocardiogram for pHTN
- Cardiac: Cardiac fibrosis → conduction defects, arrhythmias, impaired ventricular function; evaluation by echo
- Renal: Proteinuria, hematuria, & renal failure; scleroderma renal crisis is rare

Types
- **Localized scleroderma:** Dermal fibrosis w/o internal organ involvement
  - Morphea: Solitary lesions or patches on the face, scalp, or limbs
  - Linear scleroderma: Band of thickened skin (usually on legs/arms), sometimes on face
  - Tx includes high-dose steroids tapered over months along w/ MTX
- **Diffuse scleroderma**
  - **Limited cutaneous systemic sclerosis:** Skin thickening w/ calcinosis, Raynaud phenomenon, esophageal dysfunction, sclerodactyly, & telangiectasias (aka CREST)
    - Presence of anticentromere Ab associated w/ high risk of developing pHTN
  - **Diffuse cutaneous systemic sclerosis:** More acute & rapidly progressive than limited subtype; these patients have more systemic sxs; more likely to develop renal crisis & ILD
    - Diagnosis requires proximal sclerosis/induration of skin w/ ≥2 of the following:
      - Skin: Sclerodactyly
      - Vascular: Raynaud phenomenon, nailfold capillary abnormalities, digital ulcers
      - GI: Dysphagia or gastroesophageal reflux
      - Renal: Renal crisis or new-onset arterial HTN
      - Cardiac: Arrhythmias or CHF
      - Pulmonary: Evidence of fibrosis, DLCO abnormality, or pHTN
        - Presence of anti-Scl-70 associated w/ development of interstitial lung dz
      - Musculoskeletal: Tendon friction rubs, arthritis, or myositis
      - Neurologic: Neuropathy or carpal tunnel syndrome
    - Abs: ~80–100% w/ + ANA, ~20–30% w/ anti-Scl-70, 15–40% w/ anticentromere
    - Management:
      - PT/OT, splints to help prevent contractures, skin care w/ emollients, avoid extremes of temperature & sun exposure
      - No specific medication recommendations but generally includes glucocorticoids, cyclophosphamide (for lung dz), MTX (for skin dz), & ACE-Is (for renal dz)

Raynaud Phenomenon
- Episodic, self-limited, reversible vasomotor changes manifested as white → blue → red color changes in fingers/toes, but can occur around ears, nose, tongue, & lips
  - Induced by vasospasm of digital arteries that is mediated by local & systemic factors
  - Occurs spontaneously or in response to environmental cold/emotional stress
- Can be isolated (Raynaud dz) or associated w/ CTD
  - Raynaud + digital ulcers, abnl nailfold capillaries, or + ANA = ↑ likelihood of CTD
- Treatment is generally avoiding cold temperatures ± calcium channel blockers

---

MIXED CONNECTIVE TISSUE DISEASE

(Textbook of Pediatric Rheumatology. 6th ed. 2011;Ch 27)

- Has overlap features of scleroderma, SLE, & inflammatory myositis
- Needs high-titer anti-RNP Abs w/ absence of anti-Smith, dsDNA, SS-A, SS-B, & centromere

- Common sxs: Raynaud phenomenon, synovitis, swollen hands/fingers, myositis
- Major morbidity due to lung involvement like in scleroderma
- SLE features treated w/ NSAIDs, antimalarials, MTX; synovitis treated w/ steroids & MTX

SJÖGREN SYNDROME

(Curr Rheumatol Rep 2008;10:147–155)

- Characterized by slowly progressive autoimmune dz that primarily affects exocrine organs, leading to dry eyes, dry mouth, parotitis, & tooth caries
- Uncommon in children; usually present w/ other CTDs
- Need to differentiate from mumps, lymphoma, sarcoidosis, TB, & benign parotitis
- Diagnosis by lip salivary gland biopsy showing a chronic lymphocytic infiltrate

OTHER PEDIATRIC MUSCULOSKELETAL PAIN

(Nelson Textbook of Pediatrics. 20th ed. 2015;Ch 168; Rheumatology 2009;48:466–474; Pain 2011;152:729–2738; Pediatrics 2006;117:840–844)

Oncologic Bone Pain
- Red flags: Joint redness, fever, weight loss, night sweats, *night-time pain*, bone pain
- Acute leukemia, neuroblastoma, Ewing sarcoma, & lymphoma present w/ bone pain

Pain Syndromes

Characteristics of Pediatric Organic & Nonorganic Pain		
	Organic Pain	Nonorganic Pain
Timing	Day & night, during weekends & holidays	Primarily at night & on school days
Location	Typically in the joint, unilateral	Typically between joints, bilateral
Severity	Interrupts play & other enjoyable activities	Can carry out normal activities
Gait	Limp or refusal to walk	Unusual gait
Systemic signs	Fever, night sweats, weight loss, ± rash	Otherwise healthy child

Characteristics of Pediatric Pain Amplification Syndromes			
	Growing Pains	Fibromyalgia	Complex Regional Pain Syndrome
Age (yr)	Typically 4–6 yr	Adolescence	Adolescence
Sex ratio	F = M	F > M	F > M
Symptoms	Intermittent, recurrent pain in bi/l lower extremities. Worse at night. Aching or cramping at rest	Fatigue, headaches, poor sleep, dizziness, paresthesias, abdominal pain, widespread MSK pain	Superficial & deep pain in the distal part of the extremity. Exacerbated by movement
Signs	Exam is normal	Tender points	Diffusely swollen, tender, cool, & mottled extremity
Labs	Labs & imaging are normal	Labs & imaging are normal	Labs are normal; imaging may show osteoporosis
Treatment	Reassurance, massage, analgesia	PT/OT, psychosocial support	PT/OT, psychosocial support

VASCULITIS

(Textbook of Pediatric Rheumatology. 6th ed. 2011;Ch 30–36; Nelson Textbook of Pediatrics. 20th ed. 2015;Ch 161&165–167; Rheumatology Secrets. 3rd ed. 2015; Curr Rheumatol Rep 2009;11:402–409; Rheumatology 2000;39:245–252; Rheum Dis Clin North Am 2002;28:625–654)

- Inflammation of blood vessels, typically presents as a rash w/ multiorgan involvement
- Diagnosis based on characteristic clinical manifestations, lab findings of organ involvement, imaging of the vessels, & biopsy showing vasculitis
- Vasculitis characterized based on vessel size involved

LARGE VESSEL VASCULITIS

(Rheumatology 2010;49:1806–1814)

Takayasu Arteritis

- Inflammation → stenosis of the aorta & its branches (particularly the aortic arch & abdominal aorta). Can also have pulmonary artery involvement in 70% of patients leading to pHTN & cardiac involvement in 25%
- Predominantly young women (8× more common in females), median age ~25 yr, but seen regularly in pediatrics
- Common in South, Southeast, & East Asia
- **History:** Constitutional symptoms, headache, HTN, dizziness; angina/claudication possible
- **Exam:** Careful BP & pulse/bruit assessment in all 4 limbs
- **Lab:** ↑ inflammatory markers
- **Diagnosis:** Angiography needed for diagnosis, shows long-segment stenosis or arterial occlusions. Histology shows panarteritis
  - 45% of patients develop aortic aneurysms, so should perform an echocardiogram to evaluate for these & cardiac involvement
- **Treatment:** High-dose glucocorticoids w/ MTX as 1st line DMARD or w/ azathioprine, mycophenolate, cyclophosphamide; biologics if refractory to these
  - Other considerations include antiplatelet therapies

MEDIUM VESSEL VASCULITIS

(Circulation 2004;110:2747–2771; Pediatr Cardiol 2008;29:398–301;
Pediatr Rev 2008;29:308–316)

Polyarteritis Nodosa

- Necrotizing inflammation of small & medium arteries; no assn w/ glomerulonephritis or ANCA. Typical involvement: Peripheral nerves, skin, abdomen, muscle, & kidneys
- Equal sex distribution w/ peak onset at 9–11 yo in children; most cases in adults
- Unknown etiology, can be associated w/ hep B infection
- **History:** Constitutional symptoms & nonspecific abdominal pain (mesenteric vasculitis)
- **Exam:** Palpable purpura, necrotic lesions, fingertip infarcts, peripheral neuropathy
- **Lab:** Nonspecific elevation of inflammatory markers; ANCA & ANA negative
- **Diagnosis:** Biopsy w/ nongranulomatous vasculitis or angiography w/ aneurysms/stenosis
- **Treatment:** High-dose glucocorticoids & other immunosuppressants like MTX, cyclophosphamide, mycophenolate, & biologics. Antivirals if associated w/ hep B

Kawasaki Disease

- Acute febrile vasculitis of unknown etiology, fever frequently >40°C that lasts 5–25 d
- Majority of patients <5 yr, median age is 2 yr, rare after 11
- Unknown etiology, possible immune dysregulation due to infection
- Clinical criteria w/ mandatory fever for ≥5 d w/ 4 of the 5 criteria below:
  - Bilateral painless, nonexudative bulbar conjunctival injection (~90%)
  - Lip erythema, cracked lips, nonexudative pharyngitis, strawberry tongue (~90%)
  - Polymorphous exanthem, involves trunk & extremities (~80–90%)
  - Swelling of hands & feet w/ erythema of palms & soles, peels in weeks 2–3 (~70%)
  - Cervical lymphadenopathy, at least one >1.5 cm in diameter (~50%)
- Alternatively, can diagnose w/ fever + echo findings of coronary artery aneurysms
- Other clinical findings: Extreme irritability, abdominal pain, vomiting, diarrhea, arthritis of small joints, uveitis, facial nerve palsy, meningitis
- Labs suggestive of KD (can be used to diagnose incomplete KD):
  - CRP ≥30 mg/L, ESR ≥40, WBC ≥15,000, anemia, sterile pyuria (≥10 wbc/hpf), ALT ≥50, albumin <3.0, platelets after 7 d ≥450,000
- Cardiac complications: Coronary thrombosis, aneurysms, coronary arteritis, myocarditis, valvular regurgitation, pericarditis/pericardial effusion
- **Treatment:**
  - IVIG (2nd dose needed in ~15–30% if persistent fever >36 hr after 1st dose), ± steroids/infliximab if persistent after IVIG, aspirin, warfarin (if giant coronary aneurysm)

SMALL VESSEL VASCULITIS

(Textbook of Pediatric Rheumatology. 6th ed. 2011;Ch 31; Nelson Textbook of Pediatrics. 20th ed. 2015;Ch 167)

Henoch–Schonlein Purpura (HSP)
- IgA-mediated small vessel vasculitis, most common vasculitis in children
- Typical age is 2–7 yr, slight male predominance (2:1); self-limited in most, lasts ~2–6 wk
- Most w/ recent viral URI, some w/ evidence of exposure to Group A Strep
- Can have multisystem involvement, w/ triad of arthritis, colicky abdominal pain, purpura
  - Nonthrombotic palpable purpura, start as urticarial lesions
    - Typically begin on lower extremities, but can involve entire body
  - Migratory polyarthritis/polyarthralgia; typically ankles & knees, nondeforming
  - Colicky abdominal pain due to hemorrhage & edema of the small bowel, pain is diffuse, can lead to bloody diarrhea. Rarely may lead to intussusception
  - Renal dz manifests as glomerulonephritis, most significant complication (~60% of cases)
    - 5% of all children w/ HSP progress to renal failure; usually presents in 1st 2 mo
    - Persistent proteinuria = ↑ risk; follow UAs at office visits to monitor proteinuria
    - Later age of onset → worse renal dz
  - Scrotal inflammation in males
  - Pulmonary hemorrhage possible
- Poor prognostic factors: Melena, persistent rash for 2–3 mo, hematuria w/ >1 g/d proteinuria, nephrotic syndrome
- **Lab:** ↑ ESR, ↑ IgA, normal complements, normal platelet count/function
- **Treatment:** Hydration & analgesia w/ NSAIDs; steroids for renal/pulm or severe sxs
  - Severe renal dz: Azathioprine, cyclophosphamide, cyclosporine, IVIG, PLEX

ANCA (+) VASCULITIS

(Textbook of Pediatric Rheumatology. 6th ed. 2011;Ch 34; Nelson Textbook of Pediatrics. 20th ed. 2015;Ch 167; Arthritis Rheum 2009;60:3413–3424)

- Upregulation of adhesion molecules on endothelial cells cause neutrophils to bind to them & degranulate leading to endothelial injury & vasculitis
- c-ANCA (cytoplasmic) recognizes PR3 & p-ANCA (perinuclear) recognizes MPO

Granulomatosis with Polyangiitis (GPA)
- Characterized by granulomatous vasculitis of the small vessels of upper & lower respiratory tract, glomerulonephritis, & assn w/ anti-PR3 Abs (c-ANCA)
- ANCA titers not associated w/ flares
- Nephritis: Pauci-immune (vs. immune complex deposition in Goodpasture or SLE)
- Treatment: Combination of high-dose steroids, MTX, cyclophosphamide, plasma exchange

Microscopic Polyangiitis (MPA)
- Systemic necrotizing small vessel vasculitis w/o any immune deposits, characterized by focal segmental necrotizing glomerulonephritis & pulmonary capillaritis
- Present w/ rapidly progressive glomerulonephritis & pulmonary infiltrates or hemorrhage
- Requires aggressive treatment w/ similar agents as GPA

Eosinophilic Granulomatosis with Polyangiitis (EGPA)
- Granulomatous vasculitis of small & medium sized vessels, assn w/ eosinophilia
- Typically occurs in patients w/ allergic symptoms (especially nasal polyps)
  - Suspect in those w/ asthma, peripheral eosinophilia, & vasculitis
- Diagnosis generally requires tissue biopsy; treatment similar as above

Drug-Induced ANCA Vasculitis
- PTU, methimazole, hydralazine, minocycline, & levamisole (found in some cocaine)
  - Typically associated w/ anti-MPO (p-ANCA); levamisole induced classically has both

Characteristics of ANCA Associated Vasculitis			
	GPA	**MPA**	**EGPA**
Epidemiology	F:M 1:1, age range 5–78, ~16% in pediatric age group	F:M 1:1, age range 30–50, but can affect children	Rare, but possible, in children

ENT	Chronic sinusitis, nasal mucosa ulcers, epistaxis, nasal septum perf, saddle-nose deformity, oral ulcers, otitis media, hoarseness, subglottic stenosis	Uncommon	Nasal polyps, rhinitis, conductive hearing loss
Eyes	Scleritis, episcleritis, retinal artery thrombosis, retro-orbital pseudotumor	Uncommon	Uncommon
Lungs	Chronic granulomatous inflammation → nodule formation & fibrosis, can also have pulmonary hemorrhage	Alveolar hemorrhage	Asthma, patchy infiltrates, nodules, interstitial lung dz, alveolar hemorrhage is rare
Kidney	Pauci-immune focal & segmental necrotizing glomerulonephritis, often have an active urinary sediment	Pauci-immune focal & segmental necrotizing glomerulonephritis	Uncommon
Heart	Pericarditis most common	Uncommon	Heart failure
Peripheral nerve	Mononeuritis multiplex	Mononeuritis multiplex	Mononeuritis multiplex (more commonly than GPA/MPA)
Skin	Palpable purpura, ulcers, subcutaneous nodules	Palpable purpura	Subcutaneous nodules, purpura, skin infarction
Eosinophilia	Rare	None	Common (usually ≥1,500)
ANCA positivity	80–90% c-ANCA, sensitivity ~75%, w/ specificity for c-ANCA 98%	70% (p-ANCA)	<50%, p-ANCA > c-ANCA

SARCOIDOSIS

(Textbook of Pediatric Rheumatology. 6th ed. 2011;Ch 35; Nelson Textbook of Pediatrics. 20th ed. 2015;Ch 165)

- Infiltrative noncaseating granulomas of unknown etiology
- Equal male to female distribution, peak between 20–40 yr
- Before puberty, typically Caucasian; after puberty, predominantly African Americans

Evaluation

- **History/Exam:**
  - Constitutional: Lymphadenopathy, fever, weight loss, anorexia, fatigue
  - Eye: Uveitis, chorioretinitis, glaucoma, band keratopathy, synechiae, iris nodules, cataracts
  - Dermatologic: Erythema nodosum, subcutaneous nodules
  - Cardiovascular: Valvular dz, arrhythmia
  - Pulmonary: Chest pain, nonproductive cough, dyspnea
  - GI: Bowel obstruction, hepatosplenomegaly
  - Renal: Renal failure, nephrolithiasis
  - Endocrine: Pituitary dysfunction such as diabetes insipidus
  - Neurologic: Headache, seizures, CN VI, VII, VIII palsies, obstructive hydrocephalus
- **Imaging:**
  - CXR or CT: Bilateral hilar lymphadenopathy, restrictive lung dz
  - MRI: Mass lesions, periventricular white matter lesions, leptomeningeal enhancement
- **Lab:** ↑ transaminases, ↑ bilirubin, ↑ Ca (alveolar macrophages hydroxylate vit D to active 1,25 form), ↑ ACE (produced by granulomas, nonspecific), leukopenia, eosinophilia

Diagnosis

- Need biopsy showing noncaseating granulomas without another etiology
  - Differential:
    - Infectious etiologies such as TB, non-TB mycobacteria, histoplasmosis, coccidioidomycosis, brucellosis, toxoplasmosis, Blau syndrome (NOD2 mutation)
    - Noninfectious etiologies such as hypersensitivity pneumonitis, berylliosis, silicosis
    - Other immunologic etiologies such as vasculitis, malignancies

Management

- Glucocorticoids are the mainstay; DMARDs 2nd line

BEHÇET DISEASE

(*Textbook of Pediatric Rheumatology.* 6th ed. 2011;Ch 36; *Nelson Textbook of Pediatrics.* 20th ed. 2015;ch 161)

- Systemic inflammatory dz characterized by recurrent oral/genital ulcers & uveitis
- 1:1 sex ratio, median age 30, men usually present younger & w/ worse prognosis

Evaluation
- **History/Exam:**
  - Recurrent oral & genital ulcerative lesions
  - Eye lesions: Anterior uveitis, posterior uveitis, retinal vasculitis
  - Skin lesions: Pseudofolliculitis, papulopustular lesions, erythema nodosum–like lesions, pyoderma gangrenosum–like lesions
  - Vascular lesions: Phlebitis, large vein thrombosis, aneurysms, arterial thrombosis
    - Pulm artery aneurysms can present w/ PE-like sxs; anticoagulation contraindicated
  - Positive pathergy test: Hyperreactivity of the skin to cutaneous injection or needle stick
  - Pathergy, hypopyon, pulm aneurysms, & scarring genital ulcers are characteristic
  - Major complications: CNS involvement, ruptured aneurysms, bowel perforation

Diagnosis
- No characteristic auto-Abs; nonspecific ↑ of ESR, CRP, & immunoglobulins
  - IBD is the main etiology in the differential, particularly if associated w/ Fe def anemia, markedly elevated ESR (>100), & diarrhea. Other considerations are other CTDs

Management
- Mucocutaneous manifestations: Local corticosteroid creams/elixirs, topical tacrolimus, oral colchicine, dapsone, TNF-α antagonists, thalidomide, & azathioprine
- Ocular manifestations: Systemic corticosteroids, azathioprine, mycophenolate, cyclosporine, tacrolimus, TNF-α antagonists

AUTOINFLAMMATORY DISEASES

(*Textbook of Pediatric Rheumatology.* 6th ed. 2011;Ch 43–44; *Nelson Textbook of Pediatrics.* 20th ed. 2015;Ch 163; *Rheumatology Secrets.* 3rd ed. 2015; Genet Med 2011;13:487–498; Clin Exp Immunol 2012;167:369–404; J Allergy Clin Immunol 2009;124:1129–1138)

Characteristics of Auto-Inflammatory Diseases			
Syndrome	**Age at Onset**	**Duration (d)**	**Clinical Features**
FMF	<20	1–3	Erysipelas-like rash, nondestructive large joint monoarthritis, pleuritis, sterile peritonitis; responds to colchicine
TRAPS	<20	>5	Rash w/ underlying myalgias, arthralgias, conjunctivitis, peritonitis, pleuritis, monoarthritis
HIDS	<1	1–10	Rash, abdominal pain, splenomegaly, cervical lymphadenopathy, aphthous ulcers
FCAS	<1	<2	Urticaria, arthralgia, & conjunctivitis induced by cold exposure
MWS	<20	1–2	Urticarial rash, arthralgias, conjunctivitis induced by cold exposure, hunger, or fatigue; late-onset sensorineural hearing loss
NOMID	<1	Continuous	Triad of chronic aseptic meningitis, neonatal-onset skin lesions, & arthropathy; often has lymphadenopathy & hepatosplenomegaly; late onset w/ visual impairment, hearing loss, hoarseness, arthropathy

PAPA	<10	Variable	Pyogenic sterile arthritis, pyoderma gangrenosum, acne
PFAPA	Early childhood	3–6	Recurrent febrile episodes, elevated inflammatory markers, aphthous ulcers, pharyngitis, lymphadenopathy
Blau	<3–5	Variable	Polyarthritis, tenosynovitis, uveitis; similar to early-onset sarcoidosis
DIRA	<1 mo	Variable	Pustulosis, sterile osteomyelitis
CANDLE	Infancy	Daily	Erythematous annular plaques, lipodystrophy
CRMO	Early childhood	Variable	Bone lesions, anemia, rash

FMF, familial Mediterranean fever; TRAPS, tumor necrosis factor-α receptor autoinflammatory periodic syndrome; HIDS, hyperimmunoglobulin D syndrome; FCAS, familial cold autoinflammatory syndrome; MWS, Muckle–Wells syndrome; NOMID, neonatal-onset multisystem inflammatory dz; PAPA, pyogenic sterile arthritis; PFAPA, periodic fever, aphthous stomatitis, pharyngitis, cervical adenitis; DIRA, deficiency of the IL-1 receptor antagonist; CANDLE, chronic atypical neutrophilic dermatosis with lipodystrophy and elevated temperature; CRMO, chronic recurrent multifocal osteomyelitis

FETAL HEART RATE MONITORING

(Obstet Gynecol 2009;114(1):192–202)

- **Normal fetal heart rate** is 110–160 bpm
- **Tachycardia:** >160 bpm
  - Causes: Maternal/fetal infection or fever, fetal hypoxia, thyrotoxicosis, maternal medications (i.e., β-agonists or parasympathetic blockers)
- **Bradycardia** is <110 bpm
  - Causes: Hypoxia, heart block, maternal meds (i.e., β-blockers)
- **Variability:** Most sensitive indicator of fetal well-being
  - Moderate variability: Peak-to-trough amplitude range of 6–25 bpm; Marked variability: >25 bpm; Minimal variability: <5 bpm; Absent variability: Undetectable range change
- **↓ Variability:** Severe hypoxia, anencephaly, other neurologic anomalies, heart block, maternal narcotic use, $MgSO_4$
  - May also ↓ during normal fetal sleep cycles
- **Accelerations:** Fetal movement. Indicator of fetal well-being & absence of acidosis
- **Decelerations:** 3 types may occur
  - **Early:** 2/2 physiologic head compression, benign. Mirror contractions
  - **Late:** Result of uteroplacental insufficiency, indicate fetal hypoxia
    - Causes: Maternal hypotension, supine position, regional anesthesia, uterine hypertonicity, chronic HTN, postdate gestation, preeclampsia
    - HR nadir occurs after contraction peaks. Gradual ↓ HR and return to baseline
  - **Variable:** 2/2 cord compression. Typically benign, but if >60 s may indicate fetal compromise. Rapid ↓ HR and return to baseline
- **VEAL CHOP:** Variable (Cord), Early (Head), Acceleration (OK), Late (Placental insufficiency)
- **Fetal heart rate strip patterns:**
  - Category I: Normal HR, mod variability, no late/variable decels, ± early decels or accels
  - Category II: Not predictive of fetal acid–base status
  - Category III: Predictive of abnormal fetal acid–base status
    - Sinusoidal: Regular variability resembling a sine wave. May indicate fetal anemia
    - Absent variability with one of: Recurrent late decels, recurrent variable decels, brady

Neonatal Resuscitation (based on NRP algorithm)

- In neonates, most common reason to require resuscitation is respiratory failure
- When called to delivery, important to know maternal medications, prenatal history, and gestational age; assess crying, tone, and color (see APGAR below)
- High risk: <28 wk, CDH, cleft palate, CHD, AVM, shoulder dystocia, choanal atresia
- CPAP: Use T-piece resuscitator or flow-inflating bag
- Chest compressions and intubation after effective PPV given for 30 s and HR <60
  - ETT: <1 kg = 2.5, 1–2 = 3.0, 2–3 = 3.5, >3 = 3.5–4.0. Blade: <28 = 00, 28-Term = 0, Term = 1
  - If unable to intubate, place LMA until more experienced provider able to secure airway
- If HR <60 after 45–60 s of compressions, give epinephrine (preferably via UVC)
  - When placing emergent UVC in DR, only insert until blood return is achieved
- Insufficient evidence for naloxone use in neonates with maternal opioid abuse
- Monitor O_2 saturation: Goal at 5 min is 80–85% and at 10 min is 85–95%

APGAR Scoring			
	0	**1**	**2**
Heart rate	Absent	<100 bpm	>100 bpm
Respiratory effort	Absent	Weak cry, gasping, hypoventilation	Vigorous cry
Muscle tone	Flaccid	Some flexion	Active movement
Reflex irritability	No response to stimulation	Grimace	Cry or active withdrawal
Color	Cyanotic or pale	Acrocyanosis	No cyanosis

GESTATIONAL AGE AND BIRTH WEIGHT CLASSIFICATION

(Pediatrics 2004;114(5):1362–1364; Pediatr Rev 2006;27(6):224–229)

Gestational Age (GA):
- Preterm: <37 0/7 wk
  - Late preterm: 34 0/7–36 6/7 wk
- Term: 37 0/7–41 6/7 wk
- Postterm: ≥42 0/7 wk

Birth Weight (BW) Classification:
- Extremely low birth weight (ELBW): <1,000 g
- Very low birth weight (VLBW): <1,500 g
- Low birth weight (LBW): <2,500 g
- Small for gestational age (SGA): Birth weight <10th percentile for gestational age
  - Risk Factors: Maternal chronic dz, maternal HTN, preeclampsia, multiple gestations, ↑ altitude, smoking, placental abnormalities, congenital infxn (i.e., ToRCHeS), congenital anomalies
  - Symmetric SGA: Length, weight, and head circumference (HC) all <10th percentile
    - Chronic conditions or early insult, i.e., infections, chromosomal abnormalities, EtOH
  - Asymmetric SGA: weight <10th percentile with normal HC; length may be variable
    - Associated with factors causing placental insufficiency
- Appropriate for gestational age (AGA): BW 10th–90th percentile for GA
- Large for gestational age (LGA): Birth weight >90th percentile for GA
  - Risk Factors: Male, IDM, postterm, hydrops fetalis, ↑ maternal wt gain, constitutional (large parents), congenital heart dz, congenital syndromes (i.e., Beckwith–Wiedemann)

BASIC NICU MANAGEMENT

FLUIDS, ELECTROLYTES, AND NUTRITION

(Pediatr Rev 1993;14(3):103–115; NeoReviews 2011;12(3):e130–e140)

Growth
- Weight: Up to 10% ↓ from BW over 1st week then should gain 10–20 g/kg/d thereafter
- Length: Preterm should gain 0.8–1 cm/wk; term should gain 0.69–0.75 cm/wk
- HC: 0.5–0.8 cm/wk. May ↑ in premature infants for catch-up, but not >1.25 cm/wk
  - ↑ rate may indicate hydrocephalus or IVH

Fluid Requirements
- Term infant: 60 mL/kg/d
- Late preterm infant: 60–80 mL/kg/d
- Preterm infant <30–34 wk gestation: 80 mL/kg/d
- Preterm infant <30 wk gestation: 90–100 mL/kg/d
  - Insensible fluid losses ↑ w/ phototherapy, radiant warmers, RDS, stress. ↓ w/ incubators

Parenteral Nutrition:
- May give via central catheter or peripheral IV
  - If peripheral, maximum dextrose concentration of 12.5% and amino acids of 3.5%
  - If central, must add heparin to the parenteral nutrition
- **Carbohydrates:**
  - GIR (mg/kg/min) = (% dextrose × rate of infusion) / (6 × weight in kg)
  - Initial GIR goal of 4–6 mg/kg/min
  - May increase by 0.5–1 mg/kg/min daily up to goal of 10–12 mg/kg/min
    - Hypoglycemia:
      - Maintain BG >50 in 1st 48 hr, >60 thereafter
      - Initial efforts should be to improve feeding to maintain normoglycemia
      - Symptomatic: 2 mL/kg D10 bolus + continuous gtt (4–6 mg/kg/min)
      - Asymptomatic w/ BG>25: feed and start cont gtt (4–6 mg/kg/min) if needed
- **Protein:**
  - Preterm infants: Begin at 3 g/kg/d, advance by 0.5–1 g/kg/d to goal of 3.5–4 g/kg/d
  - Term infants: Begin at 1.5 g/kg/d, advance by 0.5–1 g/kg/d to goal of 3.5–4 g/kg/d
- **Fats:**
  - Begin at 1 g/kg/d, advance by 1 g/kg/d to goal of 3 g/kg/d
  - If hyperbilirubinemia present, may need to limit lipids to 2 g/kg/d
  - Monitor serum triglycerides at 1.5 and 3 g/kg/d, then weekly (normal <200 mg/dL)

- **TPN monitoring:**
  - Daily: Weight, Na, K, Cl, CO_2, Ca, Phos, and Mg until stable (then 1–2x weekly)
  - Weekly: Length, head circumference, alk phos, Hct, bilirubin, BUN, Cr, triglycerides

Enteral Nutrition:
- Term or late preterm infants that are well may start ad lib feeds
- Preterm infants should begin trophic feeds of 10–20 mL/kg/d as soon as clinically stable
  - Will require NGT or OGT if unable to take PO
- Advance feeds per institutional feeding advancement protocol
- If ↑ vomiting, abdominal distention, bloody stools, apnea/bradycardia w/ feeds, may require decreased volumes, change to NGT/OGT feeds, or formula change

Temperature Control:
- Isolette: Goal for infant temperature 36.5–37.5°C
- Dewette: Prevents evaporative heat loss in ELBW infants; start w/ 70–90% humidity & wean

PULMONARY

RESPIRATORY DISTRESS SYNDROME (RDS)

(Pediatr Rev 2014;35(10):417–429)

- Diffuse alveolar atelectasis, typically caused by ↓ surfactant in preterm infants. In late preterm or term, may be 2/2 to maternal diabetes, mec aspiration, or pulm hemorrhage
- Maternal antenatal steroids (@ 24–34 wk) will ↑ surfactant production & lung maturation
- **Clinical Manifestations:** resp failure in 1st few hours of life that worsens over 1st 2–3 d
- **CXR:** Decreased lung expansion bi/l with "ground glass" appearance and air bronchograms
- **Management:**
  - CPAP immediately after birth w/ selective surfactant administration is now recommended as alternate to routine intubation/administration in preterm infants
  - Preterm infants <30 wk who require mechanical ventilation 2/2 RDS should be given surfactant after initial stabilization
  - Consider surfactant administration for preterm infants with high suspicion of deficiency
  - Late preterm or term: Consider surfactant if not improving on mechanical ventilation

Mechanical Ventilation in the NICU
- Most common modes are SIMV + PS or SIMV-PRVC
- Initial settings: PEEP 5, Rate 30–40 bpm, PIP 16–18 (when on PC; enough to achieve chest rise and tidal volumes of 4–5 mL/kg), Vt 4–5 mL/kg (on VC), iT 0.3 s
- Goal: Provide adequate ventilation w/ lowest possible settings to prevent barotrauma & volutrauma; use lowest possible FiO_2 to prevent O_2-related morbidity (i.e., ROP)
- ETT dislodgement & mucus plugging are common causes of worsening when prev stable
  - Assess ETT position (measurement & CXR if needed) if blood gases worsening or ↓ O_2 sat
  - Suction if ETT position correct w/o chest rise or worsening

BRONCHOPULMONARY DYSPLASIA (BPD)

(Pediatr Rev 2012;33(6):255–264)

- Chronic lung disease in pts who: O_2 dependent for ≥28 d + intubated for 1st week of life or O_2 dependent for ≥28 d + persistent O_2 need at 36 wk corrected GA
- **Management:**
  - Ensure adequate oxygenation while preventing pulmonary overcirculation
  - Chlorothiazide and spironolactone (if needed) for chronic diuresis; furosemide acutely
    - Monitor electrolytes with diuretics and replete prn
      - Consider standing electrolyte supplementation if needing frequent repletion
  - Periodic echo to monitor for pHTN and/or R heart failure
  - Pulmonology follow-up recommended as outpt, especially if discharged on home O_2
  - Patients w/ BPD have ↑ caloric needs & frequently require fortification to ↑ caloric density

TRANSIENT TACHYPNEA OF THE NEWBORN (TTN)
(Pediatr Rev 2014;35(10):417–429)

- Self-limited resp distress 2/2 delayed resorption of lung fluid in late preterm & term infants
  - Typically a diagnosis of exclusion
- Usually resolves within 12–24 hr, may be present up to 72 hr
- **Risk Factors:** C section, precipitous delivery, breech delivery, macrosomia, IDM, multiple gestations, nulliparity, forceps/vacuum delivery
- **Clinical Manifestations:** Tachypnea, grunting, nasal flaring, ± retractions
- **CXR:** Normal or ↑ inflation, perihilar linear streaking ("sunburst pattern"), fluid in fissure
- **Management:** Self-resolving; if RR >60, hold PO feeds to prevent aspiration. Consider NG tube if tachypnea persists for enteral feeding. If RR >80, hold enteral feeds

PNEUMONIA
(Pediatr Rev 2014;35(10):417–429)

- **Clinical Manifestations:** Tachypnea, ↑ WOB, hypoxia, similar to RDS or TTN
- **CXR:** Normal or ↑ inflation, uni/l or bi/l streaking densities. GBS classically w/ diffuse granular appearance + air bronchograms (similar to RDS). May see pneumatoceles w/ Staph
- **Management:** See Infectious Disease section later in this chapter

MECONIUM ASPIRATION SYNDROME (MAS)
(Pediatr Rev 2014;35(10):417–429)

- Aspiration of meconium-stained amniotic fluid, 2/2 to deep gasping breaths as a result of fetal hypoxia or fetal distress in utero or during delivery
- Occurs in late pre- to postterm infants; ~5% of births w/ meconium-stained fluid
- **Clinical Manifestations:**
  - RDS/hypoxia 2/2 obstruction, surfactant dysfunction/inactivation, & chemical pneumonitis
  - 1/3 will also go on to develop PPHN (see Cardiology section later in this chapter)
- **CXR:** Diffuse patchy parenchymal opacification, hyperinflation from air trapping, may see pneumothorax
- **Management:**
  - Maintain arterial oxygen level at ≥80–90 mmHg to prevent PPHN if receiving 100% O_2
  - Consider CPAP; if hyperinflation & air trapping on CXR may ↑ risk of pneumothorax
  - If intubation required, consider surfactant administration
  - If PPHN suspected, obtain echo and consider use of nitric oxide
  - In severe cases, infants may require initiation of ECMO

CONGENITAL DIAPHRAGMATIC HERNIA (CDH)
(Pediatr Rev 1999;20(10):e79–e87)

- Lung hypoplasia due to herniation of abdominal contents through diaphragm
  - Types: Bochdalek (posterior, L-sided, 95%) & Morgagni (anterior, R-sided, 5%)
- CDH can usually be seen on prenatal ultrasounds
- Mortality estimated at ~25%; ~50% if infant requires ECMO
- **Clinical Manifestations:**
  - May have significant respiratory distress within the 1st few hours of life
  - Exam: Scaphoid abdomen, ↓ breath sounds over left chest
- **CXR:** Bowel gas in hemithorax, contralateral mediastinal shift, ipsilateral lung-hypoplasia
- **Management:**
  - Immediate intubation
  - NG tube to decompress bowel
  - If severe respiratory distress present & not improving, ECMO may be necessary
  - Surgical repair essential, preferable to delay until infant's pulmonary compliance improves

APNEA

(Pediatrics 2016;137(1):e20153757; Pediatr Rev 2003;24(1):32–34)

- Cessation of breathing for ≥20 s
- Types: Central (40%), obstructive (10%), or mixed (50%)
- May or may not be associated with cyanosis, bradycardia, or desaturation
- Etiologies: Exposure to $MgSO_4$/narcotics/anesthetics, prematurity, meningitis, birth trauma, sepsis, seizure, ICH, CHD, PDA, PGE1 therapy, NEC, anemia, inborn errors of metabolism
  - Critical to evaluate term infants for above conditions
- **Apnea of Prematurity:**
  - >50% of infants <1,500 g & 90% of infants <1,000 g will develop apnea
  - 2/2 to immaturity of central respiratory center
- **Management:**
  - Central apnea: Caffeine citrate (loading dose 20 mg/kg → 5 mg/kg daily, therapeutic range of 8–20 mg/dL), aminophylline or theophylline may be used (esp if BPD or GA >32 wk)
    - Medications may be discontinued when ≥34 wk GA, or when apnea-free × 7 d
  - Obstructive apnea: Nasal cannula, HFNC, CPAP

RESPIRATORY SYNCITIAL VIRUS (RSV) PROPHYLAXIS

(Pediatrics 2014;134(2):415–420)

- 15 mg/kg doses given monthly for a maximum of 5 doses before start of and throughout RSV season
  - Age <12 mo
    - GA <29 wk
    - GA <32 wk & required O_2 for 1st 28 d of life
    - CCHD and/or moderate to severe pHTN
    - Pulmonary abnormality or neuromuscular dz w/ impaired ability to clear secretions
  - Age <24 mo
    - GA <32 wk w/ BPD on tx within 6 mos of start of RSV season
    - Profound immunocompromise (heart, solid organ, or SCT during RSV season)

CARDIOLOGY

PATENT DUCTUS ARTERIOSUS (PDA)

(Pediatrics 2010;125(5):1020–1030)

- Defined as ductus arteriosus open >72 hr of life
- **Risk Factors:** Prematurity, RDS, ↑ IV fluid administration in the first few days of life, asphyxia, birth at high altitude, some congenital syndromes, congenital heart disease
- **Clinical Manifestations:** Harsh murmur (LUSB, 2nd–3rd intercostal space), bounding periph pulses, hyperactive precordium, hypotension, respiratory deterioration (over hours or days)
- For additional info refer to Cardiology chapter

PERSISTENT PULMONARY HYPERTENSION OF THE NEWBORN (PPHN)

(NeoReviews 2015;16(12):e680–e692)

- Severe hypoxia 2/2 to ↑ PVR, Results in R → L shunting across foramen ovale & PDA
- Hypoxemia typically out of proportion to degree of pulmonary disease
- **Clinical Manifestations:** Respiratory distress with cyanosis and hypoxemia, single S2
- **Diagnosis:** Differential sats, hyperoxia test (administer 100% O_2 for >10 min) w/ PaO_2 >100 mmHg, CXR, echo
- **Management:**
  - Pre- and postductal O_2 sat monitoring, minimal stimulation (sedation prn), avoid & correct acidosis, maintain euvolemia, mechanical ventilation, iNO
  - Goal ABG: O_2 ≥60 mmHg, CO_2 40–50 mmHg, pH 7.35–7.45
  - Systemic vasopressors (dopamine preferred, dobutamine may also be used)

Congenital Heart Disease (CHD)
Refer to Cardiology chapter

NECROTIZING ENTEROCOLITIS (NEC)

(Pediatr Rev 2017;38(12):552–559; NeoReviews 2013;14(3):e113–e120)

- Ischemic & inflammatory bowel necrosis
- Occurs in up to 10% of infants weighing <1,500 g
- Overall mortality is 12.5%. With perforation increases to 20–40%
- **Risk Factors:** Prematurity, enteral feeding (especially formula), enteral colonization with noncommensal organisms (*Klebsiella, E. coli, Clostridium, Staph epidermidis,* rotavirus, enterovirus), ↓ perfusion, CHD, polycythemia, hyperviscosity, blood transfusions
- **Clinical Manifestation:** Preterm infants typically present ~14–20 days or 30–32 wk postmenstrual age, term infants typically present w/in 1st week of life

Modified Bell Staging Criteria			
Stage	**Systemic Signs**	**Intestinal Findings**	**Radiographic Findings**
I Suspected NEC	Apnea, bradycardia, lethargy, and temperature instability	Feeding intolerance, abdominal distension, recurrent gastric residuals	Normal or nonspecific
II Proven NEC	Stage I signs plus abdominal tenderness and thrombocytopenia	Prominent abdominal distention, tenderness, bowel wall edema, absent bowel sounds, grossly bloody stools	Pneumatosis + portal venous gas
III Advanced NEC	Respiratory and metabolic acidosis, respiratory failure, hypotension, decreased UOP, shock, neutropenia, and DIC	Tense and discolored abdomen with spreading abdominal wall edema, induration, and discoloration	Pneumoperitoneum

- **Diagnosis:**
  - Laboratory: CBC/diff, CRP, blood culture, stool cultures, ABG, coags
  - Imaging: Abdominal x-ray, cross-table, & lateral decubitus radiographs
- **Management:** NPO on IVF, Replogle to LIWS, serial abdominal girth measurements, respiratory support, strict I/O's, serial x-rays
  - Abx: 10–14 d IV course. Empiric tx for late-onset sepsis pathogens as well as anaerobes
  - Surgical consult: May require necrotic bowel resection

TRACHEOESOPHAGEAL FISTULA (TEF) AND ESOPHAGEAL ATRESIA (EA)

(NeoReviews 2017;18(8):e472–e479; Am Fam Physician 1999;59(4):910–916 & 919–920)

- **Clinical Presentation:** Polyhydramnios, difficulty w/ secretions, abd distention, resp distress. Feedings with choking, coughing, and cyanosis
- **Morbidity:** ↑↑ risk of pneumonia/pneumonitis from aspiration
- **Diagnosis:** Inability to pass NG into stomach (if TEF w/ EA). X-ray to evaluate for pulmonary infiltrates, skeletal anomalies, cardiac shape for VACTERL/VATER association
- **Management:** NPO, Replogle to suction for decompression of esophageal pouch, place in 45° upright position to ↓ tracheal reflux, VACTERL/VATER work-up as above
  - Surgery: Gastrostomy frequently placed to permit enteral nutrition until 1° repair

Type	Description	Incidence
A	Isolated EA	10%
B	EA with proximal TEF	1%
C	EA with distal TEF	85%
D	EA with proximal and distal TEF	1%
E	Isolated TEF (H-type)	3%

GASTROSCHISIS

(NeoReviews 2013;14(8):e402–e411)

- Central abdominal wall defect w/o intestinal sac. Cord intact & located to left of defect
  - Rarely associated with congenital anomalies
- **Clinical Presentation:** Varying amounts of intestines protruding through defect
- **Diagnosis:** Visible upon delivery, may be seen on prenatal ultrasound
- **Management:** May deliver vaginally or via C-section. Cover bowel with moist sterile dressing w/ overlying cellophane or plastic. IVFs to replace losses, maintain normothermia, NG/OG decompression, broad-spectrum antibiotics, TPN
  - Surgery: Reduction (± silo dependent on amount of herniated contents) w/ 1° closure

OMPHALOCELE

(NeoReviews 2013;14(8):e402–e411)

- Abdominal wall defect into base of umbilical cord covered by intestinal sac. Cord stalk present on the sac, but is malpositioned; ~50% are associated with congenital anomalies
- **Clinical Presentation:** Varying amounts of intestines protruding through defect, liver & spleen may also be present in the defect
- **Diagnosis:** Visible upon delivery, may be seen on prenatal ultrasound
- **Management:** May deliver vaginally or via C-section. Regular dressings to protect sac. As long as sac not ruptured, infants have ↓ fluid/heat loss than gastroschisis as sac is protective
  - Surgery: Staged reduction with silo → abdominal wall closure

HIRSCHSPRUNG DISEASE

(Pediatr Rev 1989;10(7):207–223)

- Functional obstruction 2/2 aganglionosis of rectum and varying amounts of the colon
- ~15% of infants with delayed stool passage; 1 in 4,000 live births
  - 60–90% of infants with Hirschsprung will fail to pass meconium in 1st 24–48 hr
  - Male predominance (4:1), more common in Caucasians, present in 8% of Trisomy 21
- **Diagnosis:**
  - X-ray: Distended colon with air-fluid levels
  - Contrast enema: Transition zone w/ distal narrowed segment & proximal dilated segment
    - Barium persistence >24 hr
  - Anorectal manometry: Absent rectosphincteric reflex
  - **Full-thickness rectal suction biopsy is gold standard;** Histology: Absence of ganglion cells
- **Management:**
  - Digital rectal stim ± rectal enemas to allow passage of stool and prevent bowel obstruction
  - Surgery: Staged repair w/ colostomy vs. 1° transanal pull-through (most common)
  - **Hirschsprung enterocolitis:** ~20% of cases: Fever, distension, & hypovolemic shock
    - Tx: abx & IVFs

INFECTIOUS DISEASES

SEPSIS

(NeoReviews 2015;16(4):e221–e230; NeoReviews 2012;13(2):e86–e93; NeoReviews 2010;11(8):e426–e435; Pediatrics 2013;132(1):166–168)

- Systemic illness w/ associated bacterial infectious source
- Overall incidence of 1–5 per 1,000 births
  - In VLBW infants, rate of incidence of early sepsis is 2% and late sepsis is 36%
- Mortality rate can be as high as 25% (higher w/ prematurity)

- **Types:**
  - Early onset: Presents w/in 1st 7 d
    - Risk factors: Prematurity, PPROM, ROM ≥18 hr, GBS+ mother, maternal fever, fetal distress, chorioamnionitis, meconium fluid, fam hx GBS infxn, metabolic disorders
    - Most common: GBS, E. coli, Listeria, Staph, Strep pneumo, Enterococcus, Haemophilus
  - Late onset: after 7 d of life
    - Risk factors: Endotracheal intubation, central catheter, Foley catheter
    - Most common: CoNS, gram-negative rods, Staph aureus, GBS, fungal
- **Clinical presentation:** Temp instability, irritability, lethargy, mottling, rash, cyanosis, pallor, feeding intol, abd distention, resp distress, apnea, ↓ temp / perfusion / BG / BP / pH (metabolic), ↑ RR / HR
- Early-onset sepsis risk score (GA ≥34 wk): neonatalsepsiscalculator.kaiserpermanente.org
  - Decision re: NICU admission according to institutional policy & NICU team evaluation
- **Diagnosis:**
  - Laboratory: Blood culture (×2 if central line), CBC/diff, CRP, ± UA/UCx, ± LP
  - Imaging: CXR
- **Management:** Empiric ampicillin & gentamicin, continue for 36–48 hr. Add vancomycin if ↑ suspicion for Staph; modify/stop abx based on culture data

MENINGITIS

(NeoReviews 2015;16(9):e535–e543)

- Incidence: 0.2–0.5 per 1,000 births
  - Mortality risk: 3–13%, risk of neurodevelopmental sequelae: 20–50%
- Same pathogens, risk factors, & clinical presentation as above w/ addition of bulging ant fontanelle, seizures, and coma possible
- **Diagnosis:** Full sepsis w/u + LP (CSF cell count, culture, Gram stain, glucose, protein, ± HSV)
  - CSF studies w/ bacterial meningitis: ↓ glucose, normal or ↑ protein, pleiocytosis
- Head US to assess for IVH, ventricle size, & inflammation, ± CT or MRI later in course to assess for need for prolonged tx & identify areas of encephalomalacia
- **Management:** Empiric ampicillin & gentamicin (meningitic dosing) is classic regimen
  - Recent studies advocate for replacement of gentamicin with cefotaxime to cover ampicillin-resistant gram-negative bacteria given poor CSF penetration of gentamicin
  - Vancomycin may be added for penicillin nonsusceptible gram-positive infection
  - Duration: 21 d or 14 d after obtaining sterile CSF cultures
    - Longer courses for gram negative and/or complicated meningitis (i.e., venous sinus thrombosis, abscess, subdural empyema, ventriculitis)
  - Hearing and vision screening should be done for all infants with documented meningitis
  - Head circumference measured daily

HEPATITIS B VIRUS

(Red Book. 30th ed. 2015; Section on Hepatitis B)

- ~20,000 infants born to Hepatitis B-infected women annually
  - Neonatal exposure typically via amniotic fluid, maternal blood, or vaginal secretions
- Management:
  - **HBsAg-positive mother:** Treat infant w/ 0.5 mL IM HBIG & HB vaccine w/in 12 hr of birth
    - Will require additional testing/immunizations as outpatient
  - **HBsAg-unknown:** Give vaccine w/in 12 hr of birth regardless of weight. If weight <2,000 g, give HBIG. Test mother ASAP. If +, give HBIG to infants ≥2,000 g no later than 7 DOL
  - **HBsAg-negative:** Give vaccine at birth if ≥2,000 g or at 1 mo if <2,000 g

ToRCHeS INFECTIONS

(NeoReviews 2010;11(8):e436–e446)

Toxoplasma:
- Incidence: 0.1–1 per 1,000 births
- 70–90% asymptomatic at birth, but up to 80% develop visual or learning disabilities
- Mode of infection: Pseudocysts or oocytes present in cat feces or undercooked meat

- **Clinical manifestations:** Chorioretinitis, intracranial calcifications, hydrocephalus, microcephaly, seizures, HSM, LAD, deafness
- **Diagnosis:** Serologic testing
- **Treatment:** Combination pyrimethamine-sulfadiazine and folinic acid for 1 yr

Rubella:
- Incidence: Rare, <10 cases annually in the U.S.
- Mode of infection: Primary maternal infection
- **Clinical manifestations:** IUGR, radiolucencies of long bones, cataracts, cardiac defects (PDA, PA hypoplasia), HSM, thrombocytopenia, purpura
- **Diagnosis:** Cord blood rubella-specific IgM serology and PCR
- **Treatment:** Supportive care

Cytomegalovirus:
- Most common congenital viral infection in the U.S. (~40,000 annually)
- Most common cause of nonhereditary sensorineural hearing loss in children
- Mode of infection: Primary maternal infection or viral reactivation
- **Clinical manifestations:** HSM, "blueberry muffin" rash, SGA, microcephaly, intracerebral calcifications, chorioretinitis, dental defects
- **Diagnosis:** Viral culture or PCR of urine or saliva
- **Treatment:** 6 wk IV ganciclovir or 6 mo PO valganciclovir: Improved long-term hearing

Herpes Simplex Virus (HSV):
- Prevalence of 0.05–0.3 per 1,000 live births, and 1,500 cases annually
- Mode of infection: Primary maternal infection or reactivation
- **Clinical manifestations:** SEM & disseminated present at ~1–2 wk; CNS at ~2–3 wk
  - Localized disease: SEM (skin, eye, mouth) vesicles. If untreated, >70% will progress
  - Disseminated: Poor feeding, fever, lethargy, apnea, seizures, resp distress, hepatomegaly, jaundice, DIC. Mortality rates ~50–70% despite treatment
  - CNS disease: Seizures, lethargy, tremors, temp instability, bulging fontanelle
- **Diagnosis:** Viral cultures from mouth, nasopharynx, conjunctivae, rectum, skin vesicles, urine, stool, blood, and CSF
- **Treatment:** IV acyclovir ×14 d if local, extend to 21 d if disseminated

Syphilis:
- Incidence: 10 per 100,000 births
- Mode of infection: Primary maternal infection
- **Clinical manifestations:** "snuffles" (nasal discharge), maculopapular rash including palms & soles, osteochondritis, HSM, jaundice, LAD, hemolytic anemia, late presentation of Hutchinson triad (blunted upper incisors, interstitial keratitis, and 8th nerve deafness)
- **Diagnosis:** VDRL or RPR with 4-fold higher titer in infant than mother indicates active infection. If +, FTA-ABS (or other specific treponema antibody test) should be done
- **Treatment:** IV (Pen G) or IM (Procaine) penicillin ×10 d
  - If no sx & titer <4× maternal titer, can treat w/ 1× IM benzathine penicillin G w/ close f/u

HEMATOLOGY

Rh ISOIMMUNIZATION

(Arch Dis Child 2007;92(2):F83–F88)

- Isoimmune hemolytic anemia between Rh- mother (prev exposed to Rh [D] Ag) & Rh+ fetus
- Incidence: <1% of Rh-incompatible pregnancies 2/2 RhoGAM prophylaxis
- Risk factors: Male sex, subsequent pregnancies, fetomaternal hemorrhage, ABO incomp, C-section, traumatic delivery, Caucasian ethnicity
- **Clinical presentation:** Jaundice (unconj hyperbili in 1st 24 hr), anemia, HSM, hydrops fetalis
  - Hydrops fetalis: Progressive hypoalbuminemia, ascites, pleural effusion, severe anemia, heart failure. ↑ risk of late fetal death, stillbirth, and labor intolerance
    - Neonates p/w anasarca, cardiopulmonary distress, pulm edema, severe surfactant def, CHF, hypotension, periph perfusion defects, dysrhythmia, anemia, met acidosis

- **Diagnosis:** Blood & Rh type of mother & infant, retic ct, DAT, periph smear, fractionated bili
- **Management:**
  - Phototherapy to help ↓ unconjugated bili levels & prevent need for exchange transfusion
  - Double volume exchange transfusion may be necessary if unconjugated bili approaches exchange level; will ↓ Tbili by ~25%
  - IVIG to ↓ hemolysis by blocking Fc receptors of reticuloendothelial cells

ABO ISOIMMUNIZATION

(Arch Dis Child 2007;92(2):F83–F88)

- Isoimmune hemolytic anemia 2/2 differing blood types between mother & infant
  - Most common: Type O mother w/ type A or B baby; reaction between maternal isoAb & fetal A or B antigen on RBCs
- **Incidence:** + DAT in ~3–4% of infants, risk factors present in ~12–15% of pregnancies
  - Symptomatic disease in <1% of all newborns
- **Risk factors:** 1st born, African American race, type O mother
- **Clinical manifestations:** Jaundice in 1st 24 hr of life, unconj hyperbili, hemolytic anemia (typically more mild than Rh dz but can be severe), reticulocytosis, microspherocytosis
- **Diagnosis:** Blood & Rh type of mother & infant, retics, DAT, periph smear, fractionated bili
- **Management:**
  - Phototherapy is 1st-line, may be enough to prevent need for exchange transfusion
  - If reaching exchange transfusion bili levels, give IVIG (↓ hemolysis)
  - Typically a double-volume exchange transfusion is performed

HYPERBILIRUBINEMIA

(Pediatrics 2004;114(1):297–316; J Perinatol 2012;32(9):660–664)

Indirect (Unconjugated)

- **Incidence:** 60–70% of term & 80% of preterm infants. ↑ incidence at ↑ altitudes & in Greeks, E Asians, & Native Americans. ↓ in African Americans
- **Types:**
  - Physiologic: 2/2 to ↑ bilirubin synthesis, ↓ transport, impaired conjugation and excretion
  - Breastfeeding jaundice: Incidence ~13%, occurs in 1st wk; 2/2 ↓ intake causing ↑ intestinal bili absorption; compare wt to BW, assess hydration
  - Breastmilk jaundice: Incidence ~10–30%, occurs after 2–3 wk; unclear cause (possible enzyme in milk) and considered dx of exclusion w/ expectation of resolution by ~12 wk
  - ↑ Production: Produced through hemolysis
    - Hemolytic disease: Most common pathologic cause. RBC destruction
    - Rh and minor antigen incompatibility: Maternal IgG crosses placenta → in utero hemolysis. May result in erythroblastosis fetalis and/or hydrops fetalis
    - ABO incompatibility: See above
  - RBC enzyme deficiencies: G6PD deficiency, pyruvate kinase deficiency
  - Hemoglobinopathies: Typically do not present in newborn period. However, infant with hemoglobin H (deletion of 3 α-globin genes) may develop hemolytic anemia
  - Infection: ↑ bilirubin 2/2 hemolysis & impaired conjugation with ↓ excretion
  - ↑ RBCs: Extravascular blood collections (bruising, cephalohematomas, intracranial bleeds), polycythemia, IDM (high epo levels)
  - Bilirubin clearance disorders:
    - Crigler–Najjar, type I: AR, near-complete absence of UGT. Tbili >20 mg/dL. Treatment: Exchange transfusion → daily phototherapy. Will require liver transplant. Tin protoporphyrin & po calcium supplements may augment therapy
    - Crigler–Najjar, type II: More common than type I, typically benign. Tx: Phenobarbital
    - Gilbert syndrome: Mild unconjugated hyperbili. No hemolysis or liver disease. ↑ risk of acute or chronic bilirubin encephalopathy in neonates
  - Metabolic/Endocrine disorders:
    - Galactosemia: Unconjugated hyperbili in 1st week → conjugated during 2nd wk
    - Hypothyroidism: Deficient UGT activity → jaundice in up to 10% of affected newborns. Tx: Thyroid hormone replacement
  - GI obstruction (i.e., pyloric stenosis, duodenal atresia, annular pancreas) may cause jaundice

- Risk factors for hyperbilirubinemia:
  - Sepsis, acidosis, lethargy, asphyxia, temperature instability, G6PD, hemolytic disease, GA 35–38 wk, exclusive breastfeeding, cephalohematoma, extensive bruising, male sex, IDM, family hx neonatal jaundice, Asian race
- **Treatment**, if ≥35 wk gestation:
  - Phototherapy: Photoisomerization & photooxidation of bilirubin to aid excretion
    - Use Bhutani curves to determine "light level," or level at which phototherapy should be initiated. May also use www.bilitool.org to determine light level
  - Exchange transfusion:
    - Indications: Ongoing hemolysis, Tbili w/o ↓ of at least 1–2 mg/dL w/ 4–6 hr intensive phototherapy if already near exchange level, rate of rise indicates expected Tbili ≥exchange level within 48 hr depending on risk (i.e., infant >35 wk on high-risk curve w/ expected Tbili >17 mg/dL at 48 hr or >22 mg/dL on low-risk curve), early signs of bilirubin encephalopathy, and/or evidence of hydrops fetalis
    - Process: Double-volume exchange transfusion replaces ~85% of RBCs in circulation
      - ↓ Tbili level 50%
      - Type O negative blood typically used, must be crossmatched with maternal serum
    - Risks: Thrombocytopenia, hypocalcemia, metabolic acidosis. Mortality ~0.5–2%
- Total serum bilirubin levels for infants <35 wk gestation:

Gestational Age	Begin Phototherapy	Exchange Transfusion
<28 0/7	5–6	11–14
28 0/7–29 6/7	6–8	12–14
30 0/7–31 6/7	8–10	13–16
32 0/7–33 6/7	10–12	15–18
34 0/7–34 6/7	12–14	17–19

  - Can also consider checking serum albumin for Tbili/albumin ratio to assess unbound bili
- **Acute Bilirubin Encephalopathy:**
  - Initial phase: Lethargy, hypotonia, decreased activity, and poor suck
  - Intermediate phase: Stupor, irritability, ↑ tone. May see fever & back/neck arching
  - Advanced phase: Deep stupor, ↑ tone, inability to feed, shrill cry. ± Seizures
    - Irreversible, most will develop chronic bilirubin encephalopathy
- **Chronic Bilirubin Encephalopathy (or kernicterus):**
  - Tetrad of choreoathetoid cerebral palsy, high-frequency sensorineural hearing loss, vertical gaze palsy, and dental enamel hypoplasia. Mortality rate up to 10%

Direct (Conjugated) Hyperbilirubinemia:
- Always pathologic
- Dbili >20% Tbili or >1 mg/dL if Tbili ≤5 mg/dL
- Incidence: 1 in 2,500 infants; much less common than indirect hyperbili
- Risk factors: Congenital infections, sepsis, neonatal hepatitis, T21, TPN, ABO incompatibility
- **Clinical Manifestations:** Prolonged jaundice, pale (acholic) stools, dark urine
- Possible causes:
  - Biliary atresia: Most common cause of cholestasis & need for liver transplant in infants
  - Genetic: Alagille syndrome, progressive familial intrahepatic cholestasis [PFIC]
  - Inborn errors of metabolism: see chapter 10 for more information
  - Idiopathic neonatal hepatitis: Diagnosis of exclusion, managed supportively
  - Bacterial or congenital infections: ToRCHeS, hepatitis, gram-negative bacteremia
  - TPN-cholestasis (~40–60% of infants on long-term TPN): Reversible if TPN discontinued in timely manner
    - Enteral feeding may be protective, improvement in cholestasis in 1–3 mo
    - Use of fish oil lipids (in lieu of soy bean lipids) may reverse cholestasis and liver injury
- Treatment: Directed at underlying cause
  - Supplementation of ADEK vitamins, ursodiol, phenobarbital (↑ bile acid synthesis, ↑ bile flow, hepatic enzyme inducer), cholestyramine

INTRAVENTRICULAR HEMORRHAGE (IVH)

(NeoReviews 2011;12(2):e94–e101)

- Bleeding into cerebral ventricles from subependymal germinal matrix blood vessels
  - ↑ friability in premature infants who cannot adequately regulate cerebral blood flow
- In term infants, the majority of IVH occurs from the choroid plexus or thalamus
- May be unilateral or bilateral; bilateral IVH may be symmetric or asymmetric
- Typically a disorder of prematurity, most often in LBW and VLBW neonates
  - ~25% of neonates with BW 500–1,500 g will have IVH
  - Up to 45% of neonates with BW <1,000 g will have IVH

Classifications of IVH	
Grade	Findings on Ultrasound
I (Mild)	Bleeding confined to the germinal matrix
II (Moderate)	Bleeding occupying ≤50% of the lateral ventricles without evidence of dilation
III (Severe)	Bleeding occupying >50% of the lateral ventricles and/or evidence of dilation
IV (Severe)	Presence of infarction and/or hemorrhage in the periventricular white matter ipsilateral to a large IVH

- **Risk factors:** Prematurity (worse w/o antenatal steroids), preeclampsia, breech, resp distress, maternal chorioamnionitis, traumatic delivery, hypotension, acidosis, anemia, thrombocytopenia, genetic predisposition, extensive resuscitation, asphyxia/hypoxic event
- **Clinical Manifestations:**
  - <u>Silent presentation</u>: Up to 50%, no significant signs/symptoms, found on routine screening
  - <u>Saltatory course</u>: Happens over hours to days. Nonspecific findings: ↓ tone, ↓ spont movements, altered level of consciousness, may have eye position changes
  - <u>Catastrophic deterioration</u>: least common, minutes to hours. Findings: Coma/stupor, irreg respirations/apnea, decerebrate posturing, seizures, flaccidity, fixed pupils, hypotension, bulging ant fontanelle, bradycardia, ↓ Hct, SIADH
  - 50% of IVH occurs by 1st 6–12 hr, 75% by DOL 2, 90% by DOL 3
- **Screening:** Preferred diagnostic imaging is a cranial ultrasound (HUS)
  - Infants ≤25 wk without clinical risk factors:
    - HUS at 1–2 wk of life, PVL screen at 36 wk corrected GA
  - Infants ≤25 wk with clinical signs/symptoms:
    - HUS at 72 hr of life, repeat at 1–2 wk, PVL screen at 36–40 wk corrected GA
  - Infants ≤28 wk or ≤1,000 g without clinical risk factors:
    - HUS at 1–2 wk of life, PVL screen at 36–40 wk corrected GA
  - Infants 28–32 wk or 1,000–1,500 g without clinical risk factors:
    - Follow weekly head circumference, PVL screen at 6–8 wk of age
  - Infants ≤32 wk or ≤1,500 g with clinical risk factors:
    - HUS by 1 wk of life, PVL screen at 36–40 wk corrected GA
- **Prevention:**
  - Antenatal steroids & delayed cord clamping ↓ incidence (Neonatology 2008;93(2): 138–144)
- **Management:** No methods to reverse IVH
  - Avoid wide fluctuations in BP, manage sequelae (seizures, hydrocephalus, etc.)
  - Ppx in infants <29 wk: Consider indomethacin within 1st 6 hr of life
    - Contraindications: Ductal-dependent CHD, known grade III–IV IVH, platelets <50,000

HYPOXIC ISCHEMIC ENCEPHALOPATHY (HIE)

(Pediatr Rev 2012;33(9):387–397)

- Neurologic dysfunction 2/2 to a hypoxic–ischemic brain injury
- **Epidemiology:** Incidence ~1.5 per 1,000 live births
- **Risk Factors:** IUGR, monochorionic twin gestation, placental thrombosis, severe maternal preeclampsia, shoulder dystocia, emergency C-section, operative vaginal delivery, uterine rupture, placental abruption, cord prolapse, tight nuchal cord, maternal shock or death

- **Clinical Manifestations:**
  - Abnormal level of consciousness (may be lethargic, obtunded, irritable, or hyperalert)
  - ↓ Spontaneous movements
  - Respiratory difficulties
  - ↓ Tone ± abnormal posturing
  - Absent primitive reflexes
  - Seizure activity
  - APGAR score <5 at 5 min and 10 min
  - Fetal umbilical artery pH <7.0, base deficit ≥12 mmol/L, or both
  - MRI findings c/w hypoxic–ischemic event
- **Management—Therapeutic Hypothermia:** Protocol differs slightly at each institution. This chapter uses the NICHD NRN Whole Body Cooling Trial Protocol:
  - Inclusion criteria:
    - <u>Cardiac and biochemical criteria</u>: Gestational age ≥36 wk gestation and cord blood gas or neonatal blood gas taken at <1 hr of age with pH <7.0 or base deficit >16, **OR** history of acute perinatal event with either APGAR <5 at 10 min or need for ventilation initiated at birth and continued for at least 10 min
    - <u>Neurologic criteria</u>: Presence of moderate/severe encephalopathy defined as seizures **OR** one or more signs in 3 of 6 categories qualifies the infant for cooling

Category	Normal-Mild	Moderate	Severe
1. Level of consciousness	Normal/hyperalert	Lethargic	Stupor/coma
2. Spontaneous activity	Normal/increased	Decreased	No activity
3. Posture	Full flexion	Distal flexion/limb extension	Decerebrate
4. Tone	Normal/increased	Hypotonia	Flaccid
5. Primitive reflexes			
Suck	Normal	Weak	Absent
Moro	Normal	Incomplete	Absent
6. Autonomic			
Pupils	Normal	Constricted	Deviation/nonreactive
Heart rate	Normal	Bradycardia	Unstable heart rate
Respiration	Normal	Periodic breathing	Apnea

- Exclusion criteria: Gestational age <36 wks, unable to initiate cooling within 6 hr of birth, presence of known chromosomal abnormality or major congenital anomalies, severe IUGR (birth weight <1,800 g), infants in extremis
- Procedure: Within 6 hr of birth, eligible infants will undergo whole body cooling therapy to esophageal temperature of 33.5°C for 72 hr, then will be gradually rewarmed over 6 hr. Side effects: Bradycardia and abnormal bleeding/clotting

---

NEONATAL SEIZURES

(Pediatr Rev 2012;33(9):387–397)

- **Incidence:** Occur in 0.15–1.5% of all neonates
- **Etiology:** Infection, structural malformations, metabolic abnormalities, drug withdrawal, congenital hypothyroidism, intracranial hemorrhage, HIE, perinatal asphyxia, other genetic or neurologic disorder
- **Diagnosis:** Complete neurologic and physical examination
  - Laboratory: CBC, serum electrolytes, Mg, Phos, BG, LP, blood culture
    - Ammonia, serum/urine amino acids, & blood gas if concern for metabolic disorder
  - Imaging/others: HUS, ± MRI, EEG (spot EEG vs. LTM)
- **Treatment:**
  - Correct metabolic abnormalities, treat any underlying condition identified (i.e., meningitis)
  - Ensure airway protection and intubate if necessary
  - Anticonvulsant therapies: Phenobarbital (1st line), Fosphenytoin, Lorazepam
    - If seizures continue to persist despite above, trial of pyridoxine 50–100 mg IV while on EEG monitoring (institutional policies may vary)

BASICS OF ICU CARE

SEDATION AND PAIN CONTROL IN THE ICU

- Goal: Ensure patient safety and minimize discomfort without oversedation or delirium
- As with pain management in general, start with lowest doses and titrate up prn for effect

ICU CARE 17-1

Analgesics
- Opioids: Act at μ receptor → analgesia, respiratory depression, pupillary constriction, and euphoria

Agent	Bolus Dosing	Initial Continuous Dosing	ADRs
Morphine	0.05–0.1 mg/kg q0.5–2hr	0.05–0.1 mg/kg/hr Titrate by 1 mcg/kg/hr	Respiratory depression, histamine release
Fentanyl	0.5–1 mcg/kg q0.5–2hr	0.5–5 mcg/kg/hr Titrate by 1 mcg/kg/hr	Chest wall rigidity
Hydromorphone	0.01–0.02 mg/kg q0.5–2hr	0.005 mg/kg/hr Titrate by 0.005 mg/kg/hr	

Sedatives
- BZDs: Augment GABA-A receptor → sedation, anxiolysis, euphoria, ↓ muscle tone, anticonvulsant properties

Agent	Bolus Dosing	Initial Continuous Dosing	ADRs
Midazolam (Versed)	0.05–0.1 mg/kg q1–2hr	0.05–0.4 mg/kg/hr	Respiratory depression
Lorazepam (Ativan)	0.05–0.1 mg/kg q2–4hr	AVOID (due to propylene glycol suspension)	Respiratory depression
Propofol	0.2 mg/kg q10mo	10–200 mcg/kg/min	Hypotension, hypertriglyceridemia, Propofol infusion syndrome

- Propofol: ↑ binding affinity of GABA → hypnotic and sedative effects
  - Propofol infusion syndrome: Severe metabolic acidosis, elevated lactate, lipemia, hepatomegaly, and multiorgan failure after prolonged propofol infusion in children (BMJ 1992;305(6854):613–616)

Other Agents
- Ketamine: Works via antagonism of NMDA – Rapid acting sedative with analgesic properties
  - ADR: Emergence delirium in up to 2% of patients; abnormal dreams in up to 10% (Am J Emerg Med 2002;20:463–468)
- Dexmedetomidine: Selective α-2 agonist → mild sedative + analgesic properties
  - Offers arousable sedation with no respiratory depression – Excellent adjunct or solo therapy prior to extubation (can reduce ventilator time) (Pediatr Crit Care 2016;17(12):1131)
  - ADR: Bradycardia and hypotension

Agent	Bolus Dosing	Initial Continuous Dosing
Dexmedetomidine	N/A	0.1–0.5 mcg/kg/hr; up to 2 mcg/kg/hr
Ketamine	0.5–1 mg/kg	0.5–5 mg/kg/hr

Paralytics – Nondepolaring Neuromuscular Blockade

Agent	Bolus Dosing	Continuous Dosing
Cisatracurium	0.1 mg/kg	0.4–4 mcg/kg/min
Rocuronium	1 mg/kg	7–12 mcg/kg/min
Vecuronium	0.08–0.1 mg/kg	0.8–2.5 mcg/kg/min

VASCULAR ACCESS IN THE PICU

(Pediatric Critical Care. 5th ed. 2017:158–180)

- Central venous catheters (CVC)
  - Indications: Vasoactive medications, frequent blood sampling, TPN, monitoring CVP, multiple infusions, reliable/long-term access, dialysis, apheresis
  - Sites: Femoral, internal jugular, subclavian (less commonly used)
  - Complications: CLABSI, pneumothorax (for IJ or subclavian), arterial cannulation, bleeding, thrombosis
- Intraosseous (IO): Rapid method – Use when unable to get IV or central access quickly
  - Contraindications: Fractured or previously punctured bone, overlying infection, bone disease (osteogenesis imperfecta, osteoporosis)
  - Placement sites: **Proximal tibia**, distal femur, distal tibia, iliac crest
  - Only a **short-term** solution: Watch for extravasation, remove once other access obtained
- Arterial lines
  - Indications: Frequent acid–base monitoring, hemodynamic monitoring, need for monitoring of CPP in TBI patients
  - Sites: Radial artery (make sure to do Allen test first), posterior tibial, dorsalis pedis, femoral, axillary
  - Maintenance: Line often heparinized, usually 1 U/mL in NS @ 1–3 mL/hr (although no evidence that it changes clotting risk)
  - Troubleshooting
    - Dampened wave form: Consider kinking of line, vascular spasm (can trial papaverine – ↓ rate of failure and ↑ catheter lifetime) (Crit Care Med 1993; 21(6):825), positioning, or thrombus
  - Complications: Up to 10% of patients – Infection/inflammation (62%), mechanical (14.1%), embolism/thrombosis (7.5%), hemorrhage, hematoma, distal ischemia (rare) (Ped Crit Care Med 2008;9(4):367)
- Excellent videos on placement of all 3 types of lines are available on NEJM's website

---

PROPHYLAXIS IN THE ICU

- Stress ulcer prophylaxis
  - Reasoning: Critically ill patients are at increased risk of GI hemorrhage (up to 10%)
  - Indications: ARDS, septic shock, coagulopathy, high-dose steroids
  - Mgmt – H2 blocker i.e., famotidine (strong evidence in adults, unclear in Peds)
- VTE (venous thromboembolism) prophylaxis
  - No clear evidence to support at this point: Studies evaluating chemoprophylaxis showed mixed results (Chest 2012;146(2):e737s–e801s)
  - But RFs for VTE: Presence of CVC, OCP usage, major surgery (particularly orthopedic), burns, hx of nephrotic syndrome, inflammatory disorders, infection, prior VTE
  - Mgmt: Encourage early ambulation, early removal of lines
- CAUTI prophylaxis
  - Remove Foley catheters as soon as possible

SHOCK/CARDIAC FAILURE

OXYGEN DELIVERY/PHYSIOLOGY

(Pediatric Critical Care. 5th ed. 2017:417–429; Pediatr Rev 2005;26:451)

- Shock = acute, complex state of circulatory dysfunction → inadequate delivery of oxygen to tissues to meet metabolic demands

$$DO_2 \text{ (Delivery of Oxygen)} = CO \times CaO_2$$
$$CO = HR \times SV; \quad CaO_2 = (Hgb \times 1.34 \times SaO_2) + (0.003 \times PaO_2)$$
$$VO_2 \text{ (Oxygen Demand)} = (CO \times CaO_2) - (CO \times CvO_2)$$

- Initial evaluation
  - Labs: CBC, CMP, Lactate (looking for end-organ perfusion, anaerobic metabolism), ABG (assess oxygenation and acid–base state), mixed venous SpO₂

- Px: VS (esp tachycardia); mental status, respiratory effort, urine (concentration, output), peripheral veins (collapsed vs. distended), extremities (warm vs. cold), BP, skin and cap refill (although poor markers)
  - NOTE: Early signs of compensated shock can be very subtle (tachypnea, sluggish cap refill, tachycardia, mild alteration of mental status)
- Initial management (regardless of final etiology)
  - Start with 20 mL/kg bolus of LR or NS (most patients will be relatively hypovolemic): Be judicious until cardiogenic or obstructive shock ruled out
    - Consider 10 mL/kg bolus in children with cardiac history
  - Further management based on type of shock below
- Therapeutic endpoints: Restore age appropriate HR and BP, cap refill <2 s, adequate or appropriate UOP, restoration of end-organ perfusion (labs, mental status, and UOP)

TYPES OF SHOCK

Type	CO	SVR	Intravascular Volume
Hypovolemic	↓	↑	↓↓↓
Cardiogenic	↓	↑	↔ or ↑
–Systolic	↓↓	↑↑↑	↑↑
–Diastolic	↔	↑↑	↑
Obstructive	↓	↑	↔ or ↓
Septic (early)	↑↑↑	↓↓↓	↓
Septic (late)	↓↓	↓↓	↑ or ↔

Hypovolemic/Hemorrhagic: ↓ Preload due to internal or external losses
- **Most common cause of shock worldwide:** Signs of shock after ~25% volume lost
- Causes: GI losses (most common), hemorrhage, plasma loss (burns, nephrotic syndrome), renal losses (DM, DI)
- Management: Volume replacement (with blood if hemorrhagic), minimize ongoing losses (i.e., control hemorrhage)
  - Management of refractory bleeding: Depends on etiology – If in the setting of trauma, will require surgical management

Cardiogenic Shock: Cardiac pump failure secondary to poor myocardial function
- **Easily missed. Can appear similar to other types of shock**
- Causes: Congenital heart disease (ductal dependent lesions, single ventricles, cardiomyopathies (acquired or congenital), ischemia (ALCAPA, MI), arrhythmias, myocarditis, drugs (cocaine)
- Workup: BNP, CXR (look for pulmonary edema and cardiomegaly), echo (assess heart anatomy and function), EKG
- General management
  - Optimize preload (fluids if underfilled, diuretics if overloaded)
  - Optimize pump function: Via pressors (↑ inotropy)
  - Afterload reduction: Milrinone, nitroprusside, iNO
  - If medical therapy fails → ECMO or ventricular assist device
  - If neonate (<4 wo): Consider PGE for possible ductal dependent lesion

Obstructive Shock: ↓ CO due to direct impediment to R or L heart outflow
- Causes: Tension PTX, tamponade, PE, anterior mediastinal masses, critical coarctation of aorta, cardiac tumor
- Tx: Treat the etiology (pericardiocentesis, needle decompression, surgery); medical management is only a bridge

Distributive: Abnormalities of vasomotor tone → loss of venous and arterial capacitance
- Neurogenic: Loss of sympathetic tone due to spinal cord or brainstem injury
  - Tx: Manage similarly to septic shock but w/o antibiotics
- Anaphylactic (see page 2–3 in ED section)
- Drugs

Sepsis and Septic Shock: Unique – has elements of hypovolemic, distributive, and cardiogenic shock
- Clinical presentation: **VARIABLE** – 60% present with cold shock (↑ HR, ↓ pulses, delayed cap refill, etc.); only 20% present with classic (adult) warm shock (↑ HR, ↑ pulses, hyperpnea, flash cap refill)
- Cause: Infection (bacterial, fungal, or viral); immunocompromised patients at highest risk

- SIRS vs. Sepsis
  - SIRS (systemic inflammatory response syndrome): Clinical response to an insult (not necessary infection!): Defined as >2 of the following – Temp >38.5 or <36, WBC elevated or depressed for age, HR >2 SD above normal, RR >2 SD above normal
  - Sepsis = SIRS + source of infection; Severe sepsis = Sepsis w/ signs of end-organ injury
  - Septic shock = Sepsis w/ signs of shock
- Management of septic shock
  - Initial resuscitation: Fluid boluses (LR or NS, no difference in mortality [Pediatrics 2017;182:304]) 20 cc/kg up to x3 until improvement or fluid overload (rales, crackles, hepatomegaly)
  - **Start broad spectrum antibiotics immediately; obtain blood cultures prior to antibiotics**
    - Timing Saves Lives!: Establish access and administer fluids (within 15 min of suspected sepsis) and antibiotics (within 60 min) to ↓ mortality
  - If shock refractory → begin inotrope and establish central access
    - Cold shock → dopamine; warm shock → Epi (babies and young children) or NE (adolescents)
      - NOTE: RCT in 2015 demonstrated ↓ mortality with use of epinephrine over dopamine as 1st pressor (Crit Care Med 2015;43(11):2292)
    - Stress dose hydrocortisone 2 mg/kg (for presumed relative adrenal insufficiency)
      - Consider stress dose steroids earlier in patients with chronic steroid use
      - If possible draw cortisol level prior to steroids
      - New evidence to show that using steroids earlier in shock shortens shock time, but does not decrease mortality (Pediatr Infect Dis 2017;36(2):155)
    - Add additional pressor (cold shock w/ normal BP – add vasodilator; cold shock with low BP – add NE; warm shock – add vasopressin)
  - If not already intubated, intubation can ↓ myocardial demand (although will also ↓ preload)
  - If no improvement, make sure to r/o other etiologies of shock; consider ECMO (see page 17–11)

PRESSORS

Drug	Receptors	Effects	Dosing Range
Epinephrine	$\alpha 1$, $\beta 1$, $\beta 2$	↑ HR, ↑ inotropy Potent vasoconstriction	0.05–3.0 mcg/kg/min
Norepinephrine	$\alpha 1$, $\beta 1$	↑ HR, ↑ inotropy, Potent vasoconstriction	0.05–1.5 mcg/kg/min
Dopamine	$\alpha 1$, $\beta 1$, $\beta 2$, D1	↑ inotropy, peripheral vasoconstriction (at high dose)	3–20 mcg/kg/min
Phenylephrine	Pure $\alpha 1$	Potent vasoconstriction	0.5–2.0 mcg/kg/min
Vasopressin	V1, V2	Vasoconstriction	5–20 milliunits/kg/min

RESPIRATORY FAILURE

BASICS

- Acute respiratory failure = Sudden onset impairment of pulmonary gas exchange → inability of lungs to meet body's metabolic demand for oxygen and CO_2 exchange
- Potential etiologies by site

Upper Airway	Lower Airway	Alveolar	Pump
Croup	Asthma	Pneumonia	CNS disease
Epiglottis	Bronchiolitis	Pulmonary edema	PNS disease
Anaphylaxis	Cystic fibrosis	ARDS	Muscular disease
Retropharyngeal abscess	Bronchomalacia	PE	Chest wall deformity
Foreign body			Ant. mediastinal mass
Laryngomalacia			

- Oxygen delivery: Most dependent on effective exchange across the alveolar–capillary interface

$$A\text{–}a \ Gradient = \left[F_iO_2 \times (P_{atm}(760) - P_{H_2O}(47)) - \left(\frac{PCO_2}{0.8}\right) \right] - PO_2$$

$$\text{Normal A–a Gradient} = 2.5 + 0.21 \times (\text{Age in years})$$

- CO_2 removal: Most dependent on alveolar minute ventilation (CO_2 exchange is more efficient than O_2 exchange). Alveolar minute ventilation is determined by both minute ventilation and ratio of dead space(Vd) : Tidal volume (Tv)

Minute ventilation	Alveolar ventilation
$M_v = V_T \times RR$	$V_a = M_v \times \left(1 - \dfrac{V_D}{V_T}\right)$

- Evaluation/Assessment of gas exchange
  - VS (in particular RR and oximetry), respiratory exam, work of breathing, mental status
  - Labs: CBC, CMP, blood gases (ABG is gold standard, CBG or VBG useful if not concerned about oxygenation)
  - Imaging: Consider CXR
  - Noninvasive monitoring
    - Pulse oximetry: Measure % hemoglobin oxygen saturation
      - Sources of error: Poor perfusion, motion artifact, nail polish, pigments in blood (carboxyhemoglobinemia or methemoglobinemia)
    - Capnography: Measure exhaled CO_2 (marker of ventilation)
- Interpretation of blood gases
  - Normal ABG: 7.35–7.45 (pH) / 35–45 (pCO_2) / 22–26 (HCO_3) / 80–100 (pO_2)
  - Determine if acidosis (pH <7.35) or alkalosis (pH >7.45)
  - Determine if respiratory (primary ΔPCO_2) or metabolic (primary ΔHCO_3)

	Respiratory	Metabolic
Acidosis	↓ pH, ↑ PCO_2	↓ pH, ↓ PCO_2
Alkalosis	↑ pH, ↓ PCO_2	↑ pH, ↑ PCO_2

- Determine compensation or if mixed acid–base disorder

	Acidosis	Alkalosis
Metabolic	Winter formula Expected $PaCO_2 = 1.5*HCO_2 + 8 +/- 2$	$\Delta PaCO_2 = 0.7*\Delta HCO_3$
Respiratory	Acute – ↑ $\Delta HCO_3 = 0.1*\Delta PaCO_2 +/- 0.3$ Acute – ↓ pH = $0.008*\Delta PaCO_2$ Chronic – ↑ $\Delta HCO_3 = 0.35*\Delta PaCO_2$ Chronic – ↓ pH = $0.003*\Delta PaCO_2$	Acute – ↓ $\Delta HCO_3 = 0.2*\Delta PaCO_2$ Acute – ↑ $\Delta pH = 0.008*\Delta PaCO_2$) Chronic – ↓ $\Delta HCO_3 = 0.5*\Delta PaCO_2$ Chronic – ↑ $\Delta pH = 0.003*\Delta PaCO_2$

- If not appropriately compensated, consider superimposed secondary acid–base disorder

Hypoxemic Respiratory Failure – PaO_2 <60 mmHg – Most Common Type

- Etiologies
  - ↑ A–a gradient (indicates pulmonary process)

V/Q Mismatch	True R → L Shunt (Will not correct with O_2)	↓ Diffusion Capacity

• ↑ V/Q (pseudoshunt)
  • PE
• ↓ V/Q (physiologic dead space)
  • Pneumonia, bronchiolitis
  • Asthma
  • COPD
  • Atelectasis
  • Pulmonary edema
	• Cardiac (i.e., VSD, PDA)
	• Large AVMs (i.e., vein of Galen, pulmonary)
		• Interstitial lung disease
		• Alveolar disease
		• Pulmonary HTN
		• Idiopathic

- Normal A–a gradient (indicates no pulmonary process)
  - Hypoventilation (usually with hypercapnia, see below for details)
  - High altitude / Low FiO_2
- Mgmt – Supplemental O_2 (see section on O_2 delivery devices), if not improving consider PPV
  - If not improving, consider shunt as etiology: Requires treatment of shunt

Hypercapnic Respiratory Failure – PaCO$_2$ >50 mmHg (usually with pH <7.35)

- Sx of hypercapnia: Mild → headaches, confusion; moderate to severe → lethargy, coma
- Etiologies

"Won't Breathe" (CNS)	"Can't Breathe" (Mechanical – chest wall, muscles, upper airway; neuromuscular)	"Can't Breathe Enough" (Abnormal Gas Exchange)
• Drugs • CNS infection • Stroke • Central sleep apnea • Metabolic alkalosis • Hypothyroidism	• Neuromuscular (i.e., Guillain–Barré, MG) • Chest wall (i.e., flail chest, kyphoscoliosis) • Muscular (i.e., muscular dystrophy, myopathies) • Obstruction (i.e., bronchomalacia, epiglottitis, foreign body, sleep apnea)	• ↑ Dead space (i.e., PE, vascular disease) • Short shallow breathing (↑ ratio of Vd to Vt) • ↑ CO$_2$ production (fever, sepsis, overfeeding, meta-bolic acidosis, exercise)

- Management
  - ABCs: Ensure adequate airway (r/o foreign body or obstruction), supplemental O$_2$ and circulatory support prn
  - Assess for etiology and initiate appropriate treatment; if concern for opioid related hypoventilation trial naloxone
  - Positioning: Lie down with shoulder roll, jaw thrust, and head tilt (sniffing position)
  - Initiate NIPPV (noninvasive PPV) if no contraindications; else intubate (see refer-ence section for details) and initiate mechanical ventilation
    - Contraindications to NIPPV: Hemodynamic instability, inability to protect airway (↓ mental status), inability to comply with NIPPV

PEDIATRIC ACUTE RESPIRATORY DISTRESS SYNDROME (ARDS)

(Pediatric Critical Care. 5th ed. 2017:627–635; Pediatr Crit Care Med 2015;16(5):428–439)

- Characterized by rapid onset respiratory failure with diffuse, noncardiogenic pulmo-nary edema with significant intrapulmonary shunting and ↑ physiologic dead space
- Etiologies / triggers: Pulmonary infections, inhalations, pulmonary contusions, sepsis, trauma, blood transfusion (TRALI), severe burns, pancreatitis
- Definition/Criteria for diagnosis
  - New onset respiratory failure within 7 d of insult not explained by cardiac failure or fluid overload
  - New infiltrate on CXR (does not need to be bilateral, as opposed to adult ARDS)
  - Oxygen requirement – Via OI if on vent, P/F if on NIPPV, OSI otherwise

$$\text{SF Ratio} = \frac{SpO_2}{FiO_2} \qquad \text{Oxygen Index (OI)} = \frac{(FiO_2 \times MAP \times 100)}{PaO_2} \qquad \text{Oxygen Sat Index (OSI)} = \frac{(FiO_2 \times MAP \times 100)}{SpO_2}$$

NIPPV	Mechanical Ventilation			
	Normal	**Mild ARDS**	**Moderate ARDS**	**Severe ARDS**
P/F Ratio <300	OI <4 OSI <5	4< OI <8 5< OSI <7.5	8< OI <16 7.5< OSI <12.3	OI >16 OSI >12.3

- Management: Intubation, "lung protective" ventilation, permissive hypercapnia
  - Goals: Minimize ventilator-induced lung injury; maintain euvolemia, provide nutrition
  - Ventilator management: Low Vt (5–8 mL/kg), permissive hypercapnia and hypoxemia
    - Limit Pplat to <28 (via ↓ Vt and ↓ PEEP)
    - PEEP: Titrate for oxygenation, usually will require 8–15 cm H$_2$O
  - Permissive hypercapnia (↑ CO$_2$ ok as long as pH >7.15); permissive hypoxemia (goal PaO$_2$ >55)
  - Inhaled NO (iNO): No Δ mortality, does ↑ oxygenation
  - Prone positioning: May ↑ recruitment and ↓ physiologic dead space; ↓ mortality in adults
  - Other interventions (steroids, surfactant): No Δ in mortality
  - If failing on standard ventilator, can utilize rescue mode (HFOV or HFJV – [Crit Care Med 1994;22(10):1530]) and if necessary ECMO

- Prognosis: OI at time of intubation is predictive of mortality (Am J Respir Crit Care 2005;172(2):206)
  - Factors that ↑ mortality: ↑ OI at onset, recent BMT

ASTHMA EXACERBATION

- See page 2–2 in the ED section

OXYGEN DELIVERY AND VENTILATORY ASSISTANCE

OXYGEN DELIVERY DEVICES

Device	Flow (L)	FiO$_2$ Range
"Blow-By"	10	Up to 30%
Oxygen hood	10–15	Up to 80%
Nasal cannula	0.25–6	↑ by 4% per L, up to max of 44%
Simple face mask	6–10	5 L = 50%, ↑ 10% per additional L to max of 60%
Nonrebreather	10–15	↑ 10% per L up to 95%
High flow nasal cannula (HFNC)*	10–50	Up to 100% FiO$_2$

*At higher flows, HFNC also provides some CPAP → can help with work of breathing (Pediatr Crit Care 2014;15(5):e214)

Should humidify and heat O$_2$ when possible to minimize drying of nares and fluid loss

NONINVASIVE POSITIVE PRESSURE VENTILATION

- Indications: Hypoxemia not responding to supplemental oxygen, hypercapnic respiratory failure not requiring intubation, increased work of breathing
  - Can be useful in bronchiolitis, status asthmaticus (can prevent intubation), pneumonia, pulmonary edema, acute chest syndrome
- Delivery methods: Nasal prongs (infants, young children w/ mild disease) or face mask

Types of NIPPV

- **CPAP (Continuous Positive Airway Pressure):** Provides consistent pressure throughout respiratory cycle, acts as PEEP physiologically
  - Use: Hypoxemia and dynamic upper airway obstruction (i.e., OSA)
  - Initial settings: Can start PEEP at 5 mmHg, titrate up to 8–10 mmHg prn for hypoxemia/obstruction
- **BiPAP (Bi Level PAP)**: Delivers inspiratory (IPAP) and expiratory (EPAP) pressures
  - Uses: Increased work of breathing, hypercapnia
    - As compared to CPAP, BiPAP can ↓ work of breathing and ↑ MV
  - Initial settings: Start at ~10/5 (IPAP/EPAP or PEEP), titrate up to 20/10
    - Can also set a backup rate if concerned about apnea or hypopnea
    - Note, it is the ΔP (= IPAP – PEEP) that helps with work of breathing and ↑ MV
    - Titrating BiPAP
      - If concern is hypoxia, can ↑ PEEP but maintain ΔP (↑ IPAP by equal amount)
      - If issue with WOB or hypercapnia, can ↑ IPAP without ↑ PEEP → ↑ ΔP
- On both CPAP and BiPAP can titrate FiO$_2$ from 21–100% as needed

MECHANICAL VENTILATION

(Intensive Care Unit Manual. 2nd ed. 2014:14–30)

Review of Physiology

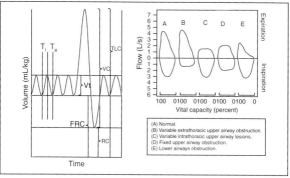

(A) Normal.
(B) Variable extrathoracic upper airway obstruction.
(C) Variable intrathoracic upper airway lesions.
(D) Fixed upper airway obstruction.
(E) Lower airways obstruction.

- Normal volume: Time Curve + Flow-Volume Loops
- Variables/Adjustable settings
  - Settings for oxygenation
    - FiO_2 – Fraction of inspired O_2: Increase as needed to achieve normoxemia
    - PEEP – End-expiratory pressure: Can increase if patient requiring high FiO_2 – Higher PEEP can help maintain recruitment of alveoli
  - Settings for ventilation (remember, ventilation is a function of MV = RR × Vt)
    - RR – Respiratory rate: Try to start at near normal rate for age, but adjust as needed to maintain CO_2 in acceptable range
    - Vt – Tidal Volume: Volume of air that ventilator will deliver with each fully supported breath – usually set to ~5–8 mL/kg
  - I:E ratio – Ratio of inspiration to expiration: For an average patient this is about 1:2, this may need to be adjusted in specific clinical situations by adjusting the inspiratory time (i-time)
- Peak and plateau pressures
  - Ppeak – Peak pressure in inspiratory cycle: Due to resistance of circuit + patient
  - Pplat – Pressure during inspiratory hold: Due to compliance of patient's lungs

Basic Modes of Ventilation *(Respir Care 2014;59(11):1747)*

- SIMV – Synchronized, intermittent mandatory ventilation: Similar to ACV, but allows for separate support of patient-initiated breaths in addition to ventilator-initiated breaths; will fully support breaths up to the RR that you have set, any additional breaths the patient takes will be supported to a lesser degree (PS). The ventilator times breaths to avoid breath stacking or patient/ventilator dyssynchrony
  - Use: Most common mode used in PICU, maximizes patient comfort
  - Variables: RR, Vt, FiO_2, PEEP, and PS
    - PS – This the pressure that the patient will get during inspiration on patient-initiated breaths: Usually set to 5–8 mmHg. The patient controls the i-time on these breaths
      - If increased work of breathing noted on nonfully supported breaths, increase either the PS (to support extra breaths more) or RR (so more breaths get full support) or consider switch to ACV
- PS – Pressure support: Instead of delivering preset TV, delivers preset pressure (similar to BiPAP). All breaths are patient-initiated, no rate is set (can set backup rate, but if concerned about bradypnea or apnea should not use PS)
  - Often used as weaning mode or as trial for extubation: Patient given enough pressure to overcome resistance of ET Tube. See "Weaning" below for more details.
  - Variables: PS, in addition to PEEP and FiO_2
- ACV/CMV – Assist/Control mode: Allows patient to control their respiratory rate and Vt, but will ensure minimum rate and minimum Vt that you set. **All breaths are fully supported, and with set i-time.**
  - Variables: RR, Vt, FiO_2, PEEP, i-time

High Frequency Ventilation (HFV)

- Modes of ventilation that utilize high frequencies with low tidal volumes: Goal is to provide adequate ventilation while maintaining higher MAP to maximize oxygenation
- Indications: Hypoxia not responding to conventional ventilation (particularly in ARDS)
- High frequency oscillatory ventilation (HFOV)
  - Mechanism: Oscillatory flow at 5–15 Hz (300–900 breaths/min) via piston pump or diaphragm with Vt of 1–3 mL/kg
  - Variables and initial settings
  - MAP (start at 4–6 mmHg above conventional vent MAP, goal to have lungs expanded to T9)
  - Amplitude (adjusted via power): Start in 30 s, titrate to patient's "jiggle"
  - Frequency (Hz): Neonate ~8–10; children ~6–8; adults ~5–6
    - ↓ by 0.5–1 Hz to ↑ ventilation after optimizing amplitude and FiO_2
  - NOTE: Both inspiration and expiration are active with HFOV
- High frequency jet ventilation (HFJV)
  - Mechanism: Delivers inspiratory gases through jet injector at 240–600 cycles/min with Vt of 3–5 mL/kg
  - Variables: Driving pressure (MAP), rate, PEEP, and FiO_2
  - NOTE: Relies on passive expiration

Troubleshooting a Ventilated Patient

- Ventilator–patient dyssynchrony: Most common – usually due to inadequate sedation, inadequate support on ventilator, trigger threshold set too high (infants), can also be due to Auto-PEEP (see below)
- Hypoxia/Sudden desaturation
  - Differential – DOPES: Displaced ET Tube, Obstruction (anywhere along circuit), Pneumothorax, Equipment (ventilator failure or disconnected), Stacked breaths (auto-PEEP)
  - Mgmt: Disconnect patient from ventilator and manually bag patient and auscultate chest to assess for ET tube displacement or pneumothorax; suction ET tube to ensure not obstructed; have your RT check the ventilator to ensure it is operating correctly and nothing was disconnected
- Auto-PEEP / breath stacking / gas trapping / intrinsic PEEP (iPEEP)
  - Cause: Expiratory time not adequate → stacking of breaths
    - Often seen in patients with bronchospasm (asthma or COPD), kinked ETT, or if RR is set too high
  - Consequences: ↑ risk of pneumothorax and barotrauma, ↓ CO and hypotension, ventilator dyssynchrony, ↑ work of breathing
  - Assessment: Some ventilators can measure iPEEP, or you can watch the flow curve on the ventilator for incomplete exhalation
  - Mgmt: Disconnect from ventilator temporarily (allow for full exhalation), can also compress chest to ensure complete exhalation; when reconnecting to vent should ↓ RR, ↓ Vt, ↓ I:E Ratio, ↑ sedation, consider switching to SIMV if on ACV

Weaning From Mechanical Ventilation (Pediatr Crit Care 2009;10(1):1)

- Readiness to extubate trials (RET): Should be done daily unless no contraindications
  - Contraindications for RET: Lack of spontaneous respiratory effort, altered mental status, hypercapnia or acidosis, FiO_2 >50% or PEEP >7, requiring any cardiovascular support
  - Methods
    - Pressure support trials (PST): Switch mode of ventilator to pressure support with low level of support (5–10 mmHg, in theory PS is to help get over resistance of ET Tube)
    - T – piece trials: Patients are removed from ventilator and connected to supplemental oxygen (no pressure support) – Not often used in Peds
    - In RCT comparing T – piece vs. PST, no difference in extubation rate, reintubation rate if passed trial, or RET failure rate (Intensive Care Med 2001;27(10):1649)
  - Trial is discontinued if any of the following: Significant tachypnea, significant ↑ in WOB, diaphoresis or anxiety, significant tachycardia, change in mental status, or hypoxia requiring ↑ FiO_2
  - Assessment for readiness to extubate
    - Able to complete trial (ideally, up to 2 hr)
    - Rapid shallow breathing index (RSBI) = RR/(Vt/Weight) – RSBI of <8 breaths/mL/kg has a 74% Se for successful extubation (Respir Crit Care 1999;160(5):1562)
    - Leak test: When cuff is deflated, ensure that there is an air leak else consider dose of steroids for possible airway edema prior to extubation
    - NIF (negative inspiratory force): If able to generate >-30 cm H_2O
      - May be worth checking in cases where there is concern for transient neuromuscular weakness

NEUROLOGIC FAILURE

BRAIN DEATH

(Philadelphia Guide: Inpatient Pediatrics. 2nd ed. 2016; Ann Neurol 2012;71(4):573–585)

- Brain death = irreversible loss of cortical and brainstem function, including respiratory drive
- Determination of brain death in children
  - Eliminate reversible causes (i.e., opioids): Obtain drug levels, EEG, imaging as appropriate, normothermia
  - Perform px as below: Assessing for coma, brainstem reflexes, apnea
  - Age specific requirements for declaring brain death
    - 6 d–1 yo: At least 2 exams
    - >1 yo: At least 2 exams 12–24 hr apart
    - Other ancillary studies (EEG, radionuclide cerebral blood flow) are used if some question remains, or parts of the exam (apnea test) could not be completed
- Px for brain death
  - Assess for normal temperature and blood pressure
  - Mental status: Coma (unresponsive to any stimulus)
  - Absent brainstem function: Fully dilated pupils, no doll's eye reflex, no vestibulo-ocular responses, no reflexes (corneal, gag, cough, suck, root)
  - Tone: Flaccid with no spontaneous or induced movements (except spinal mediated reflexes)
  - Apnea test: Give 100% O_2 for 10 min before test, remove from ventilator and allow hypercapnia to develop. Monitor CO_2 level q5min, until PCO_2 >60 or ↑ by >20 from baseline. If no respiratory effort indicates positive apnea test

STATUS EPILEPTICUS

- See page 12–1 in Neurology section

INCREASED INTRACRANIAL PRESSURE (ICP)

(Philadelphia Guide: Inpatient Pediatrics. 2nd ed. 2016:270)

- Normal ICP by age:
  - Neonate = <2 cm H_2O; <12 mo = 1.5–6 cm H_2O; Child = 3–7 cm H_2O; Adolescent = <15 cm H_2O; Adult = <20 cm H_2O
- Differential: Mass lesions, meningitis, pseudotumor cerebri, hydrocephalus, VP shunt malfunction, intracranial hemorrhage, trauma, seizure, metabolic derangement (cerebral edema)
- Clinical sx: Mental status Δ (may progress to coma), headache (particularly morning and positional), irritability, nausea/vomiting, diplopia
- Px: Cushing triad (HTN, bradycardia, irregular breathing – rarely seen), bulging fontanelle or ↑ head circumference, papilledema (rare in infants), focal neuro abnormalities
- Workup
  - Imaging: Emergent head CT (can be normal even with ↑ ICP) or US in infants with open fontanelle; VP shunt series in patients with shunt
  - Labs: BMP, serum osm, ammonia (if diffuse cerebral edema)
  - Procedures: LP if CT without any findings to measure opening pressure
- Management of ↑ ICP
  - Basics: ABCs, control seizures if present; maintain CPP (cerebral perfusion pressure = MAP – ICP; goal >50 mmHg), aggressive normothermia, normoglycemia, seizure prophylaxis or control
  - ↓ Cerebral blood volume: Elevate HOB, mild hyperventilate to $PaCO_2$ of 35–40 mmHg (if herniating can push to 25–30 for short periods of time), cerebral vasoconstricting sedation (thiopental, pentobarbital)
  - ↓ Brain + CSF Volume
    - 3% saline: Bolus or drip, titrate to serum goal of 150–160
    - Mannitol 0.25–1 mg/kg IV (effective within 10 min, last ~8 hr) – Monitor VS, lytes, serum osms (goal serum osm 300–320)
    - Acetazolamide 30 mg/kg/d IV/PO in 4–6 doses: ↓ CSF production (but can cause transient ↑ in ICP)
    - Dexamethasone 1–2 mg/kg (max 10 mg): In cases of vasogenic edema
  - Neurosurgery consult – For possible shunt vs. surgical decompression vs. placement if ICP monitor

DIABETIC KETOACIDOSIS (DKA)

- See page 5–13 in the Endocrine section

SYNDROME OF INAPPROPRIATE ADH (SIADH)

(Philadelphia Guide: Inpatient Pediatrics. 2nd ed. 2016)

- Inappropriately elevated ADH → ↑ intravascular volume and ↓ serum Osm
- Causes
  - CNS: Meningitis, encephalitis, brain tumor or infection, **head trauma**, surgery, hypoxic/ischemic encephalopathy, ↑ ICP, CNS leukemia
  - Infections: PNA, HIV/AIDS, TB, HZV, RSV, aspergillosis, infantile botulism
  - Pulmonary: Asthma, CF, empyema or abscess
  - Neoplasms: Oat cell carcinoma, bronchial carcinoid, lymphoma, Ewing sarcoma, pancreatic tumors, bladder tumors, ureteral tumors
  - Drugs: Carbamazepine, lamotrigine, chlorpropamide, vinblastine, vincristine, TCAs
- Clinical → anorexia, nausea, vomiting, headache, weakness, irritability
- Workup: BMP, ADH, TSH, cortisol
- Diagnosis: Na <135 (usually <130), euvolemic on exam, low serum Osm, high urine Na (>40 mEq/L) and urine Osm (>100, usually >300)
- Management
  - Symptomatic HypoNa → 3% Saline 1–2 mL/kg/hr (goal to increase Na of 10 mEq)
  - Chronic/Asymptomatic HypoNa → fluid restriction to 1L/m^2/d (goal to correct by 0.5 mEq/hr)

DIABETES INSIPIDUS (DI)

CEREBRAL SALT WASTING (CSW)

- Unclear if CSW is a distinct clinical entity, may instead be a variant of SIADH
- Causes: Associated classically with subarachnoid hemorrhages
- Diagnostic criteria: Similar to SIADH **EXCEPT** occurs in the setting of decreased extracellular volume
- Management: Similar to DI

ECMO/ECLS

(Pediatric Critical Care. 5th ed. 2017;302–324)

- Indications: Unresponsive shock, decompensated heart failure despite therapy, refractory respiratory failure; **must be reversible or candidate for destination therapy**
- Types of ECMO
  - V-A (Venoarterial): Provides cardiac support and pulmonary support
    - Access points: R IJ and R Carotid, Femoral A and V, Direct RA and Ascending Aorta
  - V-V (Venovenous): Provides pulmonary support without cardiac support – Acts as a "third lung", dependent on native cardiac output
    - Access: Single catheter with double lumen to RA via IJ, or two venous catheters (IJ, femoral)

- Basic ECMO Circuit + Components

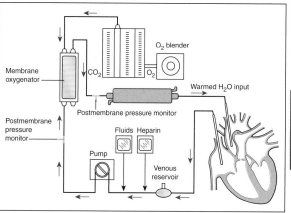

(From Nurse's 5-minute Clinical Consult: Treatments. Philadelphia, PA: Lippincott Williams & Wilkins, a Wolters Kluwer Business; 2007.)

- Pump: Determines flow rate through circuit and degree of cardiac support (if VA)
- Oxygenator: Oxygenates blood across membrane; also eliminates CO_2
- Titratable variables in ECMO + initial settings
  - Flow (RPM → L/min): Start at 50 mL/kg/min, titrate to goal depending on age
    - Infant up to 160 mL/kg/min; Children ~90 mL/kg/min; Adults up to 70 mL/kg/min
  - FiO_2: Titrate for goal arterial sats >90%
  - Sweep (L/min): Determines CO_2 clearance, titrate to achieve goal CO_2s
- Routine management
  - Regular labs: Goals as below; transfuse prn to achieve goals
    - Anemia, platelet sequestration, and coagulation or clotting are common on ECMO
    - Hgb >10, Plat >100,000
    - INR <1.5–2 (if >1.5–2 or significant bleeding, administer FFP 10 mL/kg)
    - Fibrinogen >100–150 (transfuse cryo prn)
  - Anticoagulation: ECMO has continuous UFH to prevent thrombosis – Initial bolus 100 U/kg then drip for goal ACT 180–220 (usually ~25–50 U/kg/hr) (*ELSO Anticoagulation Guidelines* 2014)
    - Can consider using anti-Xa levels (may correlate better), but take longer to obtain. Goal 0.3–0.7
    - Others – aPTT, TEG: Can use in cases when ACT or anti-Xa levels not correlating
  - Maintain fluid balance (goal net even unless overloaded)
  - Minimize ventilator barotrauma (low PEEPs and PIPs, low rates)
  - Ensure adequate sedation, consider paralytics if needed
  - In infants, perform regular head ultrasound to watch for intracranial hemorrhage (ideally get one at prior to cannulation)
  - Echo regularly
- Weaning from VA ECMO
  - Wean flow in set increments every 1–2 hr to goal of ~10% of CO; if remain physiologically stable can do clamp trial
- Weaning from VV ECMO
  - Decrease sweep gas through oxygenator to assess native lung function
- Troubleshooting ECMO
  - Acute loss of pulse pressure
    - Tamponade
    - Insufficient intravascular volume, or pump flow rate too high for patient size
    - Cardiac stun (usually in first 72 hr)
    - Arterial line malfunction
  - In an EMERGENCY the *patient* is your patient, not the pump! – Disconnect patient from malfunctioning pump, increase vent setting to optimize gas exchange, initiate PALS protocols – Let perfusionist manage pump

OVERVIEW OF CLINICAL DERMATOLOGY

Describing Lesions (*Hurwitz Clinical Pediatric Dermatology*)

Primary Lesions		
Lesion	**Size**	**Description**
Flat, circumcised, not palpable		
Macule:	<1 cm	Hypo/Hyperpigmented, e.g., lentigo, tinea versicolor
Patch:	>1 cm	Color change, e.g., port wine stain, vitiligo, dermal melanocitosis, capillary malformations
Elevated, circumcised, solid		
Papule:	<1 cm	Above skin surface, may have secondary features, e.g., verruca, molluscum
Nodule:	½–2 cm	Solid lesion, below skin surface, e.g., erythema nodosum, dermoid cyst
Tumor:	>2 cm	Deeper and solid, skin or subcutaneous, e.g., hemangioma, neurofibroma
Elevated, noncircumcised		
Plaque:	>1 cm	Broad, disk-shaped, may be a confluence of papules, e.g., psoriasis
Wheal:	Varies	Local, superficial, transient edema, e.g., urticaria
Vesicular, pustular **Elevated, circumcised**		
Vesicle:	<1 cm	Contains fluid, e.g., herpes simplex, coxsackie, varicella, contact dermatitis
Bulla:	>1 cm	Contains fluid, e.g., bullous pemphigoid, epidermolysis bullosa, bullous SLE
Pustule:	<1 cm	Contains purulent exudate, e.g., folliculitis, neonatal pustular melanosis
Abscess:	>1 cm	Deeper, walled-off containing purulent material
Other		
Comedone:	Small	Closed or open, contained within pilosebaceous follicle, e.g., acne
Burrow:	Linear	Tunneling within stratum corneum, e.g., scabies
Telangiectasia:	Varies	Persistent dilation of superficial blood vessels, e.g., spider angioma

Secondary Lesions	
Lesion	**Description**
Acute	
Crust:	Dried remains of serum, blood, pus or exudate, e.g., impetigo
Scale:	Compact desquamating stratum corneum, e.g., ichthyoses, pityriasis alba
Fissure:	Linear, chronic inflammation, loss of elasticity, e.g., angula cheilitis
Subacute	
Erosion:	Moist, vesicular or bullous, no dermis involvement
Excoriation:	Superficial loss of skin by abrasion, heal without scar, e.g., atopic dermatitis
Ulcer:	Necrosis of epidermis and dermis, heal with scar, e.g., pyoderma gangrenosum
Late	
Atrophy:	Thin, translucent epidermis, ↑ wrinkling, depression of skin with loss of skin markings, e.g., steroid induced
Lichenification:	Thickening of epidermis, exaggerated skin markings, e.g., chronic dermatitis
Scar:	Permanent fibrotic skin after damage to dermis, e.g., keloid

Select Terms to Describe Distribution of Lesions	
Acrodermatitis	affecting the hands and feet of the body, e.g., Gianotti–Crosti (viral xanthem)
Annular	or circinate, ringed, e.g., tinea corporis
Arciform	or arcuate, e.g., pityriasis rosea, erythema multiforme
Clustering	occurring in groups, e.g., herpes, contact dermatitis
Confluent	lesions that merge together, e.g., urticaria, exanthems, dermatitis
Dermatomal	lesions localized to a region supplied by one or more dorsal ganglia
Discoid	raised disc-shaped lesion, e.g., discoid SLE
Flexural	affecting flexor surfaces of the body, e.g., flexural eczema
Guttate	drop-shaped, e.g., guttate psoriasis
Gyrate	spiral-shaped, e.g., erythema annulare centrifugum
Iris	target-shaped with concentric ringed lesions, e.g., erythema multiforme
Koebner phenomen	or isomorphic response, lesions at the site of a previous injury, e.g., psoriasis, lichen
Keratosis	thickened circumscribed patches, e.g., callus formation, seborrheic or actinic
Moniliform	banded lesions, necklace-shaped, e.g., monilethrix (beaded nodules along hair shaft)
Multiform	numerous/various lesion shapes, e.g., erythema multiforme, Henoch–Schonlein purpura
Nummular	coin-shaped, e.g., nummular dermatitis
Reticular	net-shaped pattern, e.g., livedo reticularis, cutis marmorata, telangiectasia congenita
Serpiginous	serpentine-shaped, e.g., cutaneous larva migrans, elastosis perforans serpiginosa
Umblicated	lesions with a central depression, e.g., molluscum contagiosum, Kaposi varicelliform
Universal	widespread affecting entire skin, e.g., alopecia universalis
Zosteriform	lesions arranged linearly along dorsal ganglion, e.g., herpes zoster or simplex

Parts of Skin

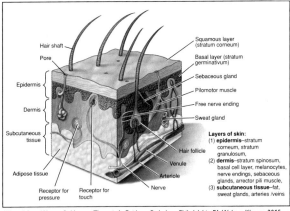

Adapted from Werner R. Massage Therapist's Guide to Pathology. Philadelphia, PA: Wolters Kluwer; 2015.

Primary Immunodeficiency Disorders	
IgA Deficiency	atopy, vitiligo, recurrent candida infections, lipodystrophy, idiopathic thrombocytopenic purpura (ITP)
Common variable immune deficiency (CVID)	pyodermas, extensive warts, dermatophyte infections, dermatitis, (autoimmune): vitiligo, alopecia areata
BTK Mutations	pyodermas, cutaneous abscesses (furuncles, cellulitis), atopic-like dermatitis, noninfectious cutaneous granulomas
Hyperimmunoglobulin	warts, oral/perianal ulcerations
Wiskott–Aldrich Syndrome	eczema
Chronic granulomatous disease (CGD)	early lesions cutaneous face/perianal *Staph* pyodermas or abscesses, purulent dermatitis, seborrheic dermatitis, acute febrile neutrophilic dermatosis (Sweet syndrome), scalp folliculitis, oral ulcers
Leukocyte adhesion deficiency (LAD)	frequent skin infections (facial cellulitis), poor wound healing, psoriasis, FERMT3 mutation cases—dermal hematopoiesis ("blueberry muffin")
Severe combined immunodeficiency (SCID)	candida infections, generalized seborrheic-like dermatosis, morbilliform eruption, exfoliative erythroderma, alopecia, Omenn syndrome—extensive cutaneous inflammation (chronic appears more lichen planus/lamellar ichthyosis), Artemis mutation—oral/genital ulcers, Adenosine deaminase deficiency (ADA)—dermatofibrosarcoma protuberans
Hyper-IgE (Job) syndrome	eczema, recurrent staphylococcal skin abscesses
Behçet Syndrome	oral/genital ulcers, folliculitis, pyoderma, acneiform lesions, palpable purpura, erythema nodosum-like lesions, pathergy (exaggerated skin injury after minor trauma)
Nutritional deficiency (i.e., Eating disorders)	xerosis, carotenemia, acne, calluses on knuckles (Russell sign), pellagra, scurvy, acral changes, hair—telogen effluvium, lanugo, dry, nails—brittle

- **Graft Versus Host Disease (GVHD) – See Image Set 1, page 18-13**
  - aGVHD: 7–10 d after exposure/transfusion, erythematous macules and maculo-papules on ears, neck, face, palms and soles, confluence, desquamate, generalization, if severe exfoliative erythroderma, toxic epidermal necrolysis
  - cGVHD: 6–18 mo, extensive cutaneous involvement, lichen planus (violaceous), xerosis, patchy dyspigmentation, sclerodermatous changes
  - engraftment syndrome: fever, vascular leak with edema

Characteristics of GVHD	
Eyes	dry, cicatricial (scar-like) conjunctivitis, keratoconjunctivitis sicca, punctate keratopathy
GI tract	chronic diarrhea, upper esophageal strictures/stenosis/webbing, hepatomegaly
Hair	alopecia
Joints/Muscles	contractures from sclerosis, fasciitis, arthritis, myositis
Lungs	bronchiolitis obliterans, interstitial fibrosis
Nails	ridging, onycholysis (separation from nailbed), loss of nails, pterygium (scar tissue in nail matrix)
Oral mucosa	lichen planus-like, keratotic plaques, atrophy, xerostomia, ulceration, mucocele, sclerosis
Skin	lichen planus-like, sclerosis, poikiloderma, ichthyosis, genital scarring, ulcers, fissures

Dermatologic Characteristics of Inflammatory Bowel Disease	
Crohn Disease	**Ulcerative Colitis**
Perianal skin tags: Occurs in 75–80% patients, correlates with colonic disease	**Pyoderma gangrenosum:** Occurs in 5% of patients
Erythema nodosum: Occurs in 15% of patients, correlates with arthritis	**Erythema nodosum:** Occurs in 3–10% patients
Oral aphthous ulcers: Occurs in >50% of patients	**Sweet syndrome:** More common in UC
Cobblestoning (buccal): Occurs in 20% of patients	**Pyodermatitis or pyostomatitis:** Pustular eruption of oral mucosa or skin folds, more common in UC, males and 20–50 yo
Granulomatous lesions: Typically lips or anogenital, dusky red, can be ulcerating	**Vitiligo** and **acquired epidermolysis bullosa** more commonly associated with UC than CD
Labial or scrotal edema	

COMMON SKIN LESIONS IN NEONATES

Normal Skin Findings (*Neonatal and Infant Dermatology; Atlas of Pediatric Physical Diagnosis*)
See Image Set 2, page 18-13, 18-14

- **Premature infants:** Stratum corneum (SC) is immature in < 28 wk EGA, consider: Dehydration/fluid electrolyte balance, excessive penetration of topical drugs, susceptibility to infections, mechanical injury, thermoregulation, light injury, scars of prematurity, and hemangiomas, maturation (keratinization) is accelerated
- **Full-term infants:** By 3 wk of age, SC is fully keratinized to adult structure and function
- **General newborn skin care:** Expect desquamation in 24–36 hr of life, expect umbilical stump to fall off 1–2 wk of life, circumcision may require moisturizer and often has yellow granulation tissue, should heal in 7–10 d and watch for adhesions
- **Benign lesions:** Blue-gray macule (Mongolian spot), physiologic cutis marmorata, harlequin color change secondary to immaturity of hypothalamic centers, bronze baby secondary to phototherapy for hyperbilirubinemia and modified liver function, should differentiate from cyanosis/carbon baby/gray baby **Sclerema neonatorum:** Rare and severe, hardening of subcutaneous tissue with minimal inflammation mostly affecting sick premature infants
- **Subcutaneous fat necrosis:** Does not have inflammation, can last for weeks to months until self resolves, may cause hypercalcemia after resolution
- **Miliaria:** Sweat retention and/or obstruction of eccrine ducts resulting in papulovesicular eruption
- **Milia:** Small cysts retaining keratin resulting in 1–2 mm pearly white papules, very common facial eruption in newborns
- **Epstein pearls:** Singular, 2–3 mm pearly white elevated papules on hard palate, similar to milia
- **Acne neonatorum:** Hormonal stimulation of sebaceous glands resulting in facial acne
- **Eosinophil pustular folliculitis:** Follicular pustules on neonatal scalp and extremities, can be associated with hyperimmunoglobulinemia E syndrome
- **Erythema toxicum:** Erythematous macules, papules and pustules on face, trunk and extremities, histology shows eosinophils
- **Pustular melanosis:** Fragile vesiculopustular lesions that can become hyperpigmented macules, found on face, neck, back and shins, rare and associated with black skin, very rarely found on scalp, palms and soles with no hyperpigmentation, Wright stain shows neutrophils
- **Vascular anomalies: (See Image Set 3, page 18-15)** Hemangiomas and other vascular tumors, Kasabach–Merritt phenomenon, pyogenic granuloma, bacillary angiomatosis,
  - Capillary: Nevus simplex (salmon patch), telangiectasia and associated syndromes, Sturge–Weber, megalencephaly, Beckwith–Wiedemann,
  - Venous: Blue rubber bleb nevus syndrome,
  - Combined: PTEN hamartoma, proteus,
  - Lymphatics: Gorham syndrome, congenital lymphomatous overgrowth (CLOVES),
  - Other: Angiokeratomas, multifocal hemangioendotheliomatosis (MLT)

See Image Set 4, page 18-15
- **Atopic dermatitis:** Severe pruritus, symmetric, erythematous papules and vesicles with exudates or crusting, associated with FHx of atopy, ↑ IgE
  - Tx: Clip nails, avoid triggers, emollients, escalate to topical corticosteroids, antihistamines and/or topical immunomodulators, bleach baths
- **Dyshidrotic eczema:** Onset <40 yo, sudden eruption of small pruritic deep-seated vesicles on hands that dry up and desquamate, can confirm diagnosis by skin biopsy or patch test
  - Tx: Avoid triggers, topical steroids, phototherapy, antihistamines, systemic immunosuppressants and antibiotics when needed, can occur after IVIG for SJS or Kawasaki
- **Lichen simplex chronicus:** Localized, circumscribed pruritic patches, caused by excessive scratching
  - Tx: Eliminate scratching: Patient education, psychotherapy, topical steroids
- **Seborrheic dermatitis:** Erythematous, scaly or crusting eruption localized to areas with high concentration of sebaceous glands (scalp, face, postauricular), self-limiting
  - Tx: Scale removal and emollients, can advance to topical steroids and antifungals
- **Id reaction:** Hypersensitivity reaction, small edematous papules or vesicles, treat by removing trigger, can be secondary to infection requiring antibiotics
- **Nummular dermatitis/eczema:** Discoid or "coin" like plaques, occur on extensor surfaces, often pruritic, associated with *Staph* infection
  - Tx: Topical steroids, may require antibiotics
- **Contact dermatitis:** Can be irritant or allergic, type IV hypersensitivity reaction
  - Tx: Remove trigger (commonly metals or *Rhus* family allergens), cool compresses first 72 hr, colloidal oatmeal baths, may require topical or IM steroids, antihistamines

COMMON CHILDHOOD LESIONS

PSORIASIS

See Image Set 5, page 18-15
- Thickened pruritic scaly plaques from excess keratinocytes, associated with inflammation and other syndromes, e.g., psoriatic arthritis, IBD, autoimmune disorders
  - **Guttate psoriasis:** "drop" like papules or plaques in children post *Strep* pharyngitis
- **Pityriasis rosea:** Herald patch followed by generalized pruritic exanthem along lines of skin cleavage forming "Christmas tree" pattern, can try emollients or topical steroids for pruritis, UV radiation hastens resolution but can result in hypopigmentation, self resolves in about 3 mo
- **Lichen planus:** Inflammatory disease causing "purple, polygonal, pruritic plaques" on flexor surfaces, genitalia and mucus membranes, treat with topical steroids and antihistamines, can have nail involvement, commonly seen in GVHD

KAWASAKI DISEASE

See Image Set 6, page 18-16
- **Kawasaki Disease (KD)** (acute febrile mucocutaneous lymph node syndrome): Vasculitis of small- and medium-sized arteries that typically affect children less than 5 yo. The etiology of KD is unknown but may be secondary to infectious agents, toxin-mediated, genetic predisposition and/or inappropriate immune activation. Most common in spring and winter.
- Most serious complications of KD are coronary artery aneurisms (occur in 5–10% of treated patients and up to 20% of untreated patients)
  - Other complications include pericardial effusions, myocarditis, congestive heart failure, arrhythmia, mitral valve regurgitation, KD shock syndrome (hypotension)

Diagnostic Criteria for Kawasaki Disease		
Classic	Fever ≥5 d	Plus at least 4 out of 5: • Bilateral nonexudative bulbar conjunctivitis • Oral mucous membrane signs, e.g., erythema, fissured lips, strawberry tongue • Peripheral extremity signs: Acute erythema or edema of hands or feet, convalescent periungual desquamation • Polymorphous rash (diffuse maculopapular, perineal accentuation, desquamating) • Cervical lymphadenopathy ≥1.5 cm (unilateral, least common feature)
Incomplete	Fever ≥5 d	Plus 2–3 criteria from classic diagnosis
Atypical	Fever ≥5 d	Meet diagnostic criteria along with clinical feature not typical or included in criteria, e.g., aseptic meningitis, urethritis, arthralgia, diarrhea

Clinical Phases of Kawasaki Disease		
Acute	1–2 wk	Fever Myocarditis Erythematous extremities Oral mucosal and conjunctival changes Cervical lymphadenopathy
Subacute	2–6 wk	Fever defervescences Arthritis Aneurysms (cardiovascular, CNS) Desquamation of rash Resolution of lymphadenopathy Thrombocytosis
Convalescent	79 wk	Nail changes Coronary artery aneurysm (rarely occur past 8 wk) Recurrent toxin-mediated perineal erythema (RTPE, can recur past this window)

- Tx: IVIG and aspirin during the acute phase to reduce inflammation and prevent damage to arteries. Ideally initiated within the 1st 10 d of symptoms.
  - IVIG 2 g/kg over 12 hr once
    - About 5–15% of patients require a 2nd dose of IVIG if suboptimal response
  - Aspirin 80–100 mg/kg/d divided q6h until patient is afebrile for 48–72 hr.
    - Ant-TNF-α monoclonal antibodies and corticosteroids have shown some effectivity but are typically used as 3rd-line therapy
- Screening for coronary artery disease:
  - Initial echocardiogram at diagnosis and 2 mo after illness
  - If coronary arteries are normal at 2 mo, no further imaging necessary
  - If abnormal, further management per pediatric cardiology specialist
- Outcomes for patients diagnosed with KD either <6 mo of >9 yr are at ↑ risk of adult vascular lesions, myocardial fibrosis and valvular incompetence.

COMMON PEDIATRIC INFECTIOUS LESIONS

(Hurwitz Clinical Pediatric Dermatology; Atlas of Pediatric Physical Diagnosis)

VIRAL

See Image Set 7, page 18-16

- **Erythema infectiousum** (Fifth disease): Caused by parvovirus B19 infection with initial viremia phase associated with respiratory symptoms then progresses to rash and arthralgias around 3 wk of illness, thus patients are not infectious at this stage, rash described as "slapped cheek" facial erythema and lacy, reticulated erythema on extremities and trunk, B19 can cause persistent bone marrow suppression in immunocompromised children, rarely can appear as pruritic papules with "glove and socks" distribution that also self-resolves

- **Roseola infantum/exanthem subitem** (Sixth disease): Caused by human herpes virus (HHV) 6 or 7 course, common in children under 3 yo, starts with high fevers that resolve with appearance of erythematous, blanchable macules and papules on the trunk eventually spreading to extremities, neck and face, exanthem self-resolves in 1 to 3 d, can also present with erythematous papules on soft palate and uvula (Nagayama spots)
- **Rubeola** (Measles): Caused by *Paramyxoviridae* virus and highly contagious (respiratory droplets), associated with "three Cs: Cough, coryza and conjunctivitis," Koplik spots: Punctuate gray or erythematous papules on buccal mucosa, lesions are erythematous or purple that become confluent and sometimes result in desquamation or coppery macules, follows a cephalocaudal spread, vaccination (twice) is key to prevention, Ribavirin can be given to immunocompromised patients, keratoconjunctivitis with vitamin A deficiency can result in blindness so supplementation is recommended, keep in respiratory isolation 4 d from onset of rash
- **Rubella** (German measles): Caused by *Togaviridae* virus and vaccination is particularly important in preventing congenital rubella syndrome, rash described as rose-pink macules and papules that become confluent and spread cephalocaudally, in severe cases there may be flaky desquamation and lymphadenopathy of suboccipital, postauricular and cervical nodes, keep in contact isolation 7 d from onset of rash
- **Varicella** (Chickenpox): Highly communicable varicella zoster virus causing both chickenpox and shingles, vaccine has been helpful in decreasing incidence of invasive GABHS infections, lesions start as red macules or papules which quickly become vesicles ("dewdrop on rose petal"), lesions start centrally and spread to extremities, concomitant lesions in various stages pathognomonic, keep in contact isolation for 5 d after onset of rash or until all lesions are crusted over, lesions heal with hypopigmentation and scarring
- **Cytomegalovirus** (CMV): Congenital CMV causes hydrops, IUGR, microcephaly with ventriculomegaly and periventricular calcifications, patients may be jaundiced, have petechiae and purpura, "blue berry muffin eruption" of maculopapular rash also seen with congenital rubella and toxoplasmosis, treat with IV ganciclovir for symptomatic CNS disease
- **Coxsackie** (hand foot and mouth disease): Benign enteroviral vesicles on palms, soles, face and buttocks, supportive care but no targeted treatment
- **Herpangina:** Caused by Coxsackie A or B, associated with fever and oral lesions (tonsils/uvula)

BACTERIA

See Image Set 8, page 18-17

Bacterial	Pathogen	Distribution	Symptoms	Treatment	Notes
Rocky Mountain spotted fever	Tick borne, rickettsial	Southeast U.S.	Fever, headache, malaise, myalgias	Doxycycline or Chloramphenicol (pregnant patients)	Petechial rash days 3–5 starts on wrists and ankles, spreads to trunk, palms and soles, face sparing
Lyme disease	*Ixodes* tick borne, *Borrelia* spirochete	Coastal Northeast U.S., 5–14 yo's	Rash, arthritis, late complications: Heart block, encephalitis, Bell palsy	Doxycycline	Early localized erythema migrans rash Coinfection with *Babesia* possible
Impetigo	*Strep* or *Staph*	2–5 yo's	Erythematous papules or pustules spread by autoinoculation	Topical or oral Abx, contact isolation	"Honey crusted" lesions on face, hands or neck

Scarlet fever	GABHS – erythrogenic toxins	5–15 yo's	Fevers, tonsillopha-ryngeal erythema or exudates, petechial macules on palate	Penicillin V, amoxicillin, or ampicillin (prevent risk of RF and heart disease)	"Strawberry tongue," "sandpaper rash," can desquamate in thick sheets, circumoral pallor
Staph scalded skin syndrome	Exotoxin release (epiderm-olytic A and B)	<6 yo's	Diffuse, painful erythroderma, fluid-filled blisters, extensive desquamation	Supportive care, IV Abx (nafcillin, oxacillin, vancomycin, clindamycin)	**NO** mucus membrane involvement
Toxic shock syndrome	*Strep* or *Staph* enterotoxin		Unstable vitals, diffuse myalgia and macular erythroderma—greater in skin folds, massive desquamation	Drain and debride source, hemodynamic stabilization, Abx including Clindamycin, IVIG	Risk factors: Postpartum, tampon use, surgical procedures, nasal packing

FUNGAL

See Image Set 9, page 18-17
- **Candida:** Congenital cutaneous candidiasis associated with widespread erythematous macules, papules and pustules on extensor surfaces and skin folds with diaper sparing, may also have pustules on palms and soles and yellow discoloration of nails, systemic candidiasis associated with VLBW premature infants between 2 and 6 wk old with or without skin involvement, thrush may present in newborn oral cavity and candida diaper rash differentiated from irritation by satellite lesions and nonresponsiveness to barrier creams, can treat with nystatin, flucanazole or gentian violet age
- **Tinea:** Caused by dermatophytosis (except tinea versicolor and tinea nigra), commonly seen in children living in warmer climates, with systemic disease or poor hygiene, presents as annular and circumscribed scaly plaques that may have a vesicular or pustular border, can coalesce to form polycyclic lesions, treat topically with clotrimazole except tinea capitis and tinea ungum (or extensive tinea corporis/tinea versicolor) which requires PO antifungals such as griseofulvin

PARASITES

- **Scabies:** Caused by *Sarcoptes* mite in children with poor hygiene, infected contact or in crowded living conditions, described as arcuate or linear (secondary to mite burrowing) pruritic lesions that spare the face and neck, treat with permethrin and washing all infected items (hot cycle or dry clean), add ivermectin for crusted lesions and expect lesions to be pruritic for weeks post therapy

INFLAMMATORY DISORDERS

(Hurwitz Clinical Pediatric Dermatology; Atlas of Pediatric Physical Diagnosis)

SYSTEMIC LUPUS ERYTHEMATOSUS (SLE)

See Image Set 10, page 18-18
- SLE is an autoimmune disease characterized by accumulation and deposition of immune complexes (type III) resulting in end-organ damage (renal, neurologic, ophthalmic, hematologic). UV light is a common trigger, especially for skin manifestations. Can be seen neonatally or within the first 20 yr of life with ↑ prevalence in female, African American and Latino populations.
- Diagnostic criteria include 4 mucocutaneous signs or symptoms (present in about 80% of cases): Malar rash, discoid lesion, diffuse alopecia (nonscarring) and oral ulcers
  - Malar rash: Flat or raised erythema sparing nasolabial folds

- Discoid lesion: Above the neck erythematous plaque or keratotic scale, may progress to atrophic scar and dyspigmentation
- Oral ulcers: Located on nasal or buccal mucosa, palate or tongue
- Alopecia: Diffuse hair thinning or fragility, other causes ruled out
- Drug-induced: Predominance of photosensitivity related lesions (livedo reticularis, urticaria, palpable purpura) and absence of malar rash, discoid lesions, mucosal ulcers and alopecia

JUVENILE DERMATOMYOSITIS (JDM)

See Image Set 10, page 18-18
- JDM is an inflammatory disorder that targets the skin, striated muscles and internal organs (GI tract, lungs and heart). Bimodal age distribution: 2–5 yo and 12–14 yo. Cutaneous involvement differentiates JDM from polymyositis.
- Characteristic skin features include heliotrope rash, shawl sign, Gottron papules, ulcers, nail malfunction, xerosis and pruritic and poikiloderma
  - Heliotrope rash: Red-purple hue, occurring on eyelids, nose and cheeks, can be asymmetric and associated with edema
  - Shawl sign: Confluent purplish telangiectasia at hairline, nape of neck, extensor surfaces and upper anterior trunk
  - Gottron papules: Flat papule and telangiectasia on dorsal interphalangeal joints
- Skin features do not correlate with muscle response and can persist despite resolution of other features. Sun protection and PO hydroxychloroquine used to treat skin manifestations

VITILIGO

(Hurwitz Clinical Pediatric Dermatology)

- Often presents prior to 20 yo, prepubertal presentation associated atopic dermatitis and with family history of vitiligo
- Acquired, patterned loss of pigmentation with variable location, size and shape of lesions
  - Well-defined macules or patches with convex borders
  - Partially or completed depigmented
  - First lesions often occur in exposed areas: Hands, face, neck
  - Common in body folds: Axillae, groin, eyes, nostrils, mouth, navel, genitalia
  - Can be associated with white hair
- Polygenic & multifactorial disorder, genes involved in tyrosinase or regulation of immune sys
  - Antigen-specific cytotoxic T cells destroy melanocytes
  - Autoantibodies often present
- Treatment: Partial repigmentation ↑ with UV light exposure and areas with ↑ density of hair follicles, potent topical steroids or topical calcineurin inhibitors can cause partial repigmentation but can result in hyperpigmentation with sun exposure, camouflage therapy can be achieved with cosmetics, aniline dye stains and quick tan formulations

DRUG REACTIONS

(Hurwitz Clinical Pediatric Dermatology; Atlas of Pediatric Physical Diagnosis)

DRUG REACTION WITH EOSINOPHILIA AND SYSTEMIC SYMPTOMS (DRESS)

See Image Set 11, page 18-18
- Commonly presents with fever, conjunctivitis, facial swelling and internal organ involvement
- Can present 1 to 6 wk after exposure to inciting medication.
  - Commonly seen with trimethoprim-sulfamethoxazole, anticonvulsants (aromatic) and sulfonamides (when patient is a slow metabolizer)
- Diffuse exanthematous eruption seen in about 75% of cases
  - Cephalocaudal spread (especially starting periorbital)
  - Erythematous and pruritic rash
  - No mucosal involvement

- Atypical lymphocytosis and eosinophilia present early in course of disease. Liver most commonly involved, associated with elevated LFTs. Late onset thyroiditis can be seen 2–3 mo after onset of symptoms
  - Full laboratory evaluation includes: CBC, LFTs, Cr, UA, and TFTs
- Treatment includes topical corticosteroids and antihistamines for pruritus in mild cases. Systemic corticosteroids (1–2 mg/kg/d) for 2–3 wk with gradual taper is indicated for cases with visceral involvement such as hepatitis, myocarditis, and interstitial pneumonitis

Stevens–Johnson Syndrome and Toxic Epidermal Necrolysis

Lesion	Description
SJS <10% skin involvement	Targetoid lesions, dusky red macules, bullae, scattered or confluent (trunk and face), dermatitis without necrolysis, prominent mucosal involvement, systemic changes
SJS-TEN 10–30% skin involvement	Similar to SJS with more confluence, interface dermatitis and necrolysis, prominent mucosal involvement, always has systemic involvement
TEN >30% skin involvement	Targetoid lesions, dusky red macules and plaques, epidermal detachment, widespread, predominantly necrolytic, less mucosal involvement than SJS, always has systemic involvement

Clinical Features of SJS and TEN

Constitutional	Fever, dehydration, sepsis, electrolyte imbalance, temperature dysregulation
Mucocutaneous	Cutaneous involvement starting in face and upper trunk, positive Nikolsky sign (sloughing of skin with light pressure), dusky blue coloration of lesions. Stomatitis with hemorrhagic crusts. Oral and genital erosions, can interfere with micturition and defecation and result in strictures. Purulent conjunctivitis with photophobia
Visceral	Hepatosplenomegaly, lymphadenopathy, occasionally pneumonitis, myocarditis, nephritis
Labs	Elevated ESR, leukocytosis, eosinophilia, anemia, elevated LFTs, proteinuria, hematuria

- Children more commonly have SJS
- *Mycoplasma* infection is most common infectious trigger of SJS in children
- If drug induced, symptoms occur within 1st 8 wk of drug exposure. Sulfonamides, penicillins, phenobarbital, carbamazepine and lamotrigine are well-known triggers of SJS-TEN
  - HLA-B 15:02 (common in Asian population) associated with carbamazepine-induced SJS-TEN, thus HLA screening should be done prior to initiating antiepileptics in these patients
  - Aromatic antiepileptics (phenobarbital, phenytoin, carbamazepine, lamotrigine) cannot be substituted for each other because of high cross-reactivity
  - Drugs with longer half-life associated with higher incidence of SJS-TEN
- Patients with defects in epoxide hydrolase-mediated detoxification, slow acetylators, and HIV-infection patients have ↑ risk of developing SJS-TEN
- SCORTEN traditionally used for adults has been shown to reliably predict pediatric outcomes (mortality, LOS, complications). Higher SCORTEN associated with ↑ morbidity/mortality should be assessed on admission to hospital

SCORTEN Scale

Risk Factor	0	1
Age	<40 yr	>40 yr
Associated malignancy	Absent	Present
Heart rate (bpm)	<120	>120
Serum BUN (mg/dL)	<28	>28
Skin involvement	<10%	>10%
Serum bicarbonate (mEq/L)	>20	<20
Serum glucose (mg/dL)	<252	>252

- Treatment is primarily supportive care: Enteral or parenteral nutrition, fluid repletion, avoidance of secondary infection and appropriate wound care for disrupted skin and mucosa, potent short-term topical corticosteroids and/or amniotic membrane application to ocular surface if ocular involvement
- Systemic steroids, IVIG, plasmapheresis and several chemotherapy medications have been studied; however, their use is controversial

Common Drug Reactions

Lesion	Drug	Description
Angioedema	ACE inhibitors, aspirin, NSAIDs	Subcutaneous and dermal edema, mucosal involvement
Acneiform	Lithium, iodides, isoniazid, phenytoin, steroids	Papules and pustules, inflammation
Drug-induced lupus	Hydralazine, isoniazid, minocycline, penicillamine, procainamide	Urticaria, vasculitis, rare mucosal involvement
Exanthematous	Antiepileptics, cephalosporins, penicillins, sulfonamides	Diffuse erythematous maculopapular lesion(s)
Fixed	Acetaminophen, barbiturates, Ibuprofen lamotrigine, loratadine, macrolides, metronidazole, phenolphthalein, potassium iodide, pseudoephedrine, quinine, tartrazine, teicoplanin, tetracycline	Erythematous, hyperpigmented plaques
Hypersensitivity	Abacavir, allopurinol, aspirin, azithromycin, carbamazepine, dapsone, lamotrigine, minocycline, nevirapine, phenytoin, vancomycin	Edema, erythematous maculopapular lesions, vesicles and bullae, mucosal involvement
Lichenoid	Allopurinol, captopril, carbamazepine, dapsone, enalapril, furosemide, gold salts, griseofulvin, HCTZ, hydroxychloroquine, hydroxyurea, imatinib, ketoconazole, NSAIDs, penicillamine, phenytoin, radiocontrast, spironolactone, sildenafil, sulfasalazine, tetracycline	Discrete flat-top red-purple papules and plaques, mucosal involvement
Pseudoporphyria	COX-2 inhibitors, furosemide, NSAIDs, tetracyclines	Photosensitive blisters and skin breakdown
Pustular	β-lactams, clindamycin, macrolides, terbinafine	Universal pustules and papules
Serum sickness-like reaction	Bupropion, cephalosporins, ciprofloxacin, fluoxetine, griseofulvin, itraconazole, macrolides, minocycline, rifampin, rituximab, sulfonamides	Urticaria, erythema multiforme-like
SJS/TEN	Acetaminophen, allopurinol, antiepileptics, dapsone, sulfonamides	Target lesions, bullae, epidermal necrosis and detachment, mucosal involvement
Urticaria	Aspirin, cephalosporins, NSAIDs, penicillins, tetracyclines, radiocontrast, sulfonamides	Superficial, pruritic erythematous wheals and edema
Vasculitis	Cephalosporins, NSAIDs, penicillins, sulfonamides	Urticaria, purpuric papules, hemorrhagic bullae, pustules, ulcers, necrosis

NEUROFIBROMATOSIS

(Hurwitz Clinical Pediatric Dermatology)

- Benign tumors with neuromesenchymal tissue including Schwann cells and neural cells
- Cutaneous marker of type I neurofibromatosis
- Presents during early adulthood as isolated, soft, flesh-colored papules or papulonodules. Can grow to become globular, pedunculated or pendulous. "Buttonhole" inward when pressure is applied to the top of the lesion
- Plexiform neurofibromas are pathognomonic for NF1 and are large, lobulated and nodular with "bag of worms" sensation on palpation
- Treatment: Depending on location and size, neurofibromas are treated with surgical excision

TUBEROUS SCLEROSIS

(Hurwitz Clinical Pediatric Dermatology)

- Autosomal dominant disorder commonly by de novo mutation in hamartin or tuberin genes involved in mTOR pathway
- Hamartomas can develop in skin, brain, eyes, heart, kidneys, lungs, and bones
- Skin manifestations include:
  - Hypopigmented macules (greater than 5 mm diameter, more than 3 macules) can be highlighted by Wood's lamp in dark room
    - "thumbprints" on back, "confetti" over pretibial areas, and "ash leaf spots" anywhere are all common descriptors
  - Angiofibromas
  - Shagreen patch, a connective tissue nevus
  - Fibrous tumors
  - Periungal and gingival fibromas
- TS likely in children with characteristic skin lesions and neurologic involvement (seizures, intellectual disability). Common causes of mortality and morbidity are seizures and bronchopneumonia
- Treatment: Seizure control is associated with lower risk of developmental delay and intellectual disability. Sun protection especially important to prevent further mutations (second hit hypothesis). Topical rapamycin (mTOR inhibitor) and surgical removal of hamartomas depending on severity

GRAFT VERSUS HOST DISEASE

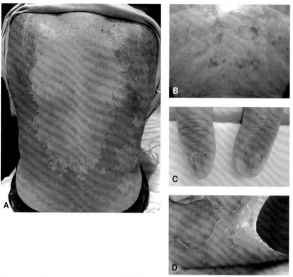

Photographs of skin graft-versus-host disease (GVHD). **A: Severe acute skin GVHD. B: Sclerodermatous chronic skin GVHD. C: Dystrophic nails in chronic GVHD. D: Oral lichenoid changes in chronic GVHD.** From DeVita VT Jr, Lawrence TS, Rosenberg SA. *DeVita, Hellman, and Rosenberg's Cancer: Principles & Practice of Oncology*. Philadelphia, PA: Lippincott Williams & Wilkins; 2014.

COMMON SKIN DISORDERS OF NEONATES

Miliaria, milia, Epstein pearls, acne neonatorum, eosinophilic pustular folliculitis, impetigo neonatorum, transient neonatal pustular melanosis, vesicular dermatosis

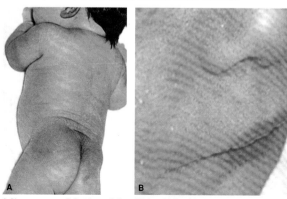

A: Blue gray macuse. B: Epstein pearls. From O'Doherty N. *Atlas of the Newborn*. Philadelphia, PA: JB Lippincott; 1979.

C: Harlequin color sign (1/2 red baby). From Jensen S. *Nursing Health Assessment.* Philadelphia, PA: Lippincott Williams & Wilkins; 2010. **D: Neonatal acne.** From Nicol N. *Dermatology Nursing Essentials.* 3rd ed. Philadelphia, PA: Lippincott Williams & Wilkins; 2016. **E: Erythema toxicum neonatorum.** From White A. *The Washington Manual of Pediatrics.* 2nd ed. Philadelphia, PA: Lippincott Williams & Wilkins; 2016. **F: Cutusmarmorata.** From Salimpour R, Salimpour P, Salimpour P. *Photographic Atlas of Pediatric Disorders and Diagnosis.* Philadelphia, PA: Lippincott Williams & Wilkins; 2013. **G: Scleremaneonatorum.** From Gru A, Wick M. *Pediatric Dermatopathology and Dermatology.* 1st ed. Philadelphia, PA: Lippincott Williams & Wilkins; 2018. **H: Fat necrosis.** From Dr. Barankin Dermatology Collection.

VASCULAR ANOMALIES

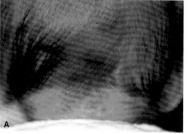
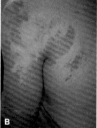

A: Salmon patch. From Prasad P. *Pocket Pediatrics.* 2nd ed. Philadelphia, PA: Lippincott Williams & Wilkins; 2013. **B: Sturge Weber.** From Nelson L, Olitsky S. *Harley's Pediatric Ophthalmology.* 6th ed. Philadelphia, PA: Lippincott Williams & Wilkins; 2013.

ECZEMATOUS LESIONS

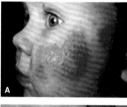
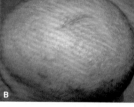
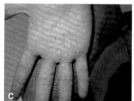
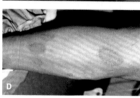

A: Atopic Dermatitis. From Sauer GC, Hall JC. *Manual of Skin Diseases.* 7th ed. Philadelphia, PA: Lippincott-Raven; 1996. **B: Sebhorrheic dermatitis.** From White, A. *The Washington Manual of Pediatrics.* 2nd ed. Philadelphia, PA: Lippincott Williams & Wilkins; 2016. **C. Dishydrotic Eczema.** From Dr. Barankin Dermatology Collection. **D. Nummular Eczema.** From Goodheart HP. *Goodheart's Photoguide of Common Skin Disorders.* 2nd ed. Philadelphia, PA: Lippincott Williams & Wilkins; 2003.

PSORIASIS

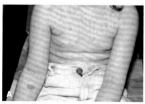
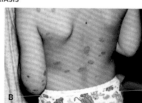

A: Psoriatic plaques. From *Circulation* 2001;103:335. **B:** From Goodheart HP. *Goodheart's Photoguide of Common Skin Disorders.* 2nd ed. Philadelphia, PA: Lippincott Williams & Wilkins; 2003.

KAWASAKI DISEASE

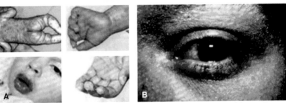

A: From *Circulation* 2001;103:335. **B:** From Goodheart HP, MD. *Goodheart's Photoguide of Common Skin Disorders.* 2nd ed. Philadelphia, PA: Lippincott Williams & Wilkins; 2003.

COMMON PEDIATRIC INFECTIOUS LESIONS – VIRAL

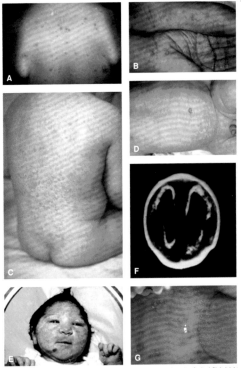

A: Varicella. From Goodheart HP, MD. *Goodheart's Photoguide of Common Skin Disorders.* 2nd ed. Philadelphia, PA: Lippincott Williams & Wilkins; 2003. **B: Rubella (German measles).** From Fleisher GR, MD, Ludwig W, MD, Baskin MN, MD. *Atlas of Pediatric Emergency Medicine.* Philadelphia, PA: Lippincott Williams & Wilkins; 2004. **C: Rash of rubella.** From *Lippincott's Nursing Advisor 2013.* From LW&W Image Library. **D: Roseola infantum (Sixth disease).** From Goodheart HP, MD. *Goodheart's Photoguide of Common Skin Disorders.* 2nd ed. Philadelphia, PA: Lippincott Williams & Wilkins; 2003. **E, F: CMV.** From Engleberg NC, Dermody T, DiRita V. *Schaecter's Mechanisms of Microbial Disease.* 4th ed. Baltimore: Lippincott Williams & Wilkins; 2007. **G: Koplik spots. The rashes of measles. Koplik spots appear as red spots along the inside of the cheek.** Reprinted with permission. Bowden V. R. , Greenberg C. S. (2014). *Children and their families: The continuum of nursing care* (3rd ed., p. 1263, Figure 24-8). Philadelphia, PA: Wolters Kluwer.

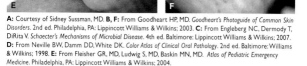

A: Courtesy of Sidney Sussman, MD. **B, F:** From Goodheart HP, MD. *Goodheart's Photoguide of Common Skin Disorders.* 2nd ed. Philadelphia, PA: Lippincott Williams & Wilkins; 2003. **C:** From Engleberg NC, Dermody T, DiRita V. *Schaecter's Mechanisms of Microbial Disease.* 4th ed. Baltimore: Lippincott Williams & Wilkins; 2007. **D:** From Neville BW, Damm DD, White DK. *Color Atlas of Clinical Oral Pathology.* 2nd ed. Baltimore: Williams & Wilkins; 1998. **E:** From Fleisher GR, MD, Ludwig S, MD, Baskin MN, MD. *Atlas of Pediatric Emergency Medicine.* Philadelphia, PA: Lippincott Williams & Wilkins; 2004.

COMMON PEDIATRIC INFECTIOUS LESIONS – FUNGAL

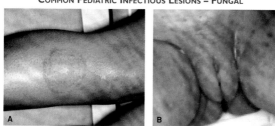

A: Tinea. From Goodheart HP, MD. *Goodheart's Photoguide of Common Skin Disorders.* 2nd ed. Philadelphia, PA: Lippincott Williams & Wilkins; 2003. **B: Candidal diaper dermatitis.** From Bickley, L. *Bates' Guide to Physical Examination and History Taking.* 8th ed. Philadelphia, PA: Lippincott Williams & Wilkins; 2002.

INFLAMMATORY DISORDERS

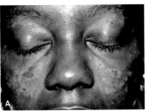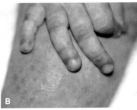

A: Systemic Lupus Erythematosus. From Goodheart HP, MD. *Goodheart's Photoguide of Common Skin Disorders.* 2nd ed. Philadelphia, PA: Lippincott Williams & Wilkins; 2003. **B: Juvenile Dermatomyositis.** From Images from Fleisher GR, MD, Ludwig S, MD, Baskin MN, MD. *Atlas of Pediatric Emergency Medicine.* Philadelphia, PA: Lippincott Williams & Wilkins; 2004.

DRUG REACTIONS

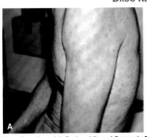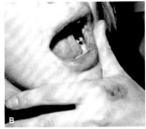

Drug Reaction with Eosinophils and Systemic Symptoms (DRESS). A: From Goodheart HP, MD. *A Photoguide of Common Skin Disorders: Diagnosis and Management.* Baltimore: Lippincott Williams & Wilkins; 1999. **B:** From Goodheart HP, MD. *Goodheart's Photoguide of Common Skin Disorders.* 2nd ed. Philadelphia, PA: Lippincott Williams & Wilkins; 2003.